The Social Importance of Self-Esteem

D1462260

The Social Importance of Self-Esteem

Edited by
Andrew M. Mecca,
Neil J. Smelser, and
John Vasconcellos

UNIVERSITY OF CALIFORNIA PRESS
Berkeley · *Los Angeles* · *London*

University of California Press
Berkeley and Los Angeles, California

University of California Press, Ltd.
London, England

© 1989 by
The Regents of the University of California

Printed in the United States of America
1   2   3   4   5   6   7   8   9

Library of Congress Cataloging-in-Publication Data

The Social importance of self-esteem / edited by Andrew M. Mecca, Neil J. Smelser, and
    John Vasconcellos
        p.   cm.
    Includes index.
    ISBN 0−520−06708−8 (alk. paper).—ISBN 0−520−06709−6 (pbk. :
alk. paper)
    1. Deviant behavior.   2. Self-respect.   3. Social problems.
4. United States—Social conditions.   I. Mecca, Andrew M.   II. Smelser, Neil J.
III. Vasconcellos, John.
HM291.S58836   1989
361.1—dc20   89−4821
                                                                          CIP

Contents

Foreword

Andrew M. Mecca

The creation of the California Task Force to Promote Self-Esteem and Personal and Social Responsibility is part of an unprecedented attempt to reframe our approaches to solving social problems. The aim of the task force is to develop an approach that actively promotes the greater well-being of the individual and of society, rather than simply reacting to an ever-growing epidemic of casualties resulting from serious social ills.

The gathering of data and testimony at public hearings, which led up to the legislation establishing the task force, built a consensus that a *primary* factor affecting how well or how poorly an individual functions in society is self-esteem. If this is the case, then, documenting this correlation and discovering effective means of promoting self-esteem might very well help to reduce the enormous cost in human suffering and the expenditure of billions in tax dollars caused by such problems as alcohol and drug abuse, crime, and child abuse.

This bold initiative was generated by veteran Democratic member of the California State Assembly John Vasconcellos, and it became a solid bipartisan program when the legislation was signed by Republican Governor George Deukmejian in September 1986. Plans for the task force attracted more than four hundred applications for appointment, more than had been received for any other state commission in the history of California. In addition, more than five thousand people have since written to express interest, join the mailing list, and become involved in this historic effort. Persons from all fifty-eight counties in California, all fifty states, and twenty-seven nations have become active.

As a result of this positive response, subsequent legislation encouraging each of the fifty-eight California counties to appoint a local task force was introduced and passed. These local councils will provide access for all at the community level and will help to sustain this work on a long-term basis. The state task force itself is committed to maximizing public involvement and has convened public hearings across the state, set up "think tanks," and invited numerous interested individuals and constituencies to contribute their views and ideas.

The work accomplished by scholars at the University of California is a significant reflection of the interest and support the task force agenda has attracted. University President David Gardner, his staff, and seven principal authors from the University of California faculty have provided invaluable support by preparing this volume, which reviews and summarizes relevant research associated with self-esteem and the pressing social problems of alcohol and drug use, teenage pregnancy, poor educational performance, crime, child abuse, and chronic welfare dependency. The chapters in this book offer for the first time a detailed summary of research relating self-esteem and these specific social concerns.

This academic work is being richly complemented by the input received from the public hearings and think tanks being held throughout California. These gatherings provide opportunities to hear personal testimony on the significance of self-esteem and to collect information from those who have pioneered programs designed to promote this quality. A central issue that has emerged from the work to date is the balance of attention devoted both to personal and social responsibility and to self-esteem. In fact, there has been considerable consensus in the public hearings and think tanks that self-esteem is a product of or is associated with character traits such as honesty, responsibility, perseverance, kindness, and self-discipline.

The investigation of self-esteem and personal and social responsibility may allow us to gain insights into more cost-effective strategies that are relevant to all citizens and that, over the next generation, can reduce the growing incidence of social problems and their related personal and economic costs. This work also challenges us to recognize the critical need for a long-term focus, for rigorous research that can evaluate the impact of strategies and programs designed to promote self-esteem.

Our modern ideas surrounding self-esteem and personal and social responsibility have a rich heritage. The language has changed, but the ideas inherent in this perspective have not. Indeed, the California task force benefits from both the wisdom and the inspiration offered by history. Leaders, poets, scholars, and historians from the earliest of times believed what we believe today: that responsibility is a manifestation of an individual's high level of self-esteem.

The scholarly work included in this volume brings academic rigor to this heritage. In addition, the various chapters pose the critical research questions that can significantly increase the depth and clarity of this investigation into self-esteem. These contributions reflect the productive work that is itself a key ingredient of self-esteem.

It is perhaps a romantic notion that self-esteem is related to concepts such as honesty, charity, dignity, faith, intellectual energy, optimism, self-acceptance, courage, and love. But our hope is that self-esteem and personal and social responsibility will be our legacy, what we leave behind for our children. In doing so, we will have brought to our community, our human family, a very great gift indeed.

Preface

John Vasconcellos

On behalf of the California Task Force to Promote Self-Esteem and Personal and Social Responsibility, I welcome your participation in our pioneering efforts to address the causes and cures of many of the social ills that plague us today. Our work and our study center on the issue of self-esteem—a quality that most profoundly affects both the lives of individuals and the life of our society.

In the 1940s, certain visionaries recognized that we could unlock the secret of the atom. Our best scientists were enlisted, and our attention, talent, creativity, and resources were focused on that endeavor. In the 1960s, other visionaries mounted the same kind of effort as we attempted to plumb the reaches and mysteries of outer space. Our remarkable success in both these enterprises reveals the power of the human vision, human capacities, and directed collective efforts.

For the 1990s, we owe it to ourselves to seek to unlock the secrets of healthy human development. It is time to plumb the reaches and mysteries of inner space and discover effective strategies that could serve to improve our communities, our personal lives, and the lives of those around us.

The issue placed before us has been clearly stated by political economist Thomas Sowell in his book *A Conflict of Visions*. He points out that the role of a vision is to inform our expectations of ourselves and of life and thereby our choice of practice in every human relationship. Every political structure and ideology, every pedagogy, every social institution, and every other endeavor is founded upon some vision of human nature.

Sowell argues that, historically and philosophically, there are only two such informing visions: a more "constrained vision," deriving from the works of Adam Smith, Thomas Hobbes, and Frederick Hayek, which proposes that human beings are basically evil, needing to be tamed and protected against ourselves and one another; and an "unconstrained vision," associated with Jean-Jacques Rousseau and John Locke, which proposes that human beings are innately inclined toward good, perhaps even perfectible.

These two visions were clearly articulated for me in two pointed comments. I heard the first in Sacramento in 1973 at a community forum on educational goals. An elderly woman rose and said to the gathering, "All this talk about goals is fine, but the real issue concerns the means we choose to attain our goals. And when you realize that little children arrive in this world as monsters needing to be tamed, you know what means to choose."

The second comment was made in 1986, when Carl Rogers, the humanistic psychologist, told a group of guests at a dinner party in Irvine, "You know, I've been practicing psychology for more than sixty years, and I have really come to believe that we human beings are innately inclined toward becoming constructive and life-affirming and responsible and trustworthy."

These two contradictory visions represent far more than a philosophical argument. Their practical implications can be seen in every sphere of life, for our choices about how we pursue any human relationship always proceed from the fundamental view of human nature that each of us holds. It is essential that we recognize for ourselves and acknowledge to others our particular personal vision.

It is the latter vision—that human beings are innately inclined toward good and that free, healthy people become constructive and responsible—which underlies the philosophy and work of what has been called the "self-esteem movement." There is within this movement an implicit (and increasingly explicit) intuition, an assumption—a faith, if you will—that an essential and operational relationship exists between self-esteem and responsible human behavior, both personal and social.

The term *self-esteem* implies a deeply felt appreciation of oneself and one's natural being, a trust of one's instincts and abilities. It is that kind of self-esteem which, instead of being narcissistic, enables us to live generously and peacefully, without delinquency or destructiveness, encouraging one another in our lives and our growth.

Our hope is that the California Task Force to Promote Self-Esteem will serve as a vehicle to focus our attention and efforts on such goals. Not only the enhancement of individual lives but the cure and prevention of some of society's most serious problems may be at stake.

Why has California taken the lead in this endeavor? Historically, California often seems to be on the cutting edge: rockets and campus activism, the tax revolt and Ronald Reagan, computers and new lifestyles, new forms of sexuality and spirituality. California is first among the states in population, with twenty-eight million residents, and more added each year. We are first in the basics of life, from agriculture, which nourishes our bodies, to arts and entertainment, which nourish our spirits. The technological revolution was born here, in Silicon Valley, and we have developed an economy that, were we a separate nation, would have the sixth largest gross national product in the world.

Standing on these foundations, Californians are also engaged in attempts to realize our higher aspirations. In doing so, we find ourselves involved in four remarkable and converging revolutions, which are breaking new ground in developing both individuality and community, as well as providing us with unprecedented opportunities and challenges.

First, California is experiencing a revolution of race and ethnicity. We are about to become the first state in the mainland United States with a majority of nonwhites. In the fall of 1988, for the first time, a majority of the children in our public schools were non-Anglo, and that change will also occur among California's general population shortly after the year 2000. California is becoming an "international" state, with the opportunity to create a truly multicultural democracy. Our ability to do so may depend on each of us developing a healthy sense of self-esteem, so that, instead of being insecure and threatened by persons who differ from us, we can appreciate one another and be enriched by persons of different races, ethnic backgrounds, and cultures.

Second, California shares with several other states a leading role in the gender revolution. In education, politics, business, labor, and religion, we are growing to recognize the inherent capacity and rights of women to be fully equal, as well as the inherent capacity and rights of men to be tender, compassionate, and cooperative. This revolution today encompasses our lives, from individual households to the boardrooms of corporate power. Again, realizing its potential may depend on the cultivation of self-esteem among both women and men, enabling us to meet one another openly and comfortably, as peers.

Third, California shares with Florida a prominent role in the revolution of aging. The fastest growing cohort of Californians is composed of people over the age of eighty-five. Instead of languishing in retirement, many of these individuals are actively bringing their experience, wisdom, and generosity to the enterprise of building society. Carl Rogers, for example, at the age of eighty-four, spent a month in the Soviet Union advising leaders there, as he had here, about ways to individualize instruction and foster creativity.

Fourth, California leads the revolution in developing human potential. From the analyst's couch to the group, and from the Center for the Study of the Person in La Jolla to the Esalen Institute in Big Sur, more of us have openly dared to wonder what it means to be human and to experiment with "becoming a person," exploring dimensions of trust, intimacy, responsibility, and spirituality.

These revolutionary developments have combined with major cultural trends—the social action movements of the 1960s, the personal growth movement of the 1970s, and the entrepreneurial spirit of the 1980s. Together, all these strands now seem to be converging in the self-esteem movement. For all the reasons discussed above, it seems somehow right that this movement should be centered in California—and perhaps it is no accident that so many of its theoretical and practicing pioneers were or are residents of our state: Nathaniel Branden, Jack Canfield, Stanley Coopersmith, Abraham Maslow, Rollo May, Carl Rogers, Virginia Satir, and others.

Why and how did the California Task Force to Promote Self-Esteem get started? Many individuals and groups had been addressing the issue of self-esteem for some time, of course, but as the author of the legislation creating the task force, I seem to have been the first public official to recognize the centrality of this issue and to propose that government pay attention to it in a systematic way. As is often the case with our choice of our life's work, my motivations proceed from my own life history. My commitment to the task force is an expression of my own converging needs and interests, both personal and legislative.

I grew up in the 1930s in a constrained, traditional, Catholic family. I was educated in both public schools and Catholic (Jesuit) schools, through college and law school. In school, I was a high-achiever, receiving awards and excellent grades. In adulthood, I became a prominent lawyer in a prestigious firm. My first campaign for a seat in the state legislature in 1966 was successful, and I have now been reelected eleven times.

Yet, through it all, I had almost no sense of my self, no self-esteem. I worked for my successes only in a constant attempt to please others. My intellect functioned superbly, but the rest of my self barely functioned at all. I had been conditioned to know myself basically as a sinner, guilt-ridden and ashamed, constantly beating my breast and professing my unworthiness. I had so little self-esteem that I lost my first election (running for eighth-grade president) by one vote—my own.

Awakening painfully to this problem, I began in 1966 to invest long and difficult years in redeveloping my self-esteem. During the past twenty-two years, I have been involved in various forms of therapy, beginning with Carl Rogers's person-centered therapy, with a priest-psychologist, and continuing today with bioenergetics therapy, all with the aim of opening up and more fully integrating myself as a whole person. My life and work have become increasingly focused on this compelling issue of self-esteem, not only in relation to my own development but also in terms of enabling others to develop a strong sense of self.

My personal experience has taught me how very central and vital healthy self-esteem is. This outlook has become so ingrained within me that it has become essential to my political views and priorities. My legislative record has paralleled and in some ways become a reflection of my personal growth. In its essence, after all, politics properly understood is nothing more than the making of policy for all of us together, the sum of our individual beings.

In 1980, I became head of the California State Assembly's Ways and Means Committee, responsible for reviewing spending legislation and the state's annual budget. Year after year, we spend ever-increasing billions of tax dollars to contain destructive behaviors, to compensate for human failures after the fact—more than a billion dollars each year for building prisons and two billion for operating them, as well as substantial sums for programs to address alcoholism, drug abuse, teenage pregnancy, child abuse, welfare dependency, and school dropouts.

It struck me that all these programs were focused on containment and remediation; almost none attempted prevention, much less cure. Most were based on the traditional assumption that we really can't hope to do much better, because people are intrinsically evil. The all-too-frequent failures were self-fulfilling prophecies, in terms of both human misery and financial efficiency. It seemed foolish and tragic to keep spending billions of dollars without ever wondering how we could get ahead of the game by searching out causes and developing strategies for prevention.

More and more frequently, I found, both the researchers studying social problems and the practitioners dealing with the individuals involved were citing self-esteem as a factor believed to be central to these problems. In light of the emerging evidence, it seemed both morally and fiscally responsible to create a formalized governmental effort to explore whether in fact self-esteem might be a "social vaccine," a quality capable of strengthening people, making them less vulnerable to problem behaviors.

Although I recognized that such a notion might sound "California-weird" and pose some political risks, my interest, my own growing self-esteem, and my supportive relationships outdistanced my caution. I consulted my long-time friend Jack Canfield—a self-esteem expert—who said, "It's time. Let's do something about it." I took the chance and introduced legislation in 1984. Somewhat to my surprise, that bill passed the assembly, although it died in the state senate.

In 1985, I reintroduced the bill, enlisting as lead coauthors Assembly Speaker and Democrat Willie Brown and two Republican legislative leaders, Minority leader Pat Nolan and Minority Caucus chair Gerry Felando, both conservatives. (Nolan had asked, "You really want to help people learn how to live without the government taking care of them?" When I replied, "That's right," he was convinced to sign on.) Again, the bill passed the assembly. This time, it also passed in the state senate by a vote of twenty-eight to eleven, but Governor George Deukmejian vetoed it, arguing that self-esteem had already been studied enough and that in any case the task could be accomplished more appropriately by the university than by the state government.

I reintroduced the bill in 1986 and focused on developing strategies to ensure its enactment. In an attempt to speak to the concerns of more conservatives, the bill's title and purpose were broadened to include the promotion of "personal and social responsibility." Its purview was limited to six pressing social issues, ones that were seen as critical by liberals and conservatives alike. I resisted much urging to abandon the term *self-esteem*, however; I believed that was precisely what we needed to address, and I wanted the legislation to be straightforward.

I personally lobbied every state senator who had voted against the legislation in 1985, and the senate finally passed the bill unanimously. Our campaign moved on, to focus on Governor Deukmejian. We enlisted key members of his cabinet and staff, as well as my Republican colleagues, to lobby the governor. With grassroots organizing, we generated more than four hundred letters, personalized and passionate, urging him to sign the bill.

The governor and I had three very intense one-on-one conversations about this bill. The turning point came during our third meeting, when he said, "I know that self-esteem is important, but why should the government get involved in this? Why not the university or somebody else?"

I responded, "First, Governor, there's so much at stake here that we can't afford to have it hidden away in a university. We need to involve the entire California public. Only the government can accomplish that. Second, think of it this way: By spending a few tax dollars, we can collect the information and get it out. If that helps even a few persons appreciate and understand self-esteem and how they can live their lives and raise their kids better, we may have less welfare, crime, violence, and drugs—and that's a very conservative use of taxpayers' money."

Suddenly the governor replied, "I've never thought of it that way before." He began raising questions about details of the bill. I immediately made a commitment to negotiate them to his satisfaction, and he promised to let me know his decision within a week. For the first time, I left his office feeling hopeful.

The next week, the governor's staff called to say that if minor amendments were made, the governor would not veto the bill. The changes were made almost immediately, and Deukmejian signed Assembly Bill 3659 into law in September. It created a twenty-five-member task force with a three-year span of activity and a yearly budget of $245,000 (the cost of incarcerating one felon for fourteen years).

The enactment of the legislation occasioned a truly astonishing outpouring of excitement and good will throughout the state. More than four hundred Californians applied for appointment to the task force. Even greater interest and enthusiasm followed cartoonist Garry Trudeau's lampoon in the comic strip "Doonesbury" in March of 1987. Ironically, his attention made us famous, providing us with a national stage and a large audience.

I wanted a task force whose work would be seen as legitimate and credible by all Californians, not a group of like-minded individuals whose conclusions could be easily dismissed. To get a well-balanced group, the power of appointing members was distributed. Four state officials—the state superintendent of schools, the cabinet secretary for health and welfare, the state attorney general, and the cabinet secretary for corrections—were named ex officio members, and each designated a departmental representative to participate in the task force. The governor made nine appointments. The Assembly Speaker and the Senate Rules Committee each made six appointments; two of these in each house came from minority party recommendations. And at its first meeting, the task force elected me and my colleague Senator Art Torres (who had carried the legislation on the senate floor) as ex officio members.

The effort to ensure diversity and balance among the group succeeded. The members of the task force are remarkably varied: men and women; members of different racial and ethnic groups; representatives of various professions, from educators and therapists to police officers and realtors; individuals from different religious backgrounds; heterosexuals and gays; thirteen Republicans and twelve Democrats. The participants have proven remarkably committed and generous, spending as much as four days a month as volunteers.

As the task force was forming, Governor Deukmejian called me to his office to discuss appointing a chairperson, pursuant to an earlier pledge. I mentioned several names, but then added, "You know, Governor, if you name one of your own appointees, rather than someone I suggest, it would add a special degree of credibility to the enterprise. I've heard several people praise your appointee Andy Mecca; it's fine with me if you appoint him." The governor looked startled, probably not expecting a nonpartisan proposal. But the next week he appointed Mecca, who has proven to be an excellent chairperson, both tough-minded and visionary.

Family therapist and teacher Virginia Satir was perhaps the most widely known and the most high-spirited of the task force members, and we owe her a great deal. Shortly before her death in September 1988, the task force voted unanimously that its final report would be dedicated to her. I was privileged to deliver this news to her less than forty-eight hours before she died. She responded by thanking the task force and asking me to tell the members what a great honor she considered their action to be.

Assembly Bill 3659 directed the task force to carry out three charges. The first was to compile research concerning the role of self-esteem as a possible causal factor in six areas of major social concern: crime and violence, alcohol and drug abuse, teenage pregnancy, child abuse, chronic welfare dependency, and educational failure. These are among the most compelling and the most lamentable social ills we face, and they are certainly problems on which we spend billions of tax dollars without seeming to make much headway. Collecting and analyzing research on the role of self-esteem in these areas could provide a foundation for designing more effective public policy strategies.

Thus the task force began negotiating with the University of California to develop summaries of academic research concerning self-esteem and the genesis of social problems. University officials recruited the most knowledgeable researchers in the relevant areas and secured their cooperation in preparing the essays in this book. Our hope is that this volume will analyze and clarify our intuition regarding the importance of self-esteem and that it will establish self-esteem at the center of our social science research agenda.

Many additional insights and proposals involving self-esteem are emerging from ongoing work in the field; some have not yet been systematically researched within the academic community. For this reason, the task force is also compiling supplementary material from operating programs in the six subject areas.

The second charge given to the task force was to compile current knowledge about how healthy self-esteem is developed, how it is damaged or lost, and how it can be revitalized. On May 4, 1988, the task force convened a brainstorming session in San Francisco, bringing together twenty practicing experts in the field of self-esteem, including Nathaniel Branden, Jack Canfield, Tom Gordon, George McKenna, Uvaldo Palomares, Scott Peck, Virginia Satir, and other men and women of various backgrounds, races, and professions. From that beginning, the task force is now developing a document concerning the "how-to" aspect of self-esteem.

The task force's third charge was to identify model self-esteem programs, including institutions to which people can turn when they need help for themselves or their families. We have begun to develop an inventory of available programs and materials and a set of criteria Californians can use to assess the legitimacy and likely value of these resources.

The state task force holds regular meetings every six weeks. After two years of meetings, our average attendance is twenty-three of the twenty-five members. We are also holding public hearings around California to give local residents an opportunity to contribute their knowledge and views to the task force's work. In addition, twenty-two departments and agencies of the state government have liaison officers who provide the task force with ongoing data about the role of self-esteem in the programs they operate.

Because of the enthusiasm and interest generated by the state task force, I introduced a resolution (coauthored by six key legislative leaders of both parties and both houses) encouraging each of California's fifty-eight counties to create a local task force on self-esteem. These local task forces are charged with connecting local experts on self-esteem with the human services programs in each county and serving as vehicles to bring the results of the state task force's work into communities throughout California. Already, forty-five counties have created such local bodies.

Individual responses to our work have also been extremely heartening. Shortly after the creation of the task force, we received a letter from a woman in Oakland which read: "Congratulations on creating the Self-Esteem Task Force. I'm eighty-seven years old, and I've been waiting a long time for the government to do something worthwhile."

But perhaps the most impressive response was an unexpected one: the task force's existence seems to have provided permission for many individual Californians to initiate their own endeavors to promote self-esteem and personal and social responsibility. The superintendent of schools in Riverside County has asked the county sheriff for the names of ten county jail inmates who can be involved in a self-esteem program that might enable them to steer their lives away from crime. Helice Bridges in San Diego plans to provide fifty thousand schoolchildren with blue ribbons reading, "Who I Am Makes a Difference." A political leader in Santa Clara County told me, "This may sound corny, but thank you. Because of your task force, I did a self-esteem weekend workshop. Since then, I'm treating my children better!"

Recently, three hundred fifty participants attended a two-day symposium, "Self-Esteem and the Community," at Humboldt State University. Two hundred people attended another conference, entitled "Multicultural Self-Esteem," at Long Beach State University. It seems clear that the self-esteem movement is becoming a broad-based social movement, engaging Californians at every level. The work of our task force has touched a deep nerve among the public, leading many individuals to enlist in this effort to look anew at who we are and how we address our problems. Nationally, reports from across the United States indicate that our endeavor has also served to legitimate the notion of self-esteem as a respectable focus of concern and analysis.

We are proud to present this volume, then, as an integral part of our work. We hope that it will serve to move the concept of self-esteem to center stage in social science research, to lay a solid foundation for future research, and to inspire other researchers to become involved in these efforts.

Perhaps most important, however, we also hope that it will, in conjunction with the other work of the task force, help to educate and encourage many individual Californians in the development and practice of self-esteem in their everyday lives. Research and science can discover the trail and point the way, but it is left to each of us to make the importance of self-esteem a reality in how we lead our lives and improve our society.

My father, who was an educator, early on taught me a lesson whose significance I recognize more each day: "You can't give what you haven't got." Virginia Satir, in her characteristic way, stated the same lesson positively: "What each of us most profoundly teaches is not 'what I say,' but 'how I model.'" By the character of your own presence, you will either encourage or discourage others' sense of themselves. Your own self-esteem and practice of responsibility inevitably affects these qualities and actions in others. Developing self-esteem and responsibility—a potential "vaccine" against the social problems we face—may be the most compelling of human ventures.

Self-Esteem and Social Problems: An Introduction

Neil J. Smelser

The well-being of society depends on the well-being of its citizenry. This is the central proposition on which the chapters in this volume—as well as the work of the California Task Force to Promote Self-Esteem and Personal and Social Responsibility—are based. This proposition is somewhat unorthodox, because a great deal of Western social and political thought would have it the other way around. Classical economic theorists, for example, regarded the productive and market arrangements of capitalism as an apparatus by which the greatest good for the greatest number could be realized; classical democratic theorists regarded the perfect democratic polity as the set of arrangements that would bring forth the best and most rational choices from an informed electorate.

The more particular proposition that informs our enterprise here is that many, if not most, of the major problems plaguing society have roots in the low self-esteem of many of the people who make up society. It is supposed that those citizens who appreciate themselves and have a sense of personal empowerment will cultivate their own personal responsibility and will attend to the tasks that are necessary for the welfare of the community and the society. It is further supposed that those in society who are burdened with the conviction that they are not worthy will take refuge in behaviors that are unproductive, costly, deviant, and dangerous to society and will, by that measure, contribute disproportionately to serious social problems. Bearing these two propositions in mind, it becomes essential for the leaders of society, first, to establish social conditions that will maximize the development of self-esteem among the population and, second, to establish social arrangements that will rescue and rehabilitate those who have emerged from families and communities with a sense of diminished self-worth. That is the agenda of the California Task Force to Promote Self-Esteem, and that is the agenda that we in this special volume on self-esteem and social problems are putting to the best critical test in light of the best social scientific literature available to us.

My task in this introductory essay is to develop a statement that synthesizes the issues raised and discussed, the knowledge compiled, and the conclusions assessed by the individual contributors to this volume. This will mean covering some of the same ground they do, but from a more general point of view. To that end, I will consider several major questions:

- What constitutes a social problem?

- How do we define the nature of a social problem, and how do we define self-esteem?

- What are the linkages between individual self-esteem and the generation of a social problem?

- How do we measure both of these?

- How do we go about establishing scientifically that connections exist between diminished self-esteem (cause) and the kind of behavior that constitutes a social problem (effect)?

- What are the scientific findings relevant to those connections?

- How do we intervene in a way that will attack the causes of the identified social problems and prevent the loss of self-esteem of those who are part of them?

What Constitutes a Social Problem?

In our accepted ways of thinking, a social problem is a kind of carbuncle on the social body, a tear in the social fabric that signals some kind of malfunctioning in society and sets up demands for its own amelioration. A social problem is some kind of tangible, identifiable, unwanted thing in society.

This conceptualization of a social problem, which treats the existence of a problem as a matter of verifiable fact, is, I argue, unrealistic. Before an empirical state of affairs can qualify as a social problem, it must be linked with a whole range of cultural and ideological phenomena. Let me illustrate:

First, behavior that we identify as constituting a social problem must be relevant to some institution that we endow with *cultural value*. Pregnancy out of wedlock, for example, is a problem in large part because it stands in violation of the value we place on the family as the legitimate locus for childbearing and child-rearing. Dropping out of the educational system is a problem because of the value we place on learning, both in itself and as preparation for entering the occupational structure. Chronic welfare dependency is a problem in part because it involves not participating in an established job or career; it is an interruption of involvement in that valued social role.

Second, behavior that becomes defined as a problem is also regarded as *deviant* in relation to some role expectation. This is clearest with respect to violence and crime, which are deviant because they are against the law; the same can be said for the use of illegal drugs. Dropping out of school also may be illegal because it deviates from the established code calling for compulsory schooling up to, say, age sixteen. Other behaviors, such as excessive alcohol consumption, teenage pregnancy, and being out of work, are not illegal, but they violate social norms relating to substance dependency, premarital sexual and childbearing behavior, and holding a job. A social problem thus involves some kind of social deviance.

The necessity of these value and normative references means that even though a certain kind of behavior may be prevalent in society, it is not considered a social problem unless and until these linkages are established. Child labor, for example, has always existed, but it did not come to be viewed as a social problem until moral crusaders holding humanitarian values deemed it one, and until child labor legislation supplied norms against which it could be considered deviant. The same is true of child abuse: only with the rise of humane values relating to parental discipline, and only with the rise of new expectations about punishment and degradation, did this widespread practice become a social problem. It follows that social problems may become such by virtue of value and normative drifts in society as much as by virtue of the appearance of new kinds of behavior. It is the *linkage* of a behavior to relevant value and normative considerations that gives it its character as a social problem.

An additional ingredient in the definition of a social problem—an empirical ingredient—is that the behavior in question must have a great enough incidence or prevalence to be regarded as significant; there must be some numbers of people perpetrating such behavior. The isolated occurrence of mass murders by snipers, for example, is not customarily defined as a social problem; rather, it is seen as a matter of individual psychopathology. The fact that almost all authors in this volume begin their expositions by referring to "the scope of the problem" also emphasizes the importance of incidence. A further ingredient, though not always an essential one, is evidence that the kind of behavior in question—drug dependency, mental illness, dropping out of school, child abuse—has been on the increase in the recent past. And a final part of this "numbers" aspect is that in order for a behavioral phenomenon to be considered a social problem, a sizable number of people have to be able to successfully define it as such and to make the required symbolic linkages to the relevant cultural and normative references; otherwise, it will not be perceived as a social problem, but only as the private and perhaps idiosyncratic preoccupation of a few.

Another element that goes into identifying a social problem is that it must be regarded as involving some economic or social cost. Crime is a good example: paying for the long-term incarceration of convicted criminals is an expensive proposition, to say nothing of the cost in human lives and private property that crime involves. The social cost of premarital pregnancy—defined in terms of welfare costs for mothers and the psychological costs to the children—is another ready example. It is the cost component of chronic welfare dependency that really endows that phenomenon with its characterization as a problem. Absenteeism, inefficiency, and low worker morale are among the high economic costs of alcoholism and drug dependency.

Finally, another necessary part of what defines a social problem is that we believe we can do something about it. It has to be something at which we can successfully throw resources; something we can ease by getting people to shape up; something that can be cured through social policy legislation and decisions and the application of knowledge; something that can be ameliorated. Otherwise, it is seen as one of those ineradicable scars on the social body that we have to live with, a necessary evil, one of those inevitable frailties of human nature. Better put, a social problem is something that we believe we have a way of dealing with; and if a significant number of people succeed in defining a social phenomenon as something we can do nothing about—it is "in the genes," it is in the nature of social life—it loses its status as a social problem.

This faith that we can do something about a social problem rests on two frequently unspoken assumptions about causality: first, that we understand what the main causes of the social problem are and therefore can target them in order to ameliorate the problem; and second, that we know that the recommended legal, policy, reformative, and therapeutic interventions will have an effect on those causes and thus will achieve that amelioration. It goes without saying that these assumptions are frequently not verified and that they are often not much more than matters of faith on the part of social diagnosticians and social reformers. Nevertheless, they are always present as part of a concern with social problems.

This discussion demonstrates that, in the last analysis, the existence of a social problem is a matter of persuasion and a matter of politics. To get a social problem on the agenda, sufficiently visible and powerful people have to persuade those who officially name social problems that a kind of behavior exists that is costly to society and that it has a high incidence in society—an incidence that is perhaps on the increase. Furthermore, they have to be persuasive in arguing that the problem constitutes an erosion of some institution we consider valuable or sacred, that it involves behavior that is deviant in light of some established law or norm, and that it is a problem we can do something about with the right social policy and the right investment of resources. All kinds of groups in society are forever jockeying with one another in attempts to have their favorite societal ill officially defined as a social problem and thereby placed on the table before the legislature or other concerned body; but of course only some of them succeed. For this reason, it is highly problematic—and it is the outcome of a complicated political process—that a social problem ever gets to be defined as such, much less gets the public attention it may deserve.

One final observation emerges from this discussion of social problems. The California Task Force to Promote Self-Esteem—and the scholars who have contributed to this volume—have focused on certain major concerns in American and California society that seem to qualify as social problems, that is, they include all the ingredients identified above. These social problems are child abuse, crime and violence, teenage pregnancy, academic failure, alcohol and drug abuse, and chronic welfare dependency. Obviously, these are only a few of the problems that could have been selected; an equally good case could have been made for including ecological and environmental threats, risks from nuclear power, threats to international security, the complex of sexism-racism-ageism, divorce and separation, and, above all, physical and mental health. We could easily have expanded the list to several hundred; in fact, there is no end to the catalogue. The problems considered here must be regarded as illustrative only, constituting but a small fraction of society's ills.

A Plausible Case for the Link Between
Self-Esteem and Social Problems

As an intuitive matter—based on our own personal experiences and our observations of others—we know what it is to experience high self-esteem. It means, fundamentally, that we appreciate ourselves and our inherent worth. It also means that we have a positive attitude toward our own qualities; that we evaluate them highly; that we are imbued with a sense of our own ability, competence, and power to do what we want; that we compare ourselves favorably with others; and that we can organize our daily round of activities and performances in keeping with these feelings of self-worth. We also know what it means to experience diminished self-esteem; it means the opposite of all those positive elements just described, and it results in self-deprecation, helplessness, powerlessness, and depression.

Also as an intuitive matter, we know how we are likely to behave, depending on whether we think well or poorly of ourselves. If the former is the case, we can take command and control of our lives; can consistently behave responsibly and well toward our duties and to others; and can do this on our own, without relying on any kind of psychological or social crutches. If we are down in the dumps, however, the tendency is to withdraw from performance into passivity; to seek some ready way to pick ourselves up or to have someone else do so; to seek out some activity that will make us feel better about ourselves, at least in the short run. As often as not, that kind of behavior is likely to be antisocial and deviant from some point of view: we take several drinks too many; we find a way to get high; we quit work; we drop out of school; we take our depression or hostility out on someone else; or we thrash around for some momentary impulse gratification, whatever that might be. This withdrawing, self-defeating, and deviant behavior is the stuff of which social problems are made, because it involves getting out of responsible, expected behavior patterns and getting into just the opposite. When this kind of behavior is aggregated, it becomes a social problem, and it gains the attention of those who care about how society is faring.

We are intuitively aware of what it takes to turn high self-esteem into low, and what it takes to turn low self-esteem into high. In the former instance, constant failures and a constant bombardment with the message that one does not count as a person or with others gradually add up to the feeling that one is a cipher in this world. In the latter case, the first step is acknowledging that one regards oneself as worthless or helpless or in the grips of self-abasement, combined with a sense of personal suffering and a desire to drag oneself out of the hole. When this is linked with a personally meaningful experience—perhaps finding a mate, perhaps getting a new job, perhaps entering psychotherapy, perhaps finding a new social or religious identity—the individual finds a new sense of capability, power, and self-control; a liking for oneself and who one is; and a capacity to get out of the realm of behavior that is damaging to oneself and to others and to reach toward the realm of responsible and pro-social behavior. Moreover, it is this significant turnaround from low to high self-esteem—and its behavioral consequences—that allows the ebbing away of those kinds of behavior that constitute social problems.

Intuition also tells us that both benign and vicious cycles characterize various levels of self-esteem and their supposed behavioral consequences. This is particularly true when we consider self-esteem in its interpersonal reference. As for the benign cycle, consider the appearance of a respected and admired role model in the life of a young and disadvantaged schoolchild, a model who, by giving encouragement and support and being a good mentor, fills that pupil with a sense of value, competence, and power. These feelings are reflected in the superior academic and social performance of the child; this feeds positively into the child's self-perception and turns into an upward spiral that may continue throughout life. Consider also the confirmed and self-abased alcoholic who finally acknowledges to friends and supporters in Alcoholics Anonymous that he or she is completely helpless in the face of alcohol dependence, who through membership and assistance from alcoholic colleagues is able to find strength through abstinence, and who builds from this a greater involvement and achievement in work, marriage, and friendship. As for the vicious cycle, we need consider only that dynamic described in this volume by Scheff, Retzinger, and Ryan: one partner in an interpersonal relationship is subtly but tangibly shamed by the other and does not acknowledge this debasement but instead lashes out in a violent rage toward the other person. The violence sets off a frenzy of greater shame and guilt, which can find expression only in another bout of destructiveness.

In this case, the causal link is clear: low self-esteem is the causally prior factor in individuals seeking out kinds of behavior that become social problems. Thus, to work on social problems, we have to work directly on that which deals with the self-esteem of the individuals involved. Or, as we say in the trade, diminished self-esteem stands as a powerful *independent variable* (condition, cause, factor) in the genesis of major social problems. We all know this to be true, and it is really not necessary to create a special California task force on the subject to convince us. The real problem we must address—and which the contributors to this volume address—is how we can determine that it is scientifically true.

Further intuitive reflection, however, should convince us that citing diminished self-esteem as an independent variable in the generation of social problems is only a partial diagnosis. We know equally well that diminished self-esteem is often the product of something outside the individual, something in one's personal and social environment. If a child is singled out as the family dummy, is the one voted least likely to succeed, or is abused by parents and siblings, that child is a poor candidate for having high self-esteem throughout any part of life. If a child in school is continually identified by teachers as stupid, is made to sit in the corner with the dunce cap on, or is relegated to the inferior academic track, he or she is a good candidate for developing a poor self-concept. If a child is continually scapegoated by peers and is always the follower and never the leader, he or she may don that role throughout life. Or if individuals are members of a group in society—usually a minority group—that is routinely abased, thought to be inferior, and denied access to chances for advancement and a share of the good things in life, those individuals may pick up and wear the image that they do not count for much or deserve much. In short, self-esteem is as much an effect of psychological and social causes as it is a cause of social problems. Or, as we say in the trade, it is an *intervening variable* in the genesis of social problems. Those who would ease social problems, moreover, would have to have social reform on their agenda—that is, the effort to reshape the practices and institutions in society that make for human suffering, degradation, and injustice. In this conception of social problems, such problems are ultimately the product of culture and society, and efforts at amelioration involve social transformation, not only individual therapy and rehabilitation.

In practice, of course, the diagnosis of and assault on social problems involve working on both theories at once—that social problems are the products of individuals with psychological dispositions who act out or act up in society and thus create the problems, *and* that they are the products of imperfect social institutions that generate the dispositions in individuals to act this way. Many social problems seem almost intractable; they do not go away easily; and they call for a multifaceted attack, an attack that involves both many kinds of therapy and the rehabilitation of individuals, on the one hand, and the reform of practices and institutions, on the other.

The big issues facing those social scientists and policymakers who wonder about social problems and their causes and cures are to formalize this intuitive knowledge: to develop the proper definitions of what behaviors constitute social problems and what factors constitute their causes; to develop proper measures of those behaviors and those factors; to find associations or correlations between the behaviors and the factors; to assign causal significance to those associations; and to devise interventions that will modify the factors and thus change the behaviors. To these difficult issues we now turn.

Defining Self-Esteem and Its Consequences

Two theoretically minded colleagues of mine in West Germany undertook a major research project about two years ago. It concerned the topic of "the major social crises in postmodern Western society." After two years of concerted work, they submitted their conclusion: "We have been able to determine that we can neither define nor measure either 'major social crises' or 'postmodern Western society.' That concludes our research report." Things are not quite so bad in our case, but it has been found—and it is reported by the contributors to this volume—that we encounter a number of conceptual problems in getting at the essence of self-esteem and its various behavioral consequences.

As suggested before, we have a fairly firm grasp of what is meant by self-esteem, as revealed by our own introspection and observation of the behavior of others. But it is hard to put that understanding into precise words. Often, when we try to describe something we are uncertain about, we flounder around with a number of different words, not one of which captures its essence. In addition to self-esteem, our authors have identified the ideas of self, self-concept, self-respect, awareness, identity, image, congruence, and consciousness. None of these hits the nail on the head. Neither do the negative opposites, such as lack of self-concept, powerlessness, helplessness, ineffectiveness, inefficacy, self-derogation, anxiety effects, depression, or lack of self-esteem. Is there anything we can salvage from this definitional maze?

One starting point is to identify the almost universally accepted components of the concept. There is first a cognitive element; self-esteem means characterizing some parts of the self in descriptive terms: power, confidence, agency. It means asking what kind of person one is. Second, there is an affective element, a valence or degree of positiveness or negativeness attached to those facets identified; we call this high or low self-esteem. Third, and related to the second, there is an evaluative element, an attribution of some level of worthiness according to some ideally held standard.

What that standard is is another feature of self-esteem. Sometimes the standard is an absolute sense of self-regard, measured against an ego ideal that one holds out for oneself. Or it may be a relative standard, measuring one's sense of self-worth in relation to an internal aspiration or desired level of attainment. Sometimes the standard or point of reference is mainly internal or psychological; sometimes it involves measuring one's self-worth in relation to another person or group. The latter case is particularly important for members of minority groups, who compare their own group's fortunes to the situations enjoyed by other groups in society.

Greater definitional difficulties arise when we consider the stability of the concept of self-esteem. Should it be regarded as some kind of global attribute, one that enjoys a constant strength and level of organization for the individual? Or should it be treated as largely situational? All of us know that we feel good about ourselves at one moment, bad about ourselves at another, depending on mood and social situation. Add to this complication the fact that high self-esteem is sometimes experienced as an inherent set of feelings, but at other times as a defensive reaction against feelings of inferiority or inadequacy. In the latter case, high self-esteem is better described as vanity, arrogance, or egotism. All these definitional difficulties will come into play when we consider problems of measurement or try to arrive at operational definitions of the concept.

With respect to the supposed behavioral consequences of high or low self-esteem, we are somewhat better off conceptually, but not too much so. Definitions are most easily formulated in the areas that are clearly marked off behaviorally from their opposites. For example, we know what it is not to be enrolled in school, because of the institutional character of that attachment; it is more difficult to determine when one is not learning, however. It is relatively easy to define when one is out of work, though the phenomena of part-time work, seeking or not seeking employment, and unpaid labor complicate that definition. It is relatively easy to define teenage sexual activity, and quite easy to define teenage pregnancy. It is easy to define what we mean by the ingestion of some drug substance, much more difficult to define the ingestion of "too much." We know fairly well what we mean by "crime," but we are often hard put to come up with a clear definition of what constitutes violence. In the area of child abuse, we find the greatest difficulties. Bhatti, Derezotes, Kim, and Specht cite legal, medical, sexual, and psychological definitions of abuse, each of which yields a different range of meanings.

It is particularly important to raise these questions of definition, because we want to be certain that definitions of supposed causes (e.g., low self-esteem) are kept separate from definitions of their supposed behavioral consequences (e.g., psychological stimulation by drugs or alcohol). Otherwise, we will be caught naming the same things twice, thereby making it difficult to argue that they are independent from one another and difficult to avoid circular reasoning.

Measuring Self-Esteem and Its Consequences

In measuring what we have conceptually defined, it is customary to ask two kinds of questions: Is the measure we adopt reliable (that is, is it a consistent measure of some definite phenomenon)? Is the measure we adopt valid (that is, does it constitute a measure of what we think we are measuring)?

In assessing self-esteem, we have been supplied primarily with measures designed by professional psychologists, and we are short on other kinds of measures. The typical psychological measure is arrived at by posing a question or set of questions to a group of people, asking them how they describe themselves, how effective they believe themselves to be, or how much in control of things they are. Or the questions may be framed to get at how people feel about themselves, for example, how positively or how negatively they regard themselves. Or the questions may be devised to discern how people compare their own well-being with that of some comparison group. Several true-false questions from the Tennessee Self-Concept Scale may serve as an example:

1. I have a healthy body;
2. I am satisfied with my moral behavior;
3. I have a lot of self-control.

This set of questions touches the internal or psychological aspect of self-esteem and the individual's sense of self-competence. From this list, we already can see one measurement problem, namely, that one set of questions (self-descriptive) may be getting at something entirely different from what another set of questions (self-evaluative) addresses, thus tapping different facets of the mental set we define as self-esteem. Be that as it may, the "measure" of self-esteem is usually taken to be the kind of response evoked by administering the questions in an interview or experimental setting. The responses are usually recorded, averaged, and given some quantitative representation. The object of seeking these sorts of measurements is to identify some index that we can compare and correlate with the supposed behavioral consequences of the measured attribute.

Two measurement problems are associated with this kind of self-report procedure. First, no measure of self-esteem taps more than one or two of the facets of that phenomenon (cognitive, emotive, evaluational, or interpersonal), and for that reason any measure will yield an incomplete representation. Second, most of the measures assume that self-esteem is global, not situational, and does not vary over time. This assumption is questionable. It is true that with many measures of reliability (split-test, inter-judge, repeated administration over time) the phenomenon of self-esteem seems to have some integrity; it seems to be something that can be tapped on a fairly consistent basis. Yet investigators have discovered that measurements of children's self-esteem fluctuate over time and from situation to situation and that measurements of children's self-esteem yield results that are different from those found by measurements of adults' self-esteem, even when the instruments designed to measure the one kind are adapted to measure the other. When it comes to assessing the validity of these measures, the concept of self-esteem often becomes slippery and elusive. Validity of such a measurement is usually assessed by holding it up against some other kind of measure of self-estimation or of performance (e.g., on intelligence tests) or some other kind of self-assessment (e.g., depression, feelings of empowerment or self-control). These measures of validity are very erratic, suggesting either that the phenomenon of self-esteem is not very stable or that its measures are imperfect representations of something else.

Measuring the behavioral consequences of self-esteem also poses some difficulties, which parallel the definitional difficulties outlined above. We can measure welfare dependency by checking with various welfare agencies or by asking people whether and how long they have been out of work, but these measurements of "spells" often do not record erratic or short-term work. We can also track rates of school attrition or dropout rates by consulting school enrollment records, but these too may be inaccurate; it is often not known whether dropouts have left school altogether or are in school somewhere else, because they are not usually tracked after they drop out. We can measure whether a teenager is sexually active (although the line between sexually active and inactive is difficult to draw, because level of activity may differ over time), and we can determine medically if a teenager is pregnant. We have consistent measures of crime (although police arrest records, self-reports of victims, and self-reports of perpetrators yield a wide range of figures, especially for major crimes). Measures of violent behavior, however, are difficult to come by, largely because violence appears in so many psychological and social forms. With respect to one form of violence in particular—child abuse—the measurement problems mount, because of the vagueness of the line between nonviolent and violent behavior and because one kind of violence is often indistinguishable from another. We have good medical and behavioral measures on the intake of drugs and alcohol, but we do not have any consensus on what it takes to declare someone "dependent" on these substances. Thus, when attempting to determine the "scope" or incidence of the problems posed by these behaviors, all our authors found themselves referring to various measures; but all of them also took refuge in discussing the difficulties that stem from "unrecorded" or "invisible" occurrence and thus confound any consistent effort to measure prevalence, much less changes in prevalence over time.

There are good sociological reasons why measures of the supposed behavioral consequences of self-esteem are so elusive. Many of these behaviors are either illegal or deviant from some point of view. Both the perpetrators and the recorders of such behaviors may have a vested interest in keeping a low profile. This secrecy is well understood by the perpetrators, who keep their behavior "in the closet." As for the recorders, police, attorneys, physicians, and insurance companies often keep the lid on various kinds of behavior (alcoholism, for example) to avoid stigmatizing individuals or blemishing a person's official record.

As we will indicate later, the main purpose of social science investigations of the phenomena we have been discussing is to establish meaningful correlations between one set of reliable and valid indicators and another set and to work out the best ways to establish causal relations between them. But if the measures are not independent from one another, and if they are not reliable and valid, we have to assume that the measures of association are bedeviled with an unknown amount of error.

Establishing Associations and Causes

We now move from the intuitive models of high self-esteem and low self-esteem and their consequences—representations of which make great sense—to the adoption of scientific procedures that will establish relations among these variables and permit the inference of causal priority. In this operation, we must first establish what our expectations are with respect to causal priority. For most of the social problems listed in the legislative charge to the California Task Force to Promote Self-Esteem, the expected causal direction is fairly clear: low self-esteem (and perhaps the tendency to abuse) on the part of the abused; depression leading to alcohol and drug abuse; low self-esteem leading to quitting school or work; and so on. In some cases, however, the logic is only half-plausible. For example, because so much unemployment is involuntary and so many of these unemployed people are chronically dependent on welfare, we can hardly expect that the causally prior condition for chronic dependence is low self-esteem. It might be the case, however, that such dependency causes low self-esteem, because chronic dependency is stigmatized in our society and because it contributes to feelings of helplessness and powerlessness.

The next step is to identify a population that scores low on self-esteem and to see if these low scores can be related to one or more suspected behavioral consequences, particularly as this relationship is compared with that of another population that scores "normal" or "high" on self-esteem measures (often referred to as the "control group"). Or, to take another and more indirect tack, the investigator may take a group that is assumed to be low in self-esteem because of its disadvantaged economic or social position (for example, blacks) and ask whether members of this group engage in the behaviors predicted, again in relationship to members of other groups (for example, Asian Americans or Anglos).

The procedures by which these plausible relations are tested for correlation are highly standardized. We need first a quantitative measure of self-esteem, gathered by administering one of the many measures designed to tap that variable, and a quantitative measure of the problem behavior in question. These measures are converted into scales (how much of the time do I feel dissatisfied with myself? how often do I take drugs?), and a standardized measure of association (correlation coefficient) is applied. Often, this is combined with an estimate of how much of the variance in the dependent variable (e.g., drug-taking) is accounted for by scores on the independent variable (e.g., low self-estimation). A further test of the strength of association is made by estimating, by standardized statistical procedure, how often this association might have been expected to occur by chance alone (say, 5 percent of the time).

One of the disappointing aspects of every chapter in this volume (at least to those of us who adhere to the intuitively correct models sketched above) is how low the associations between self-esteem and its consequences are in research to date. In some cases, consistent relationships are found. Substantial numbers of studies show a low level of self-esteem among socially isolated parents who abuse their children; high self-esteem is associated with the use of contraceptives by teenage girls; measures of high self-esteem correlate positively with achievement in the classroom, and, as self-esteem decreases, so does academic achievement; *within* different sociocultural groups, drug and alcohol abuse are positively correlated with low self-esteem.

With respect to the sources of low self-esteem, the results also appear to run in the expected directions. Children with alcoholic parents have lower self-esteem than other children; children who have been abused by their parents show low scores on self-esteem measures; adults who have been on welfare for long periods show low self-esteem; and students who fail in competitively based school situations suffer from blows to their self-esteem.

Sometimes, however, the associations run in unexpected directions. For example, the use of psychoactive drugs seems to have a positive effect on self-esteem (though the association is questionable, because other changes in consciousness appear to take place as well). In a curious report on intervention, Bhatti, Derezotes, Kim, and Specht describe a TV ad developed by the National Committee on Child Abuse that seems designed to convince abusive parents that their behavior is reprehensible (and thus to lower their self-esteem), which suggests—strangely— a positive association between high self-esteem and child abuse!

The news most consistently reported, however, is that the associations between self-esteem and its expected consequences are mixed, insignificant, or absent. This nonrelationship holds between self-esteem and teenage pregnancy, self-esteem and child abuse, self-esteem and most cases of alcohol and drug abuse. The question naturally arises:

why are the correlations so low? The following possibilities come to mind:

• As often as not, an association between self-esteem and its behavioral consequences is not found because the variable of self-esteem is never even measured or brought to bear. That is the case in most of the studies of drug and alcohol abuse among different minority groups. And self-esteem or other psychological factors as independent variables are almost never represented in studies of chronic welfare dependency.

• The anticipated relationships may be valid but are counteracted by a counterassociation that arises from actually engaging in the problem behavior. For example, a teenage girl, plagued by feelings of low self-esteem and loneliness, may engage in sexual behavior (and even become pregnant) because she needs love and affection at any cost. But through the mechanisms of reinforcement and anticipatory association, she may experience feelings of increased self-esteem from the sexual relationship or the pregnancy. Lonely, dispirited, and depressed individuals may abuse their bodies by ingesting too much drink or too many drugs, but they may receive temporary boosts to their self-esteem through those actions. These feelings may be reinforced by rewards from supportive peers. Through the vicious cycle of shame, guilt, and self-disgust, an individual may strike out in rage at an intimate, but the temporary relief experienced may generate stronger feelings of self-worth and self-realization. In all these cases, the causal priority is reversed, and the positive association is washed out by the negative one.

• Another reason why posited or predicted associations may be low has to do with the character of the variables being related. Self-esteem is represented as a global, dispositional variable with a great many possible behavioral outcomes, including substance abuse, crime and violence, compulsive seeking for social support, and a variety of withdrawal behaviors, including dropping out of school and quitting work. Because there are multiple consequences, it stands to reason that self-esteem will be correlated with many outcomes, but that correlation will be weak in any given case. From a state of self-esteem alone, in other words, it is not plausible to expect a high correlation with any of these consequences.

• The main reasons for low correlations are probably methodological; that is, the measures of self-esteem do not tap that variable reliably or validly, and the measures of the behavior in question are similarly flawed. The error built into associations (or nonassociations) between variables is always unknown, because its magnitude is always a mystery. The logic that intuitively links self-esteem with some kind of outcome does not correspond with the logic that leads us to construct quantitative indices of dispositional qualities such as self-esteem and quantitative indices of actual behavior; thus the link that we all know exists is shrouded in error.

• Potentially positive associations are not found because additional plausible factors are not held constant. If level of intelligence is controlled, it, rather than self-esteem, may turn out to be the major determining factor in academic performance. The availability of contraceptives may be an opportunity factor that confounds the link between low self-esteem and both teenage sexual behavior and teenage pregnancy. Crockenberg and Soby report that because race and ethnicity may affect teenage sexual behavior and pregnancy, any association between those behaviors and psychological dispositions may be clouded. Also, in a given cohort of teenagers (for example, in the 1970s and 1980s), all of the young people may have been sexually active at an earlier age than in the past (because of more lenient sexual mores); certainly it is difficult to assume or demonstrate that increased incidence was caused by a jump in the incidence of low self-esteem.

If the association between self-esteem and behavior is so often reported to be weak, even less can be said for the causal relationship between the two. Why, we ask next, must this causal relationship be regarded as so weak?

The first answer to this question is based on the common scientific knowledge that correlation does not establish cause. This has been acknowledged ever since John Stuart Mill demonstrated it in his discussion of methods of scientific proof and ever since Émile Durkheim was forced to concede, much against his methodological preferences, that concomitant variation (association or correlation) cannot be taken as evidence for positing a causal connection.

The second answer is found in the specific limitations of the studies reported in the various chapters. As each author indicates, most of the research on which the findings and interpretations are based has been done with small samples, with relatively simple psychological measures of self-esteem held against some outcome, with simple correlational methods, with no control groups or control variables taken into account, and with temporal priority of variables not taken into account. Thus, each author uses well-advised caution in assigning causal signifi-

cance to whatever associations were observed. In several chapters, longitudinal designs—which are one of the best means of gaining insight
into causal priority of one variable over another—are discussed. In one
case, there appeared to be a longitudinally based, causally significant relationship between length of time on welfare and the variable of learned
helplessness (low self-esteem). In another case, Crockenberg and Soby
report the results of three longitudinal studies relating self-esteem and
subsequent pregnancy; two studies found a relationship between the
two variables, and the third reported no association between self-esteem
and pregnancy. The strength of these studies lies in the fact that measures of self-esteem were taken before the reported or observed pregnancies, but even here there was little effort to control for the intervention of other variables.

New Research

The main conclusion to be drawn from this extended discussion of
definition, measurement, and association is that the social-psychological variable of self-esteem is simultaneously one of the most central and
one of the most elusive factors in understanding and explaining the behaviors that constitute major social problems. It is central because it is
the omnipresent variable that intervenes between personal and institutional histories of individuals with productive, responsible, and self-
realizing behavior, on the one hand, and deviant, self-defeating, socially
costly behavior, on the other. Furthermore, it is a variable that is not
reducible to those personal and institutional histories, because we can
produce both instances of well-endowed, well-loved, and well-supported
individuals who move through life with the gloomiest assessment of
themselves and instances of children who are disadvantaged and abused
from almost every standpoint but who manage to tough it out and pre-
serve a high estimation of themselves and their capacity for personally
and socially responsible behavior. The variable of self-esteem is elusive,
however, because its precise role in the drama of self-realization is difficult to pinpoint scientifically; by using the conventional kinds of scientific methods we possess, it is difficult to arrive at strong associations
between self-esteem and its supposed causes, on the one hand, and self-
esteem and its supposed outcomes, on the other. Or, to put the matter
more simply, the scientific efforts to establish those connections that we
are able to acknowledge and generate from an intuitive point of view do
not reproduce those relations.

When we are confronted with the situation I have just described—an evidently important variable or set of variables whose importance is nevertheless not readily discernible in the available research—a multifaceted attack is usually called for. Some of the necessary work must be mainly theoretical, directed toward recasting the definition, meaning, and behavioral significance of the concept. Perhaps the global concept of self-esteem should also be disaggregated conceptually into isolable subvariables. More reliable and valid measures should be sought. And above all, our scientific procedures need to be improved; we must have more ambitious and better-devised scientific investigations if the state of our knowledge in the several areas in which self-esteem plays a role is to be advanced. The new kinds of research I have in mind should have some particular characteristics.

First, the samples studied should be large. The research reviewed in the following chapters has been carried out primarily with small, ad hoc samples generated by researchers who have pulled together the sample from groups that were available to them through some personal or institutional contact. Small samples yield relations that cannot be regarded as statistically significant; when uncovered, these relations cannot permit causal inferences; and, above all, small samples do not permit the holding constant of other variables suspected of affecting the relationships between self-esteem and some outcomes.

Second, major control variables should be taken into account in the design of the studies and samples. Researchers should draw separate samples from populations of low-income, middle-income, and high-income groups; from populations of children with low intelligence and children with high intelligence; from children of intact families and from children of broken or one-parent families; from children in minority groups and children in the majority group; and so on. All these group factors are of obvious significance in the development of self-esteem and its consequences; but if representatives of these groups are mixed indistinguishably in the same samples, the finer play of the individual and the institutional histories of the persons studied cannot be traced.

Third, the research must involve more than simple correlational studies. The imposition of controls described above is one way of going beyond simple correlations and controlling for variables. In addition, research designs should take into account that both the factors affecting the genesis of self-esteem and the behavioral consequences of self-esteem are multiple. This calls for imposing methods of multiple regression, partial correlation, path analysis, and the like, so that the relative strength of each of those factors is singled out, identified, and assigned an appropriate designation.

Fourth, the studies must be longitudinal. Samples can be drawn either prospectively—that is, from groups of those whose "career" outcomes with respect to some kind of behavior (crime, substance abuse, educational persistence) are not yet known—or retrospectively—that is, from groups of individuals who have "arrived" at one or another of these outcomes and groups of individuals who have not. In the samples drawn prospectively, the task is to track the subjects over time, recording the distinctive features of their family circumstances (e.g., birth order, divorce history of parents, kinds of abusive behavior); the parade of successes and failures they experience in school, and the treatment they receive from teachers; their history of experiences with peers in the classrooms and on the sports fields; their encounters with advisers, scoutmasters, camp leaders, and other potential mentors; the brushes they have with police and juvenile authorities. In samples drawn retrospectively, histories should be rewritten "backwards," as it were—reconstructed to take into account the same sorts of variables that impinge on individuals' lives. When possible, experimental or quasi-experimental designs should be devised, so that proper controls can be attained over third factors; and the administration of survey and other instruments should be supplemented by in-depth interviews and direct observations of the subjects, so that the meaning-context of the events to which they are exposed through their developmental years can be ascertained. Above all, these studies should document the vicissitudes of the subjects' self-esteem in its various measurable facets.

A model for these kinds of studies is found in the beginning efforts to study criminal careers, in which there is systematic examination of large samples of those who seem destined for a life of crime or those who have become involved in such a life, as contrasted with those who have never committed crimes or those who became involved as juveniles but later "dropped out" in favor of more law-abiding lives. Important events in the lives of these subjects are family experience (including discipline and nurturance), school experience, work history, marital history, and experiences in prison. These are the same variables, moreover, that affect those who engage in various kinds of self-abuse, those who end their schooling early, those who are unable to hold a job, and so on.

Such longitudinal, controlled studies should involve every kind of sample and group available. It is apparent, however, that from the standpoints of urgency and policy relevance the most careful and well documented study should be devoted to those groups who tend to contribute most to social problems and whose self-esteem appears to be at greatest risk (disadvantaged minorities, low-income groups, children from poverty-stricken and single-parent families, for example).

Fifth, the research must be adequately and substantially funded. Launching large-scale, longitudinal study involves both the expenditure of much greater sums of research money than have been available heretofore and the mobilization of the finest research talent available. Supporting such research means changing our basic assumptions about empirical investigation, because it involves funding research projects that will be based on an investment of money over many years; moreover, this investment will have to be renewed periodically, so that the long-term tracking of the samples can continue. Only ample funding of this sort can produce an understanding of the development of the social problem behaviors that concern us. It seems fair to conclude that failure to provide such support for sound, policy-related research may prove far more costly in the long run, both in terms of dollars and in terms of human suffering.

The Problem of Intervention Strategy

It follows from this brief overview of scientific research that the guidelines for intervention and policies aimed at rehabilitation, prevention, and institutional reform will be as murky as the state of our knowledge of the phenomena concerned. And so they are. The authors who have assessed the state-of-the-art knowledge of factors important in the genesis of many social problems have been unable to uncover many causally valid findings relating to that genesis—and they have therefore been correspondingly unable to come up with systematic statements relating to cure or prevention. Most settled for reviewing that portion of the literature that discussed possible interventions and evaluated these studies as best they could.

In their review, Bhatti, Derezotes, Kim, and Specht identify several possible theoretical explanations of the increase in child abuse in recent generations. These include the weakening of taboos against the exploitation of children, the continued existence of poverty and economic stress, men who are intimidated by "liberated" women (men who subsequently strike out at their children to regain a sense of their own manhood), and the growing prevalence of those types of families in which child abuse may result from insufficient bonding (stepfamilies, adoptive families, single-parent families, and families in which both parents are working). Policy interventions based on this range of possible causes should be correspondingly varied, including psychotherapy, police action to prevent abuse, and punishment of abusers, as well as institutional changes that would ameliorate the conditions that contribute to abuse, such as poverty and family frailty. Yet the authors are able to identify only two kinds of intervention that have been tried: psychotherapy of various sorts that aims to restore self-esteem to those who have been abused, and limited sorts of prevention aimed at protecting children from being abused. Neither intervention has produced more than inconclusive results, and no efforts whatsoever seem to have been directed at any of the possible underlying institutional causes of child abuse. Crockenberg and Soby argue that the family and the school are the most logical focus of policy interventions to affect the incidence of teenage pregnancy, but the basis of their argument appears to be little more than that these institutions are the most important sources of control over impulsiveness in the teen years.

Other possibilities for intervention are mentioned in the various chapters, but in many instances the form of intervention appears to involve certain other social costs that we may be unwilling to pay. One line of research—actually, some of the best research—has shown that black children who experienced their early years of schooling in integrated school settings appear to exhibit lower self-esteem than do black children who have been taught in schools that remained effectively segregated. Does this mean that we wish to turn back the clock and return to a system of segregated schools? Few would argue that that policy is worth the social cost. Covington suggests that primary schools should maximize what he calls equity systems, in which all students are provided with equally attractive incentives for pursuing academic goals and are not subjected to the zero-sum competitive school settings in which few students are winners and most students compete mainly to avoid failure. But such a system appears to run the risk of minimizing the competitive, individual-achievement basis for incentives, which runs through most of the institutions of our society. Do we want to scrap the competitive principle in schools, only to revive it in later occupational settings and thus make schooling irrelevant to later life? Many would agree that the negative effects on self-esteem that schooling almost inevitably involves should be conditioned by humane practices, but few would argue that the deeply institutionalized competitive principle can be realistically minimized in school settings in the short run.

Wisdom appears to suggest caution, then, in the area of policy. Certainly we should encourage interventions and public expenditures that could strengthen rehabilitation and construct institutional arrangements to rescue or bolster self-esteem. But these interventions should be cautious, with experimentation, model programs, and continuous evaluation the order of the day. As scientific findings become more reliable, however, and as the involvement of self-esteem in the causes of social problems becomes better understood, policy interventions can profitably become correspondingly bolder.

The Association Between Child Maltreatment and Self-Esteem

Bonnie Bhatti, David Derezotes,
Seung-Ock Kim, and Harry Specht

The problem of child maltreatment is currently receiving a great deal of public attention, accompanied by a vast array of programs to prevent child abuse and to punish and treat child abusers. Many of these efforts are directed at changing in one way or another the self-esteem of abusers and high-risk parents. A popular TV spot developed by the National Committee on Child Abuse, for example, is directed at lowering the self-esteem of people who abuse their children; the intent is to prevent abuse by making parents feel that abusive behavior is insensitive and reprehensible. In contrast, psychotherapeutic intervention often attempts to *increase* the self-esteem of abusive parents.

People use the term *child abuse* to mean many things, ranging from mild physical restraint to emotional rejection to sexual assault. Similarly, the term *self-esteem* can mean the sense we have of ourselves (regardless of how others see us) or the sense of how we believe others regard us (despite our own inner sense of worthiness). The association between child abuse and self-esteem is exceedingly complex. In this chapter, we will describe the knowledge available in social science literature about the relationship between these two phenomena. We will also attempt to clarify some of the terminology used in debates on these issues, as we focus on the following questions:

1. What is the current scope of the problem of child abuse?
2. How is child abuse defined and measured?

3. How is self-esteem defined and measured?

4. What factors appear to be associated with child abuse, and, specifically, to what extent is one's degree of self-esteem associated with child abuse?

5. In what ways does society attempt to treat (that is, to change the behavior of) child abusers?

6. What evidence is available to assess the effectiveness and efficiency of these treatments?

The Scope of the Problem

Recent statistics on child maltreatment * indicate a continuing rise in the number of reported cases. One national study revealed almost 2 million reported cases of child abuse in 1985 (American Humane Association 1987). This figure represents 30.6 abused children per 1,000 children in the United States. Of the cases reported in the study, 43 percent were substantiated. The authors of this national study caution against inferring that the remaining 57 percent of the reported cases were false allegations; rather, there simply was insufficient evidence at the time of the report to substantiate the allegation.

The American Humane Association (AHA) also conducted a study of abuse cases in Florida, Illinois, New York, and Texas. Of a total of 225,360 abused children in the four states, 21.7 percent were physically abused, 11.7 percent were sexually abused, 55.7 percent were physically and/or emotionally neglected, 8.5 percent were emotionally abused, and 10.2 percent experienced other forms of abuse such as abandonment (AHA 1987). As in other studies, these various forms of abuse overlap one another, resulting in multiple counting of cases. (For example, a particular child may suffer from all forms of abuse and therefore be counted more than once.)

The AHA reports that the numbers in its nationwide study represent an increase of 11.6 percent from 1984 to 1985, and an increase of 100 percent since 1976. These findings are consistent with many other studies showing an increase in the reported incidence of child maltreatment. There is much debate among child abuse experts over what ac-

---

* The term *child maltreatment* will be used interchangeably with the term *child abuse* in this discussion; the former term is currently used by experts to describe the many forms of abuse that children can suffer, including physical abuse, sexual abuse, neglect, and psychological maltreatment.

counts for this increase. In a review of the literature, four perspectives emerge that offer plausible explanations.

The first view argues that there has been a weakening of the taboo against the exploitation of children, particularly the taboo against sexual abuse (Russell 1986; Sgroi 1982; Butler 1978; Rush 1980). This view was introduced by feminist writers and is now a predominant theme in theories of sexual abuse. Feminist theorists hold that public acceptance of child pornography has resulted in the sexualization of children. Groups such as the René Gunyon Society are emerging, with slogans such as "Sex by age eight, or else it's too late." Russell (1986) and others believe that this attitude originated, in part, in the sexual revolution of the 1960s, which promoted a nondiscriminating, "anything goes" attitude toward sexual activities. This perspective suggests that increases in child maltreatment are largely the result of changes in cultural values and beliefs.

A second perspective holds that increased economic pressures result in increased social problems, one of which is child abuse. This perspective not only is supported by feminists but also is popular with other abuse experts such as Gil (1978), Garbarino and Gilliam (1980), Kempe and Kempe (1984), and Justice and Justice (1979). Some experts believe that external pressures such as dissatisfaction in the workplace or lack of financial resources serve as catalysts for many forms of violence in the family (Dietz and Craft 1980; Kempe and Kempe 1984). This argument suggests that child maltreatment is essentially an economic and political problem.

Proponents of a third view link the increase in child abuse to the struggle of women to gain equal rights. Men, they argue, have traditionally been raised to expect deference and admiration from women and to feel a sense of power over them. When men fear losing this power and admiration and feel intimidated by women, they may reach out to or abuse children to satisfy their needs for power and control. A related phenomenon involves the profound changes in the makeup of modern families, particularly the increasing number of stepfamilies, adoptive families, single-parent families, and families in which both parents are working. Some argue that in such families adults often do not experience the bonding that usually occurs between infant and parent, making children in these families more vulnerable to abuse. This perspective suggests that child maltreatment is fundamentally a problem of social structure.

A fourth perspective holds that there has actually been no significant increase in child abuse. Rather, there has simply been an increase in reporting, because public education has enhanced public awareness both of the problem itself and of child abuse reporting laws, such as those that make reporting the simple suspicion of child abuse mandatory in many states. Some experts believe that child abuse, both in and out of the home, has always existed, but that only recently has the problem been recognized and taken seriously. This perspective suggests that increased child abuse is in fact a statistical phenomenon.

A major problem with incidence studies is that they are based on *reported* cases. Many researchers believe that such studies do not accurately reflect the extent of the problem. Incidence rates are usually based on the number of reported cases, but there is continuing evidence that much abuse goes unreported. This is particularly characteristic of incest, because of the taboo against discussing it. One study showed that only 6 percent of extrafamilial sexual abuse and 2 percent of intrafamilial abuse experienced by the respondents had been reported (Russell 1984). A study of convicted child molesters indicates that the number of molestations they had actually committed was five times greater than the number of incidents for which they were apprehended (Groth, Longo, and McFaddin 1982). A study conducted by the National Center for Child Abuse and Neglect estimates that in 1981 only 33 percent of the known cases of child maltreatment in the United States had actually been reported (Westat Development 1981).

Because incidence studies focus only on those cases receiving professional attention, they are not very useful in determining the scope of the problem in the general population. Prevalence studies are more useful for acquiring this type of information. (*Incidence* refers to the number of people who "come down" with a condition—for example, the number admitted to mental hospitals each year. *Prevalence* refers to the number of people who suffer from a condition—for example, those who are mentally ill at a given time.) Samples in incidence studies are often biased, because professionals may label the respondents as "abused" prior to the sample selection process. Prevalence studies seem to give a more accurate picture because they are based on a proportion of the population rather than on a clinical sample. Although more studies have begun using random samples, few of them examine all forms of abuse, and most study a limited geographical area.

Definitional inconsistencies also complicate the process of data collection. Methodical comparison of incidence studies is difficult, because definitions of child abuse in the various studies are often not comparable and may be so imprecise as to be useless. This is often the case in studies of sexual abuse; definitions of incest, for example, vary from fantasies involving the sexualization of a child (Rosenfeld, Nadelson, and Krieger 1979) to very restrictive definitions in which the act involves only heterosexual intercourse between postpubescent children and family members (Bixler 1981). The diagnosis of child maltreatment also presents problems. For example, the *Diagnostic and Statistical Manuals of Mental Disorders I, II, and III* do not include separate categories for certain forms of child abuse, such as incest. Thus, data collection is hindered because many cases of incest or other abuse may be disguised under labels such as "parent-child problem," or "adjustment reaction of childhood." This categorization skews the incidence rates.

Despite the many pitfalls, national incidence studies are useful in generating public discussion. The fact remains, however, that child abuse research lacks a solid empirical base of information about the extent of the problem, which limits our ability to make sound, effective policy decisions. We may not be able to eliminate the methodological problems of determining the incidence of child maltreatment, but nationwide prevalence studies could certainly add to our knowledge.

Perspectives on Child Maltreatment

Defining child maltreatment is problematic. First, definitions vary across cultures, races, and times (Gelles and Lancaster 1987). These definitions are essentially value-based, and values differ among various peoples, times, and circumstances. Second, definitions may have different purposes. Parton (1979) identifies three approaches to child maltreatment: *penal, medical,* and *social.* The *penal,* or *legal,* approach is concerned both with protecting the child victim and with the punishment of offenders. The protective component is emphasized by the child protective service (CPS) system, which includes social workers and law-enforcement staff who receive, investigate, and intervene in child abuse cases. The punishment of offenders involves the court system (which can also protect children through removal and placement), in particular the superior courts, which can prosecute offenders.

In the *medical* approach, child maltreatment is perceived as a result of external conditions, and the emphasis is on cure and prevention. The *social* approach may incorporate one of two perspectives: the radical view defines child maltreatment as the result of social processes and emphasizes social reorganization; the traditional view is more concerned with therapeutic rehabilitation of the offender, who is seen as psychologically damaged and socially inadequate. Zigler (1983) provides, in addition, a sociological definition in which he considers the idea that certain practices are socially acceptable and that child abuse should be defined according to the standard of social acceptability.

In many professional settings, definitions of child abuse become operational through guidelines written as specific policies for particular objectives. Thus both explicit definitions and guidelines for professional practice must be considered when examining the relationship between self-esteem and child maltreatment. The question of the specific versus the general concerns both lawmakers and child abuse specialists. An extremely broad definition of abuse could result in a huge number of maltreatment cases flooding an already overburdened CPS system and could generate skepticism among the public. A very narrow definition, however, could result in overlooking serious cases and failing to protect some children who are at risk. A workable definition must fall between these extremes, difficult as it is to pinpoint.

Although a fairly specific definition may be established for a particular professional group, some discretion for the individual professional to determine the nature of child abuse always remains. Professional discretion is necessary because no single definition can include every possible factor that should be considered. Therefore, the training, personal background, characteristics, and—perhaps most important—the values of the individual professional all have significant impact on the selection of cases that are eventually defined as child maltreatment.

Finally, as Calam and Franchi (1987) point out, any particular definition may focus the attention of professionals away from certain kinds of damage that children suffer at the hands of their caretakers. Calam and Franchi argue that definitions should not obstruct the primary goal, which is to protect the child. Such questions as children's rights, child development, and alternative methods of caretaking should be considered when assessing and defining child maltreatment cases.

Using the typologies suggested by Parton (1979), we will next examine the various definitions of child maltreatment in more detail.

Social Definitions

According to Navarre (1987), definitions of child maltreatment have three dimensions: *action, outcome,* and *intent. Action* refers to caretaker behavior that has a high probability of an adverse effect on the child. *Outcome* refers to the results of child maltreatment experienced by the victims. Unfortunately, research cannot consistently and reliably predict adverse outcomes, because outcomes are related to many other variables, such as developmental age of the child, environmental and familial circumstances, duration and intensity of the maltreatment, and the child's characteristics. *Intent* refers to the motivation behind the offender's action. Analysis of intent should include not only the intent of the caretaker but also the intent perceived by the child. As Navarre admits, intent is the most difficult of the three dimensions to measure, and therefore its use in an operational definition by the legal or social service system cannot be justified.

Burgess and Garbarino, in their evolutionary analysis of child maltreatment, suggest a definition that includes both caretaker behaviors and damage to the child: "Child abuse refers to any nonaccidental injury sustained by a child under eighteen years of age resulting from acts of commission or omission by a parent, guardian, or other caretakers. . . . Such acts range from violent, impulsive, extreme physical assault to nonimpulsive, seemingly deliberate torture of a child to intensive psychological deprivation" (1986, 88).

Giovannoni and Becerra (1979) describe child maltreatment from what they call a *social deviance* perspective. This sociological term essentially implies that the meaning of child abuse is determined by taking account of the social system in which it occurs. Giovannoni and Becerra consider the social deviance perspective more useful than the diagnostic perspective of medical professionals, because the former considers significant social and cultural factors that shape how societal groups care for their children.

Gil uses a macro-level perspective to describe child abuse, because of his strong concern for children's economic, social, civil, and political rights. Gil refers to child maltreatment as "any act of commission or omission by individuals, institutions, or society as a whole, and any conditions resulting from such acts or inaction, which deprive children of equal rights and liberties, and/or interfere with their optimal development" (1976, 130). The Child Welfare League of America, in contrast, defines child abuse and neglect from a familial, micro-level perspective: "The child on whose behalf protective services should be given is one whose parents or others responsible for the care of the child do not provide . . . the love, care, guidance, and protection a child requires for healthy growth and development; and whose condition or situation gives observable evidence of the injurious effects of failure to meet at least the child's minimum needs" (1973, 12).

Giovannoni and Becerra argue that these kinds of social work definitions rest "in part on an implicit assumption that requirements for 'healthy growth and development' are known and that beliefs about children's needs are shared" (1979, 88). They note that even if most professionals were to agree on a definition of sexual abuse, other areas of child maltreatment, such as those involving other issues of morality, would remain controversial—for example, some might raise questions of sexual morality concerning family nudity and bathing practices.

Giovannoni and Becerra conclude that professionals have significant disagreements about the kinds of caretaker behaviors that are abusive and the degree of harm that such behaviors cause. These authors believe that such disagreements stem more from differing professional values and ideologies than from conscious or unconscious intrapsychic processes. However, they also find considerable consensus among both professionals and the public about the seriousness of sexual abuse and extreme forms of physical abuse and physical neglect. Giovannoni and Becerra describe nine forms of child maltreatment: sexual abuse, physical injury, lack of supervision, failure to provide material support, fostering delinquency, emotional maltreatment, educational neglect, harmful parental sexual mores, and parental substance abuse.

Medical Definitions

Medical approaches formulated by physicians tend to focus on the psychopathology of abusive parents and the evidence of physical injury, observed directly or with X-rays (O'Toole, Turbett, and Nalepka 1986). Some attention is given to the importance of stress and the intergenerational "cycle of violence." O'Toole and his colleagues note that nursing texts often have a broader perspective on defining child maltreatment than do texts written by physicians, because the former give greater emphasis to child and parental behaviors as indicators of abuse and to the relative importance of family dynamics and the child's behavior. Although some authors, such as Justice and Justice (1976), assume that physical abuse is generally the easiest form of maltreatment to define, O'Toole, Turbett, and Nalepka suggest that medical professionals often use vague concepts such as "normal" and "abnormal" injuries to shape the definition of physical abuse and may ignore information from the family, community, and school, as well as racial, cultural, and socioeconomic factors.

Giovannoni and Becerra (1979) describe the medical approach to child maltreatment as a "diagnostic perspective," characterized by an emphasis on the processes of pathology, symptoms, and cure; medical professionals may use symptoms to categorize cases of child abuse, for the purpose of forming diagnoses and planning interventions. The work of Kempe and Helfer (1977) is cited as an example of a medical definition of child maltreatment; their focus, though broad, is primarily on parental characteristics.

Legal Definitions

In most states, there are three sets of laws that use definitions of child abuse (Giovannoni and Becerra 1979); California is typical in this regard. One set of laws covers how and when mandated reporters of child maltreatment must report (California Penal Code, section 11161). A second set of laws defines criminal child maltreatment (California Penal Code, section 273). A third set is included in the California Welfare and Institutions Code, chapter 1068, and describes the grounds for making a child a dependent of the court. In all three sets, vague language such as "mental suffering" and "suitable home" is used in describing various forms of child maltreatment. Giovannoni and Becerra suggest that these definitions are useful to social workers and other professionals only if they are complemented by clearly written, more specific guidelines. As Nagi (1977) reports, social workers find that a large proportion of the cases reported to child protective services fall within an "area of doubt"—that is, although the children may be suffering, there is often insufficient evidence of abuse to satisfy the requirements of child maltreatment guidelines and definitions.

The state of California, in its guidelines for professionals, defines child maltreatment to include physical abuse, physical neglect, sexual abuse, and emotional maltreatment (Office of the Attorney General 1985, 5–13). These definitions do not specify degree of injury, but they do consider caretaker behaviors and their effects on victims: "The act of inflicting injury or allowing injury to result, rather than the degree of injury, is the determinant for intervention." Physical abuse is "any act which results in a nonaccidental physical injury." Physical neglect is the "negligent treatment or maltreatment of a child by a parent or caretaker under circumstances indicating harm or threatened harm to the child's health or welfare." Sexual abuse is defined as "acts of sexual assault on and sexual exploitation of minors." Sexual assault includes rape, rape in concert, incest, sodomy, lewd or lascivious acts upon a child under the age of fourteen, oral copulation, penetration by a foreign object, and child molestation. Sexual exploitation includes child pornography and child prostitution. Emotional maltreatment is defined as "excessive verbal assaults (belittling, screaming, threats, blaming, and sarcasm), unpredictable responses (inconsistency), continual negative moods, constant family discord, and double-message communication." In the guidelines, the state also provides specific behavioral indicators of abusive caretakers and of child victims.

In other states, the degree of specificity in definitions of child maltreatment varies greatly. In her fifty-state survey of child welfare, conducted for the National Conference of State Legislatures, Smith (1986) found that every state except Texas (where legislation is pending) provides statutory definitions of abuse and neglect.

In summary, a very wide range of meanings can be attached to the term *child maltreatment*. These definitions, of course, affect how we perceive the problem. If we use a medical definition, for example, we deal with a smaller universe than if we use a definition that includes all of the perspectives reported above. The "size of the universe" under consideration is obviously a factor in any analysis of the relation between self-esteem and child maltreatment.

The Concept of Self

The self can be defined as "the totality of a complex and dynamic system of learned beliefs that an individual holds to be true about his or her personal existence and that gives consistency to his or her personality" (Purkey and Schmidt 1987, 32). At first glance, the concept of self may appear ill suited for a central place in the study of *social* problems, for, as Rosenberg writes, "in its essence, nothing is more quintessentially psychological; an unequivocally subjective phenomenon, its home is located in the inner world of thought and experience" (Rosenberg 1981, 593).

But the relevance of self-concept to the study of social problems is not difficult to grasp. The self develops out of the individual's social experiences and interactions in the different social contexts of the life course—the family, the school, the workplace, and the community. Although the individual's perception of self is experienced internally, that perception is a product of social interaction.

The concept of self is by no means a simple one. One must attempt to sort out those features of the self that are stable and enduring and those that are "situated" (i.e., those parts of the self that are adjusted to social interaction). As James noted, on the one hand, "there is a certain average tone of self-feeling which each one of us carries about with him, and which is independent of the objective reasons we may have for satisfaction or discontent." But, on the other hand, a person also "has as many different social selves as there are distinct *groups* of persons about whose opinion he cares. He generally shows a different side of himself to each of these different groups" (James 1890, 294; emphasis in original). Thus, we may be restrained with our parents and teachers, and silly and adolescent with our friends. We do not reveal ourselves to clients and employers in the same way as we do to our colleagues and intimates.

There is an enormous amount of literature and a good deal of empirical research on the ways in which self is affected by social context. Much research has focused on the relation between social esteem and self-esteem. For example, it is commonly believed that minority children develop low self-esteem because they compare themselves unfavorably with the white majority in terms of social class and family structure (traditional nuclear families versus single-parent families). Research offers little support for this conclusion, however. Wylie's review of the research finds that minority group members do not have significantly lower self-esteem (1979, 57–116). Rosenberg's research suggests that all children and adolescents tend to compare themselves with those in their immediate interpersonal environments; when minority children compare themselves with their minority peers, there is a normal distribution of self-esteem. It is only when social circumstances place minority children in situations in which whites are the majority that their self-esteem may suffer (Rosenberg 1981, 605). This research should remind us that situations must be viewed from the perspectives of those who experience them and not just from the perspective of an observer. Findings of this sort are extremely useful in assessing such questions as the effects of school busing, the causes of poor academic achievement, and other problems related to race and ethnicity.

The concept of self has been a central theme of social psychology for the past thirty years. As Stryker (1977) points out, there are two major traditions in social psychology—the *psychological* and the *sociological*. The *psychological* tradition (Rogers 1965; Epstein 1973; Bandura 1977) focuses on the consequences of the self-concept for individual functioning, that is, how feelings about one's self affect one's behavior and social interactions. In this tradition, Epstein defines the self-concept from an attribution perspective, as a self-theory that a person constructs as an experiencing, functioning individual in interaction with the world. He also points out that the self-theory is a mechanism that serves to "optimize the pleasure/pain balance of the individual over the course of a lifetime" (1973, 407). Thus, one of the important functions of self-theory is to help maintain self-esteem and to organize experience in a manner that enables one to cope with it effectively.

The *sociological* tradition in social psychology (Rosenberg 1979; Burke 1980) emphasizes how social-structural and contextual factors influence individuals' perceptions of self. The sociological perspective seems to see the structuring of self as developing throughout life, whereas the psychological tradition tends to see the self becoming structured in the earlier years of life. Rosenberg's work is primarily sociological, concentrating on the development of self-evaluative behavior in terms of how social milieu affects behavior (Rosenberg 1965, 1979).

The perspective from which the concept of self is seen obviously influences the ways in which we attempt to deal with social problems. Using the psychological perspective, we will tend to intervene at an individual level; that is, we will favor interventions that alter a person's perception of self in order to change his or her behavior and social interactions. Using the sociological perspective, we will be more likely to intervene at the social level; that is, we will favor interventions that alter social arrangements in order to change the individual's perception of self and his or her behavior and social interactions.

Dimensions of Self-Esteem

Most research on the self-concept focuses on self-esteem, and the self-concept is frequently equated with self-esteem. But self-esteem appears to occupy only a small part of our thoughts about ourselves. McGuire and Padawer-Singer (1976) report the interesting finding that when people are allowed a high degree of freedom in describing themselves, fewer than 10 percent of their responses deal with self-evaluation. Among sixth-graders who were asked, "Tell us about yourself," almost a quarter of all responses were devoted to habitual activities such as recreation and daily routines. The second most frequently mentioned category involved significant others—mostly parents, siblings, and friends. The other categories mentioned were one's attitudes (17 percent), school (15 percent), and demographic characteristics (12 percent). Self-evaluation accounted for only 7 percent of all responses.

A distinction can be made between *self-conception* (identity), and *self-evaluation* (self-esteem). Self-conception usually refers to the concept that individuals hold of themselves as physical, social, and spiritual or moral beings. In Rosenberg's terms, the self-conception is broadly defined as the "totality of an individual's thoughts and feelings having reference to himself as an object" (1979, 7). Self-esteem, however, has been referred to as an individual's overall self-evaluation, the self as "an object of knowledge." James (1890) viewed self-esteem as the ratio of our actualities to our supposed potentialities, that is, the ratio of success to pretensions.

According to Gecas, "identity focuses on the meanings comprising the self as an object, gives structure and content to the self-concept, and anchors the self to social systems. Self-evaluation or self-esteem refers to the evaluative and affective aspects of the self-concept" (1982, 4). These aspects of the self-concept are closely interrelated: self-evaluation is typically based on substantive aspects of the self-concept, and identities typically have evaluative components.

Increasingly, aspects of self-esteem have been differentiated: inner and outer self-esteem (Franks and Marolla 1976), self-evaluation and self-worth (Brissett 1972), and sense of power and sense of worth (Gecas 1971), for example. Franks and Marolla use a two-dimensional approach, distinguishing inner self-esteem and outer self-esteem. The sense of inner self-esteem derives from feelings of one's own efficacy and competence—that is, the effects that one's actions have on the environment account for inner self-esteem. In contrast, outer self-esteem is bestowed by others; it deals with approval or acceptance by significant persons. Outer self-esteem refers to our desire to be connected affectively with others. One's sense of power and potency (inner self-esteem) can be quite independent of a sense of being accepted and liked by others (outer self-esteem). Social comparisons become very important in this context. It should be noted, however, that both the inner and outer dimensions of self-esteem can be seen as belonging in a sociological frame of reference (Franks and Marolla 1976). For example, minorities may worry about being accepted by white co-workers, but they may not be concerned about acceptance from whites with whom they have no relationship.

As Franks and Marolla (1976) show, two dimensions of self-esteem often seem to parallel each other: those situations in which one evaluates oneself highly are often those situations in which one experiences a sense of mastery. The distinction between self-evaluation and self-worth, though conceptually important, tends to blur at the experiential level.

Knapp (1973) raises questions about the stability of self-esteem at different developmental stages in childhood, noting that it may seem to vary dramatically even within short periods of time. Little is known about whether self-esteem can, in fact, be changed and, if it can, the forms of intervention that are effective. The influences of culture, race, and sex-role identification on self-esteem are also relatively unknown.

Martinek and Zaichkowsky (1977), along with Knapp, suggest that the self-esteem of young children may be very unstable until about the age of seven. (Piers [1969] has confirmed this in her extensive investigations with elementary school and secondary school children.) Martinek and Zaichkowsky refer to Jersild's (1969) findings that certain emotional tendencies, feelings for others, and character traits are globally related to the self.

Battle (1981) reports that children's self-esteem has a weak, but statistically significant, positive relationship with intelligence. (Other researchers, such as Coopersmith [1967], have reported similar findings.) Teachers' ratings of students' self-esteem and students' self-reports correlate highly, but, as Piers (1969) and Coopersmith (1967) also found, teachers' ratings and students' school self-esteem (related to academic achievement) are not significantly related. Battle concludes that "one's self-esteem is not dependent on any particular factor (e.g., academic achievement), but on a combination of factors" (1981, 16). Battle also found, as did Coopersmith (1967), that among both adults and youths self-esteem is negatively correlated with depression. Finally, the self-esteem of academically successful students was significantly higher than that of less successful children with learning disabilities.

Sources of Self-Esteem

The difference between a sense of competence based on self-evaluation and a sense of value based on self-worth is important, because each arises in a different process of self-concept formation. Briefly, the process of reflected appraisal contributes to the formation of self-worth, whereas competency-based self-evaluation is associated with self-attribution and social comparison.

There are four sources for the formation of self-esteem. The first is reflected appraisal, which is grounded in Cooley's concept of the "looking-glass self" (1902) and in Mead's idea of "role-taking" (1934). Cooley's concept of reflected appraisal is the notion that our sense of self is derived largely from our perceptions of how others regard us. In Cooley's view, self-esteem may be more strongly associated with the *perceived* appraisals of others than with actual appraisals. For example, Rosenberg (1979) found that the association between self-perception and reflected appraisals or social comparisons was stronger if the significant other was highly valued by the subject. Mead (1934) noted that self-image arises in social interaction as an outcome of the individual's concern about how others react to him or her. The "generalized other" serves as a source of internal regulation to guide and stabilize the individual's behavior in response to certain actions.

A second influential source of self-esteem is the social comparison process (Festinger 1954, 117–140), by which individuals assess their own abilities and virtues by comparing themselves to others. Social comparisons are most likely to occur in situations where information and standards are ambiguous or uncertain.

Self-attribution is a third source of self-esteem. It refers to how individuals explain their behavior (e.g., "I did poorly on the test because the teacher doesn't like me"). The notion of self-attribution suggests that self-esteem is tied not so much to an individual's behavior as to his or her interpretation of the behavior. As Gecas (1982) points out, attribution theory is, in general, more appropriate to consideration of self as a causal factor in social interaction than to explanations of the development of self.

Finally, social identity is also closely tied to self-esteem. Social identity refers to socially recognized belonging, such as one's social class and status, race, religion, or organizational affiliations. Low prestige in terms of social stratification does not necessarily produce correspondingly low self-esteem, however. According to Rosenberg's notion of "psychological centrality," the impact of any given stimulus depends on its centrality in the individual's cognitive structure. Thus, individuals must first become aware of their lower status in respect to significant others in the environment, as in the example of minority children in majority-dominated educational settings cited earlier (Rosenberg 1981; Rosenberg and Pearlin 1978).

Instruments for Measuring Self-Esteem

Instruments that measure self-esteem generally fall into one of four categories, each with certain limitations: behavioral trace reports, direct observations, projective techniques, and self-reports (Knapp 1973). Behavioral trace reports attempt to base judgments on concrete behaviors, such as grades and teachers' comments, thereby eliminating observer bias; problems with memory (e.g., the teachers') and validity (e.g., grades) do exist, however. Direct observations are used with very young children who are not yet able to communicate effectively on a verbal level; but it is possible that the values, feelings, and attitudes of the observer may bias the results. Projective techniques can reveal unconscious processes in children and adults, but scoring procedures are difficult and may be neither objective nor valid. Self-reports are practical and easily scored, but respondents may manipulate their self-reports to obtain desirable results (e.g., to elicit sympathy from the observer). Of course, techniques can be combined in various ways to achieve reliability, but this makes assessment more expensive.

Hughes (1984) reviewed the nineteen most-used instruments for evaluating self-esteem among children aged three to twelve, concluding that although therapists working with children and adults frequently cite changes in self-concept and self-esteem as goals, there is no widely adopted, coherent theory of self-esteem and the self-concept. She believes the Piers-Harris Children's Self-Concept Scale to be the best for clinical application with children aged nine to twelve, because of its high reliability and validity, but she found no measure equally adequate for use with younger children. The McDaniel-Piers Scale was recommended for children aged six to nine because of its reliability and popularity. Hughes also recommends the Behavioral Academic Self-Esteem Scale as the best "teacher report" measure. She notes a distinction made in the literature between self-concept, as "the descriptive perception of the self," and self-esteem, as "the evaluative assessment of those descriptions" (1984, 659).

The Martinek-Zaichkowsky Self-Concept Scale for Children (Martinek and Zaichkowsky 1977) is designed to measure the "global self-concept of children from first grade through eighth grade." Children are given a self-report instrument that utilizes pictures instead of words.

The authors claim that the instrument is "culture-free." Although they have not yet established validity and reliability measures for this scale, as Wylie (1979) indicates in a review of the literature, there is a critical need for a well-validated scale that measures the self-esteem of younger children and that does not require the ability to read or understand English.

The Self-Observation Scale (Katzen and Stenner 1975) also utilizes a self-report instrument in assessing the self-esteem of children at the primary, junior high, and senior high school levels. The authors have completed a fairly extensive validation study of their instrument, and they maintain that it emphasizes the healthy and positive aspects of self rather than the more negative and pathological ones.

Katzen and Stenner use a "practical decision-making orientation" instead of the more traditional orientation of theory and research. According to the authors, the emotional development of children has not received enough attention; the emphasis in research has traditionally been on cognitive development. Their instruments are designed to help educators and psychologists attend more effectively to emotional development in this age group. Their instruments use written questions that are organized into seven scales: self-acceptance, self-security, social confidence, self-assertion, peer affiliation, teacher affiliation, and school affiliation. The forms developed for the primary school level use pictures for student responses, whereas the other forms use a verbal format.

The Culture-Free Self-Esteem Inventory (Battle 1981) provides instruments for use with children from grades one through twelve, as well as with adults. These instruments are designed both to help identify children, youths, and adults who are in need of psychiatric help and to provide general information for the professional helper or researcher. The author claims to have developed inventories that are useful with clients of all cultures and races.

The Coopersmith Self-Esteem Inventory (1975) is designed for subjects aged nine years and older. This instrument is based on a widely known study of self-esteem and has demonstrated a degree of reliability and validity that has made it very popular with researchers. Respondents are asked to check various columns of responses to questions.

The Tennessee Self-Concept Scale (TSCS), developed by Fitts (1965), is one of the most widely utilized self-esteem scales. It is also one of the few well-developed measures of self-esteem for use with adults. Using self-reporting, it measures self-concept across many subareas, providing both an overall self-esteem score and a complex self-concept profile.

The ninety statements (evenly balanced for positivity-negativity) fall into one of five general categories: physical self, moral-ethical self, personal self, family self, and social self. Each category is divided into statements of self-identity, self-acceptance, and behavior. There are also ten items from the Minnesota Multiphasic Personality Inventory (MMPI) lie scale. Each question has five response categories, from completely true to completely false. The TSCS yields an overall self-esteem score, a total positive score, along with self-esteem subscale scores related to different dimensions of perceiving the self.

The Rosenberg Self-Esteem Scale (1965), originally developed for use with high school students, measures the self-acceptance aspect of self-esteem. The scale consists of ten Guttman-type items with four responses, from strongly agree to strongly disagree, which are, however, scored only as agreement or disagreement. The scale is designed with brevity and ease of administration in mind.

Factors Associated with Child Abuse

As concern about child abuse has grown in recent years, a variety of explanations have been proposed to account for the etiology of this problem. Some have argued that child abuse is triggered by stress and psychological disturbance in parents (Oates, Forrest, and Peacock 1985; Morris, Gould, and Matthews 1964; Melnick and Hurley 1969; Steele and Pollock 1974), whereas others have argued that abuse-eliciting characteristics of children (Oates and Forrest 1985; Martin and Beezley 1976; Green 1978; Kinard 1980a), dysfunctional patterns of family interaction (Burgess 1978; Green, Gaines, and Sandgrund 1974), stress-inducing social forces (Gelles and Lancaster 1987), or abuse-promoting cultural values (Gil 1987) are primarily responsible for abuse and neglect.

Research on the relationship between culture and child abuse is still in beginning stages. (See, for example, Spearly and Lauderdale 1983.) Wide differences in the definitions and methods used in studying child abuse make it difficult to assess the impact of racial and cultural factors on an international basis (Gelles and Cornell 1983). Evidence exists, however, that both racial and cultural influences (Korbin 1981) and economic factors (Spearly and Lauderdale 1983) can shape parenting practices. Complicating these findings is the fact that differences *within* any racial, cultural, or economic group are at least as broad as the differences generally found *between* such groups.

Belsky (1980) provides a system of analysis that draws heavily on

Bronfenbrenner's (1979) ecology of human development. This framework consists of four levels of analysis: *ontogenic development,* the *microsystem,* the *exosystem,* and the *macrosystem.* Ontogenic development involves personal characteristics that individual abusive parents bring with them to the family setting and to the parenting role. The *microsystem* refers to the family setting itself, that is, the immediate context in which child maltreatment takes place. The *exosystem* represents the social structures (e.g., the world of work, the neighborhood, and informal social networks) that encompass the microsystems of the individual and influence what goes on there. The *macrosystem* refers to cultural values and belief systems that may foster child maltreatment.

On the ontogenic level, Belsky stresses that abusers have repeatedly been found to have histories of maltreatment in their own childhoods. Belsky argues that, within the microsystem of the family, child abuse should not be considered as merely a function of the characteristics of either parent or child, but must be seen as an interactive process, with characteristics of both child and parent (e.g., how the child responds to how the parent behaves) becoming factors in the level of risk of child abuse. Within the exosystem, research evidence links maltreatment with unemployment, which is associated with lack of financial resources, a sense of powerlessness and isolation, and increased parent-child contact. The most significant elements in the macrosystem are society's attitudes toward violence and corporal punishment, particularly a general acceptance of physical punishment as a means of controlling children's behavior; the belief that children are their parents' chattel, property to be handled as the parents choose; and a narcissistic "me first" approach to life in contemporary American society.

Finkelhor (1986) tried to find commonalities in all forms of family violence, including both caretaker actions and outcomes for victims. He argues that child maltreatment is similar to other forms of violence inasmuch as it represents an abuse of power by a child's caretaker. But although caretakers do have obvious power over children, most abusers also perceive themselves as powerless. According to Finkelhor, the victims of child maltreatment are typically "brainwashed" into accepting low self-esteem and a distorted view of reality that legitimizes the abuse.

Self-Esteem of Abusive Parents

Several studies report that abusive parents have lower levels of self-esteem than members of control groups (Shorkey 1980; Oates and Forrest 1985). But many of the studies on this subject do not provide clear definitions of self-esteem or child abuse. Moreover, it is not possible to determine the extent to which poor self-esteem actually results from a parent's abusing a child or being identified as an abusive parent.

Mothers who abuse their children are said to have low levels of self-esteem and often have histories of emotional deprivation in their own childhoods. Steele's study (1980) shows that it is common for abusive or neglectful caretakers to have histories of significant neglect, with or without physical abuse. From his experience, he stressed the importance of the parent's identification with a harsh, rejecting mother and with a bad childhood self-image.

Most of the earlier studies (Morris, Gould, and Matthews 1964; Steele and Pollock 1974) tend to be based on clinical judgments rather than on empirical evidence, but there have been several empirical studies of the self-esteem of child abusers. Melnick and Hurley (1969) compared ten abusive mothers with ten control mothers. They found that abusive mothers differed significantly from control-group mothers, as revealed by lower scores on the California Test of Personality (CTP) Self-Esteem Scale. Abusive mothers also differed reliably from control mothers in scoring higher on the Thematic Apperception Test (TAT) dependency frustration and Pathogenic Index, and lower on the TAT need to give nurturance and on the Manifest Rejection portion of the test.

Schneider, Hoffmeister, and Helfer devised a predictive screening instrument as part of a program to identify parents who were likely to be abusers. They found that the IM ("I'm no damn good") item cluster was particularly important, and they concluded that "in order to love oneself, one has to first be loved, approved of, and nurtured by parent figures. Lacking this parenting, the high-risk parent cannot develop high self-esteem" (1976, 405).

Green, Gaines, and Sandgrund, comparing a group of thirty abusive parents with an equal number of neglecting parents and a third group of normal parents, found that abusers are likely to develop poor self-concepts as a result of their own experiences in childhood. The authors characterize the abuse-prone mother as follows: "The mother passively re-enacts with the abused child the rejection and humiliation she originally experienced with her own mother. The resulting anxiety, guilt, and loss of self-esteem threaten the mother's fragile, narcissistic equilibrium" (1974, 885). Anderson and Lauderdale (1982) report identical results. They found not only that abusive parents have low self-esteem as measured on the Tennessee Self-Concept Scale, but, more important, that their sense of self is in conflict and they are confused. Overall, these parents have poorly integrated personalities, as evidenced by a high level of personal maladjustment.

Shorkey (1980) analyzed data from a study of fourteen abusing mothers and an equal number of control mothers, using three personality scales: the sense of personal worth scale of the California Test of Personality, the Srole Anomia Scale, and the Rosenberg Self-Esteem Scale. The abusing mothers did not rate themselves as having lower self-esteem, based on the Rosenberg Scale. In contrast, their ratings on the sense of personal worth scale indicated that they perceived others' evaluations of them as lower than the nonabusing mothers perceived such evaluations to be.

Oates and Forrest (1985) compared thirty-six abusive mothers with thirty-six matched-group mothers. Abusive parents in this study had lower self-esteem and less regard for their partners, as judged by their desire that their children should not grow up to be like themselves or their partners. Also, they were less likely than the comparison mothers to discuss problems with other people.

Self-Esteem of Abused Children

The fact that abused and neglected children experience low self-esteem is well documented; maltreated children have measurably lower levels of self-esteem than children who are not abused (Sturkie and Flanzer 1987; Oates, Forrest, and Peacock 1985). Children with low self-esteem are also more likely than their peers with higher self-esteem to have behavior problems. There is considerable evidence that lowered self-esteem is one result of child sexual abuse, particularly as a long-term effect. Finkelhor (1986), in his review of the literature, found four forms of impact on child victims of sexual abuse: traumatic sexualization, stigmatization, a sense of betrayal, and feelings of powerlessness. Stigmatization includes lowered self-esteem, as well as guilt, shame, and a sense that one is different from others. A number of studies have shown negative effects on the self-esteem of sexually abused children— some effects that were short-term (DeFrancis 1969) and others that were long-term (Brière 1984; Bagley and Ramsay 1985–1986; Courtois 1979; Herman 1981).

Based on behavioral observations, Green (1978) reports that abused children exhibit a depressed affect with low self-esteem as the result of chronic physical and emotional abuse. Sturkie and Flanzer (1987) found that members of abusive families (twenty-four individuals) were more depressed than the forty members of a cohort of comparison families, although in this case both maltreated adolescents and comparison adolescents were more depressed and had lower self-esteem than their parents. Dembo et al. (1987), studying the relationship between self-esteem and different kinds of maltreatment, found that physical abuse seemed to cause greater feelings of self-derogation than did sexual abuse. That is, child victims of physical abuse often perceive themselves as bad, worthless, and deserving of the "punishment" they receive. This is less the case with sexual victimization, because these victims are frequently valued as "love objects" by their abusers, who may themselves often suffer from early economic deprivation or a history of emotional impoverishment.

Gecas (1971) points out the importance of certain parental behavior patterns—primarily parental support and control—for the development of a child's self-evaluation. He finds that parental support is strongly and consistently related to various measures of adolescent self-evaluation. On the two scales of self-evaluation, support is more strongly related to Self-Esteem(SE)-Worth than to Self-Esteem(SE)-Power. SE-power refers to "the person's feeling of competence and effectiveness," and SE-worth refers to "personal influence and feelings of personal virtue and moral worth" (Gecas 1971, 468). Maternal support has a strong effect on SE-worth, whereas paternal support is more strongly related to SE-power. In general, the relation between parental support and self-esteem is stronger for girls than for boys, and the influence of parental support is stronger for the same-sex child than for the opposite-sex child. Further research may increase understanding of the relationship between abusive parents' behavior patterns and their children's self-esteem. Current interest in the etiology and effects of psychological maltreatment of children may lead to studies that link lack of parental support and control to children's self-esteem.

Oates, Forrest, and Peacock (1985) investigated the self-esteem of abused children through structured interviews with children and use of the Piers-Harris Children's Self-Concept Scale. Thirty-seven abused children were matched with thirty-seven nonabused children. The results show that abused children see themselves as having significantly fewer friends than do the comparison children. Abused children were also significantly lower in self-concept, as well as having less ambitious occupational goals.

In contrast, several other studies have not shown any differences in self-concept between abused children and control-group children. Elmer (1977) compared seventeen abused children with seventeen matched children who experienced accidents. The majority of the children in both groups were lower-class. Analysis of responses on the Piers-Harris Children's Self-Concept Scale showed no group differences on any of the subscales or on the overall scores. The researchers concluded that membership in lower classes may have as powerful an effect on child development as abuse.

Kinard (1980a, 1982) found conflicting results. On the Piers-Harris Children's Self-Concept Scale, there were no differences between the mean scores of the abused group and those of the nonabused group, even though the abused children were more likely to have scores indicating negative self-concepts. On the Tasks of Emotional Development (TED) Self-Concept Task, the two groups differed significantly on mastering the task of establishing a positive self-concept, as indicated by less mature responses. These results suggest that children's sense of identity is not well formed.

The research findings discussed above are summarized in Table 2.1.

Table 2.1.   Summary of Research Findings

Authors	Sample Size[a]	Lower Self-Esteem Found Among Abusive Parents or Abused Children?	Scale
Melnick and Hurley 1969	10(10)	Yes	CTP
Shorkey 1980	14(14)	No/Yes	RSES/CTP/ Srole Anomia Scale
Green, Gaines, and Sand-grund 1974	30(30)	Yes	Interviews
Anderson and Lauderdale 1982	111	Yes	TSCS
Oates and Forrest 1985	36(36)	Yes	Interviews
Sturkie and Flanzer 1987	24(40)	Yes	Hudson Package
Elmer 1977	17(17)	No	Piers-Harris
Kinard 1980a	30(30)	No/Yes	Piers-Harris/TED
Oates, Forrest, and Peacock 1985	37(37)	Yes	Piers-Harris

[a]Size of experimental group listed first; size of control group given in parentheses.

Interventions

Our discussion now moves to the broad range of intervention strategies used to deal with child abuse. Most intervention programs emphasize psychotherapeutic treatment, although the strategy of prevention through education is becoming increasingly important.

Three levels of intervention have been identified by Hart and Brassard (1987): *macrosystem, exosystem,* and *microsystem.* Intervention on the *macrosystem* level involves changing societal values and social policies through political action. Examples of such strategies include raising the standard of living of single-parent families, ensuring that various children's services are priorities in federal and state budgets, creating a national health insurance plan (including mental health insurance), establishing affordable housing and full employment, and providing child care and respite care services for single and working parents or salaries for parents who stay at home with their children. Intervention on the *exosystem* level is oriented toward community and societal institutions. These interventions might include banning corporal punishment in schools, modifying the scope of legal interventions, and improving the training of child care personnel. Finally, intervention on the *microsystem* level focuses on the individual and the family, perhaps reducing the levels of stress and isolation of families, intervening with high-risk parents before their children are born, or providing various forms of psychotherapy and education to family members.

On the macrosystem and exosystem levels, some interventions are intended to affect child abuse directly. For example, media spots on television may be designed specifically to describe what psychological maltreatment is and how to prevent it. Other types of intervention may be designed for another primary purpose but may nevertheless have a beneficial, indirect impact on the problem of child abuse. A new policy that establishes free child care for all children may be intended to improve the economic status and the opportunities available to women in society; yet the policy may also result in dramatic reductions in child maltreatment as many women are relieved of the stress of having constant responsibility for their children.

Although exosystem intervention strategies are usually not expressly intended to enhance self-esteem, they may well have a significant effect on the self-esteem of family members. Psychotherapy is emphasized as a treatment strategy in most intervention programs for child abuse. For example, in a survey of child abuse prevention services in Oakland, California, conducted by the Family Welfare Research Group (1986), about 50 percent of the services had counseling programs. Only 14 percent had parent education classes, 17 percent had in-home intervention services, 11 percent had therapeutic day care, 14 percent offered respite care, and 26 percent had case-management services. Many therapists believe that the most effective counseling programs should include many of these other kinds of services. Nonetheless, psychotherapy seems to be a preferred approach in dealing with family and parenting problems, as well as many other issues, throughout our culture (Garfield and Bergin 1978).

Psychotherapy and Self-Esteem

Freedman, Kaplan, and Sadock define psychotherapy as a "form of treatment for mental illness and behavioral disturbances in which a trained person establishes a professional contact with the patient through definite therapeutic communication." They define the goals of the treatment as an activity in which the therapist "attempts to alleviate the emotional disturbance, reverse or change maladaptive patterns of behavior, and encourage personality growth and development" (1980, 1324). Garfield and Bergin define psychotherapy as "an interpersonal process designed to bring about modifications of feelings, cognition, attitudes, and behavior which have proven troublesome to the person seeking help from a trained professional" (1978, 3). Generally, psychotherapy is a one-on-one approach to alleviating emotional and social problems through verbal interaction between therapist and patient.

Research in the past fifteen to twenty years shows that some forms of psychotherapy are effective, at least for some types of problems. Studies examining outcomes report that psychotherapy yields positive results when compared with no treatment, pseudotherapies, and wait-list and placebo treatments (Garfield and Bergin 1978). The well-known Temple study (Sloane et al. 1975) compared the effects of behavior therapy with those of psychotherapy. Two-thirds of the patients were diagnosed as neurotic; one-third were diagnosed as having personality disorders (N = 90). A third group (the control group) consisted of people on a waiting list. Although all three groups showed some improvement, 80 percent of those in the behavior therapy and psychotherapy groups showed improvement. The Pennsylvania study (Rush et al. 1977) was conducted with outpatients who exhibited depressive symptoms. Again, psychotherapy had a significant effect, in contrast to pharmacotherapy (involving the use of drugs in treatment). The Malan group, who conducted the Tavistock studies (Malan 1976), concluded that psychoanalytically oriented psychotherapy was very effective with certain types of patients, such as psychoneurotics and those exhibiting psychophysiological problems.

Although there is a history of inconsistency in the results of research on psychotherapy outcomes, most reviews now conclude that the effects of psychotherapy are indeed positive. There are some major flaws in the methodologies used in this research, however, and this is likely the reason for the inconsistency (Morris, Turner, and Szykula 1988). A key problem has been the lack of standardization of intervention techniques. It is virtually impossible to have a standardized form of psychotherapy, and this of course leaves much room for therapist variables to confound findings.

Although the specific technique used is significant, some of the strongest predictors of successful psychotherapy are interpersonal and intrapersonal characteristics of the client. Clients who have high self-esteem may have more positive outcomes in psychotherapy. In their review of research on psychotherapy with children, Barrett, Hampe, and Miller (1978) conclude that response to treatment varies with the nature of diagnoses rather than with the treatments themselves. That is, some disorders show more positive outcomes with particular treatments than do others.

Measuring the effects of psychotherapy on self-esteem raises some unique problems. Most studies of psychotherapy outcomes tend to focus on specific illnesses and the rate of improvement by examining "remission" as an outcome; however, remission per se may not be an adequate measure of changes in self-esteem. Most of the current self-concept measurement scales, such as the Tennessee Self-Concept Scale (Fitts 1965), rely on self-report, which leaves room for reporting bias. The most appropriate method would be to apply some type of standardized measurement at pretreatment, posttreatment, and follow-up.

Regardless of the lack of clarity about the definitions and effectiveness of psychotherapy, it is widely used in many different forms in our culture. Garfield and Bergin note that "from a form of medical treatment for 'nervous and mental disease' in the nineteenth century, psychotherapy in our time has become the primary secular religion, its goals ranging from heightened self-fulfillment, serenity, emotional and spiritual well-being . . . to the traditional objectives of mitigating neurotic and psychotic disturbances" (1978, 17).

Psychological Approaches to Treatment

Various approaches are currently being used in psychotherapy with high-risk and abusive parents. Wodarski (1981) describes five models of treatment for abusive parents. The first, the *psychopathological* model, emphasizes direct services to parents. Specific goals include development of insight, increasing social skills, raising self-esteem, and building relationships. Second, the *sociological* model emphasizes change in social values and conditions: increasing the value the community places on parenting, as well as increasing financial and social support for day care and respite care, parent education, housing, recreational facilities, and children's rights.

The third model, called *social-situational,* is most concerned with the interaction among members of abusive families. Parents are taught how to modify their children's behaviors more effectively, with methods such as time out, positive reinforcement, and explanation. Fourth, the *family-systems* model emphasizes the organization and structure of the family. This model appears similar to the social-situational one, but the family-systems approach emphasizes inventing new roles for family members and reinforcing the parent as the source of control in the family. Fifth, the *social-learning* model utilizes behavioral changes in family members, as does the social-situational model, but it emphasizes a more formal social-learning methodology that includes definition of goals, selection of reinforcers, and implementation. Wodarski criticizes all of these approaches as being singular in focus. He advocates a comprehensive treatment approach that includes child management, marital enrichment, vocational skills enrichment, and interpersonal enrichment programs.

Shorkey (1979) describes a similar grouping of interventive methods. In Shorkey's view, the parent's behavior is an important element in the assessment process. Supportive social services are seen as a complement to therapy, with the goal of decreasing family stress and increasing life satisfaction. Finally, evaluation of the treatment is a critical step in all of these methods.

Justice and Justice (1976) provide an outline of models representing the kinds of therapeutic approaches currently used in treating child abuse. The first seven models are called *psychodynamic* (dealing with the past history of the parent); *personality/character* (focusing on current traits of the abuser); *social learning* (increasing parenting skills); *family structure* (managing the dynamics among family members); *en-*

vironmental stress; social-psychological (relieving stress factors and changing social norms); and *mental illness* (which applies to the fewer than 5 percent of abusive parents who suffer from psychoses or other major psychiatric disorders). Justice and Justice have themselves developed an eighth model, the *psychosocial,* which examines the interactions between the child, the parent, and the environment and which incorporates the seven approaches described above.

Each of the traditional therapeutic approaches has potential contributions to make to the treatment of child abuse. Given the limitations of this chapter, only some brief comments can be made regarding selected theories.

Freud's (1963a, 1963b) *psychoanalytic* approach to psychotherapy is the theoretical foundation for many therapists who work with abusive and high-risk parents. Freud's structural model of the id, ego, and superego, the stages of psychosexual development, and his ideas regarding defense mechanisms all have useful applications in this area. Freud's most fundamental contribution to understanding the abusive parent is his emphasis on examining the client's past; as Covitz explains, "most therapeutic treatment will involve some analysis of childhood experience and the relationship with parents" (1986, 156). The stages of psychosexual development provide practitioners with a framework to explain the etiology of a parent's psychological state and level of functioning.

Freud believed that psychoanalysis could help clients eventually become more sensitive to their own children: "Parents who have themselves experienced an analysis and owe much to it, including an insight into the faults of their own upbringing, will treat their children with better understanding and will spare them much of what they themselves were not spared" (1932, 150). Many people believe, however, that mere insight into the past will not necessarily lead to a reduction in child maltreatment. The parent must develop new skills, attitudes, and knowledge in addition to the insight gained in the counselor's office. It has not been demonstrated, for example, that parents who develop insight into their past have higher self-esteem or are more effective in enhancing the self-esteem of their children.

Most *humanistic* approaches in psychotherapy are based on the work of psychologist Carl Rogers (1965), who believed in the individual's natural tendency to self-actualize. Self-actualization is most likely to occur when the person experiences "unconditional positive regard." The therapist's role is to support the client unconditionally as the client resolves the incongruence between subjective (self) and external (others) reality. As with other phenomenological approaches, Rogers's *client-centered therapy* emphasizes building awareness and improving one's decision-making ability in the here and now. Many abusive and high-risk parents did not receive unconditional positive regard from their own parents during childhood. Rogers's humanistic approach provides nurturing for these parents and perhaps helps to improve self-esteem, which is a common need of abusive parents. The goal of self-actualization is also an important addition to the psychoanalytic approaches, which tend to be oriented toward the past rather than the present. Maslow (1971) described self-actualized people as honest and devoted to some calling or vocation. Such people may be less likely to abuse their children; research seems to indicate that unhappy, unemployed, and irresponsible parents tend to be more abusive.

Similar approaches have been developed by other humanistically oriented psychotherapists. *Gestalt therapy* (Perls 1969) emphasizes increasing the clients' awareness of their current needs and internal conflicts. A number of techniques are used to achieve this awareness, including group psychodrama and the famous "empty chair" individual exercises. The working through of projections and retroflections, as well as other defense mechanisms, is encouraged. Clients are urged to be honest and assertive (Polster and Polster 1973). The self-esteem of abusive parents, as well as that of children who have been abused, is one dimension of awareness that is dealt with by Gestalt therapists.

The *rational-emotive* approach, as developed by Ellis (1962), assumes that people have the ability to become rational by changing their way of thinking. According to Ellis, changes in thinking lead to changes in behavior and emotions. He believes that this technique works best with intelligent clients who are neither psychotic nor extremely disturbed or confused (Patterson 1973). For Ellis, the outside world (stressful events, children acting out, and so on) is not the cause of emotional and behavioral changes in the client. Rather, the client's own beliefs about the world cause such changes (Association for Advanced Training in the Behavioral Sciences 1986). Ellis tries to help the client change irrational beliefs that create destructive emotional and behavioral reactions such as child abuse. For example, Ellis might choose to show an abused child that her poor self-esteem is based on irrational assumptions about herself and others.

Yalom (1975) noted that *group therapy* is effective when cognitive learning is combined with self-disclosure and learning through watching others. Other important elements of group therapy include helping others in the group (altruism), experiencing group cohesiveness, learning that others have similar problems (universality), giving and receiving feedback, expressing feelings (catharsis), and increasing one's hopefulness about life. Group therapy may therefore be particularly helpful with abusive parents, because they often need information about such questions as child development and home safety, as well as needing opportunities to develop themselves. The opportunities for growth in areas such as altruism, universality, and catharsis are also useful to the abusive parent, who is likely to be isolated, to lack social skills, and to have poor self-esteem.

Group therapy is popular with those who provide treatment for abusive parents. Groups are most appropriate for those individuals who have difficulty expressing feelings in individual treatment but can sometimes express sadness and anger readily when they hear other group members express similar feelings (James and Nasjleti 1983). In their work with abusive mothers, Oates and Forrest (1985) helped build the self-esteem of their clients by using lay therapists to provide mothers with practical emotional support. Self-help groups have become common in the treatment of abusers; some child abuse experts consider groups such as Parents Anonymous and Parents United to be quite effective in both treatment and prevention (Giaretto 1982; Lieber and Baker 1977).

In such self-help groups, parents are encouraged to help one another through a mutual support system. The group support system decreases the demands on the therapist to meet the clients' dependency needs (McNeil and McBride 1979). Through group reinforcement, parents can improve their self-esteem by learning that they should not look to their children or therapist to satisfy their needs. Some experts caution, however, that therapists in self-help groups must learn to defer to the clients' needs and beliefs only when it is beneficial to the treatment process (Ryan 1986).

A major advantage in using groups to develop self-esteem is that it enhances socialization skills, as a "community" forms among the group members. Phelan (1987) believes that such a community can provide a sense of common experiences, values, beliefs, and social solidarity for abusive parents and abused children. Another effect of the group process on self-esteem is the way in which group dynamics encourage confession, responsibility for self, and individual psychological growth.

Most adolescent parents may be considered high-risk by definition, for they are actually children raising children. Unfortunately, many adolescent parents come from homes that were abusive (Daro 1987), and thus they are not only immature but also often psychologically damaged as they begin parenthood. Daro names four treatment approaches used with adolescent parents: parent skill training, crisis intervention, job training, and shelter-oriented care. She believes that effective psychotherapy with adolescent parents incorporates interventions meeting all the needs represented by these four approaches. Kaufman (1986) argues that treatment in groups is the preferred form of psychotherapy with adolescents.

This survey of various methods of psychotherapy has identified some specific intervention strategies that are used in preventing and treating child abuse. Each of the psychological approaches described is also potentially useful in the development of self-esteem. More research is required both to determine the circumstances under which each approach (or combination of approaches) is indicated and to determine the relative effectiveness of each approach in treating child abuse cases and in improving the self-esteem of family members.

Techniques Used to Treat Low Self-Esteem

In individual, group, and family treatment, various techniques are used to enhance self-esteem. Some of the goals of treatment include improving the client's capacity for self-mastery, individuation, empowerment, assertiveness, and the use of social support systems. These goals are accomplished through using techniques such as guided imagery, body awareness exercises, problem solving and rehearsing, assertiveness training, role modeling, role playing, peer-group support, and art therapy.

Self-mastery can be achieved through the therapist's use of guided imagery, body awareness exercises, problem solving and rehearsing, sex education, and the practice of defiance and self-protection (James and Nasjleti 1983). Many experts suggest focusing on positive rather than negative behavior to begin building self-esteem. Gambrill (1981) stresses the importance of building on available skills rather than trying to decrease negative behavior. She also suggests increasing self-management skills so clients can feel that they have a greater effect on their environment. It is advisable to focus clients on the positive traits in their families and backgrounds when they first start therapy. Giaretto (1982) argues that before efforts to increase personal and family growth can succeed, individuals must believe that they and their families are worth the effort. Only from this positive stance can clients focus on the negative aspects of their lives. Porter, Blick, and Sgroi (1982) suggest the use of role modeling, role playing, peer-group support, and positive peer pressure. They suggest that treatment should focus on accountability, behaving responsibly toward one's self and others, and individuation from one's family of origin. Their treatment plan includes structured opportunities for clients to make choices and be responsible for their own actions. Involving the family in the treatment plan is believed to enhance the client's sense of mastery over future plans.

A major consideration in treating clients with low self-esteem is helping them gain some sense of control or power. Thus therapists commonly apply the principles of "empowerment" in such cases. The development of an effective support system is the first step in this process (Solomon 1976). The client must then identify blocks to power and develop strategies to reduce the effects of these indirect and direct blocks. Brickman (1984) "empowers" clients by encouraging them to take a stand, to say no effectively, and to speak up more. In treating an abusive family, she recommends reversing the traditional family roles by first asking the victims to give their account of the family situation. This opportunity for the victim to define the situation increases the child's sense of importance.

Clients also need the opportunity to acquire socialization skills and test the mastery of such skills. Contact with other children or adults is often established through activities such as parents' groups, day care, community programs, mothers' and toddlers' programs, family agencies, preschool co-ops, and postnatal care—activities that can help to build a solid social support system.

In another approach used to counsel mothers who have physically abused their children, Feshbach (1980) enhances the mother's self-concept by teaching her to separate her child's behavior from her own sense of self-worth. The goal is to help parents develop an individuated identity, to differentiate between the success and failure of the child and their own successes and failures. Feshbach states that "to the extent that the parent's self-esteem is independent of the child's behavior, the parent is less likely to react with extreme anger when the child does not conform to parental instructions and expectations" (1980, 55). A parent's unrealistic expectations of a child play an important part in lowering the child's self-esteem (Oates, Forrest, and Peacock 1985); thus, decreasing the parent's dependency on the child's achievement as a source of self-esteem can in turn have a positive effect on the child's self-esteem.

Children who are abused often feel a loss of nurturance, which can contribute to low self-esteem. Through the use of groups, therapists can provide role models to show parents that they can be nurturing, accepting, encouraging, and loving individuals (McNeil and McBride 1979). Encouraging the parent or caretaker to provide intense nurturing will give the child a greater sense of security (Porter, Blick, and Sgroi 1982).

Low self-esteem can also hinder the appropriate release of anger. Art therapy can help to release feelings of anger and hostility, improving one's self-concept. Art therapy can be a healthy and safe way not only to vent negativity but also to explore alternatives. A child who is depressed and withdrawn can learn to open up through art therapy and ultimately improve self-esteem (Porter, Blick, and Sgroi 1982; Axline 1969; Moustakas 1969).

Assertiveness training is also considered an effective method of enhancing self-esteem. Assertiveness is increased through identifying needs and desires, formulating realistic expectations of self and others, and, finally, developing and implementing adequate plans to accomplish goals. Such training is particularly useful in helping people identify strengths and receive positive feedback when deserved (Sgroi and Dana 1982). Positive reinforcement such as verbal praise for appropriate behavior can significantly increase a person's sense of self-worth.

As noted above, efforts to prevent child abuse through education are an increasingly important part of intervention strategies. Over the past decade, concerns about child abuse led first to development of experimental efforts and then to communitywide prevention programs. These programs, which generally began with elementary school curricula, gradually became designed to include preschool, middle school, and high school students as well. Currently, at least fifteen states have child abuse prevention programs that are supported by state funding.

In California, the enhancement of self-esteem in children is seen as a major goal of child abuse prevention efforts. The California Child Abuse Prevention and Treatment Act (CAPTA) now provides $11.5 million each year for child abuse prevention efforts with children from preschool through high school, making CAPTA the largest program of its kind in the nation. Enhancement of self-esteem is a common objective of CAPTA-funded primary prevention programs at all age levels.

Evaluations of Intervention Programs to Increase Self-Esteem and Reduce Child Abuse

Most professionals engaged in treating abusive families would support the premise that low self-esteem is a significant characteristic of such families. Most therapists would agree that improving the self-esteem of members of abusive families, including victims, abusers, and nonabusive parents, is an integral part of the therapeutic task. There are, however, several problems pointed out in child abuse research pertaining to the treatment of self-esteem.

First, although child abuse experts often discuss the usefulness of treatment and prevention efforts, they fail to describe the methodology used to improve clients' self-esteem. The therapeutic objective is often described in the literature simply as "increasing self-esteem" (Oates, Forrest, and Peacock 1985). Guidelines for treatment and intervention rarely provide any details about the specific steps an abusive family needs to take to improve self-esteem. It may be that therapists are indeed working to increase self-esteem, but there is a dearth of knowledge about *how* this occurs.

Second, research on the effects of therapeutic intervention to increase self-esteem is also limited. Few follow-up studies have been conducted to verify whether treatment and prevention programs actually affect self-esteem. Follow-up studies tend to measure the success of treatment or prevention by measuring the change in one or two variables, such as continued abuse or family reunification (Giaretto 1982). Empirical tests of treatment efforts rarely indicate changes in the self-esteem of clients (Abel, Becker, and Cunningham-Rather 1984; Tracy et al. 1983). Thus, we do not know, for example, whether abuse decreases because abusers develop better self-control, learn techniques for dealing with emotional tensions, or increase their self-esteem.

A third problem lies in the lack of control or comparison groups in studies of child abuse treatment, which makes it very difficult to measure treatment effects. The use of a control group in evaluating child abuse treatment is rare, as it would require the withholding of treatment. Because such a test would be highly unethical, a true experimental design is rarely used in child abuse treatment research.

Finally, many types of interventions are used in treating child abuse; however, the question of self-esteem seems to be addressed only in research that focuses on psychotherapeutic methods. Interventions such as parenting groups, day care services, employment counseling, and financial aid may be very effective both in reducing child abuse and in increasing self-esteem, but we were unable to locate any studies that specifically examine the effect of these kinds of intervention on self-esteem.

The Characteristic to Be Treated

It is not clear that the direct treatment of low self-esteem is the most effective way to deal with the problems of those involved in child abuse. Self-esteem cannot be viewed in isolation from other problems in abusive families. A low level of self-esteem may contribute to or be caused by other problems, such as social isolation, inadequate parenting, a sense of helplessness, poor body image, an inability to trust others, and an inability to express one's feelings. A low level of self-esteem in adolescents has been found to manifest itself in thoughts about suicide, depression, and substance abuse (Porter, Blick, and Sgroi 1982). Parents with low self-esteem tend to draw on their children to meet their emotional needs (Summit 1983). In a review of nine studies, Kinard (1980a) reports that abused children exhibit a sense of depression and unhappiness and a poor self-concept.

People with low self-esteem are often believed to have a poor body image, and this is especially common in abusive families, specifically for victims of abuse (Brickman 1984; James and Nasjleti 1983; Porter, Blick, and Sgroi 1982). Body image can be improved by helping clients overcome inhibitions through discussing feelings of discomfort and inadequacies. Victims' self-esteem can be rebuilt by helping them to reclaim their bodies through nourishing, nurturing, and exercising their physical selves.

Parents' low self-esteem can contribute significantly to other life problems. The sense of worthlessness experienced by many abusers contributes to the act of abuse. The abusive relationship may compensate for a parent's feeling abused or rejected by others. It may serve to restore a sense of power and control to individuals who have felt a lack of control in their marital relationships and childhood experiences. Abusing a child may gratify a need for attention and recognition. It may meet a need for affiliation and temporarily strengthen the adult's sense of identity (Sgroi 1982). Treatment of all these problems will contribute to the building of self-esteem.

Treatment Modalities

Several treatment modalities, such as individual psychotherapy, behavior modification, group therapy, and family treatment, have been used in the field of child abuse. Individual treatment is often the first phase, where victims of abuse are encouraged to identify and express negative feelings they may have about themselves. The self-esteem of all the family members may be even lower when they contemplate how the abuse could have occurred. Feelings of guilt and responsibility can overwhelm any of the family members, including the offender, the victim, and others.

Tsai and Wagner (1978) found that these feelings of guilt contribute to the low self-esteem of women who were sexually molested as children. A six-month follow-up study of the women in their sample revealed that alleviating this guilt resulted in a corresponding increase in self-esteem. It is important to help each family member understand the abusive pattern and how this cycle can be broken. Once an individual has progressed in treatment, the group forum is encouraged as the next step in therapy.

Prevention

Most of the literature on preventing child abuse describes programs designed for children (Helfer 1982; Schmitt 1980; Finkelhor 1986). The main emphasis of prevention efforts is helping children learn to protect themselves from abuse. Programs are based on the principles of "empowerment" and focus on teaching children how to be assertive, how to recognize abusive behavior, how to say "no," and how to detect the potential for abuse.

One can speculate that acquiring these skills builds self-esteem. But one study measuring the effectiveness of prevention found that children who had high self-esteem before intervention derived greater benefits from prevention efforts than did children with low self-esteem (Fryer, Krazier, and Miyoshi 1987). Thus the correlation between prevention programs and increases in self-esteem remains questionable.

Building self-esteem is a recurrent theme in treatment and prevention interventions, but empirical tests of the effects of current programs on self-esteem are minimal. Most of the existing research is speculative and anecdotal. The few studies that have been conducted appear to evaluate only psychotherapeutic interventions and overlook the effectiveness of other types. This oversight in research continues to pose a problem for child abuse professionals and should be a major focus of future research endeavors.

Conclusion

Having reviewed the social science literature on the relation between self-esteem and child abuse, we find that we can draw only one firm conclusion: that considerably more knowledge is needed to guide development of social policy and programs to deal with problems of self-esteem and problems of child abuse. There is a good deal of literature and research on the subject of self-esteem, and, similarly, there is a sizable literature on the subject of child abuse. Relatively little of this work, however, deals with the connection between the two.

Public concern about child abuse is relatively recent, and there have been continual changes in ideas about the cause of the problem. Many problems of definition arise when one attempts to describe the nature and scope of child maltreatment. Development of interventions and public policies to reduce child abuse is determined, to some extent, by the public's understanding of the problem, by whether a legal, psychological, medical, or social perspective prevails, for example. Thus, if child abuse is perceived as primarily a psychological problem, the public is more likely to support psychotherapeutic interventions; if it is perceived as primarily social, there is likely to be strong support for social service and educational programs. There may also be ideological ties to other social concerns, for example, among some feminists who see child abuse as part of women's oppression.

We have also noted that there are many different conceptions of self-esteem—some primarily psychological and others primarily sociological—all dealing with different dimensions of the phenomenon. As with the concept of child abuse, various perspectives on self-esteem lead us to emphasize one or another policy direction. The sociological perspective tends to support policies and programs that will increase self-esteem by reducing environmental pressures on vulnerable persons (e.g., provision of child care for single teenage parents); the psychological perspective tends to support policies and programs that will increase self-esteem by changing individuals (e.g., counseling and psychotherapy).

Many factors appear to be associated with child abuse: age and marital status of the parent(s), income, employment, and emotional and personal characteristics of both parents and children, among others.

Self-esteem appears to be related to child abuse, that is, abusing parents and abused children tend to have lower self-esteem. But self-esteem is also related to all of those other factors—unemployed parents and poor school achievers suffer from low self-esteem, for example. It is not entirely clear whether the low self-esteem of child abusers precedes (i.e., causes) or follows (i.e., results from) the abusive behavior. Thus, self-esteem may be both a causal variable and an intervening variable with respect to child abuse.

As one reviews the literature, however, one factor associated with child abuse fairly leaps out: we refer here to *social isolation*. Child abusers tend to be people who are lonely and isolated—single, teenage parents or unemployed, poorly educated people who are, from a social-contextual viewpoint, out of joint, cut off from opportunities to fulfill appropriate social role expectations, and lacking social support.

Interventions to deal with child abuse range from the societal (changing laws and values) to the social (providing social and practical supports to vulnerable parents) to the individual (psychotherapy to increase self-esteem). Most programs that are explicitly intended to treat child abusers are psychotherapeutically oriented, and some of these programs explicitly attempt to increase the self-esteem of abusing parents.

There is some evidence that such intervention programs do result in reduced child abuse. But there is not any empirical evidence in any follow-up of treated parents that their self-esteem was in fact increased as a result of the intervention. Moreover, we find no research that deals with the effects that nonpsychotherapeutically oriented intervention programs might have on both self-esteem and the incidence of child abuse (for example, finding that a child care program for single teenage parents resulted in increased self-esteem for parents and children and in a reduced incidence of child abuse).

Given the current paucity of knowledge about these questions, we must conclude the following:

• There is insufficient evidence to support the belief in a direct relation between low self-esteem and child abuse.

• Low self-esteem should not be perceived as the *primary* cause of child abuse, especially in light of other factors such as age, employment status, availability of child care, and economic insecurity.

• There is no solid evidence that counseling and psychotherapy increase self-esteem.

• There is no basis on which to argue that increasing self-esteem is an effective or efficient means of decreasing child abuse (by comparison with other interventions).

• There is strong evidence that the *social isolation* of parents is a significant factor in causing both child abuse and low self-esteem. Social isolation may be caused by circumstances such as unemployment or being a single teenage parent. This finding suggests the need for social interventions rather than psychotherapeutic interventions. (This does not diminish the possible relevance of self-esteem in the prevention of child abuse. It does suggest, however, that the *psychological* factor of self-esteem may be changed indirectly, as the result of a *social* intervention.)

• Policy interventions to reduce child abuse that involve increasing self-esteem should be encouraged and should include interventions at the individual, family, group, community, and societal levels.

• All such programs should be evaluated using systematic methods of research to assess their effectiveness and efficiency.

Bibliography

Abel, G. G., J. V. Becker, and J. Cunningham-Rather. 1984. "Complications, Consent, and Cognitions in Sex Between Children and Adults." *International Journal of Law and Psychiatry* 7(1): 89–103.

Adler, A. 1958. *The Practice and Theory of Individual Psychology*. Paterson, N.J.: Littlefield, Adams.

American Humane Association (AHA). 1987. *Highlights of Official Child Abuse, Neglect, and Abuse Reporting in 1985*. Denver: American Humane Association.

American Psychiatric Association. 1980. *Quick Reference to the Diagnostic Criteria from DSM III*. Washington, D.C.: American Psychiatric Association.

Anderson, S. C., and M. L. Lauderdale. 1982. "Characteristics of Abusive Parents: A Look at Self-Esteem." *Child Abuse and Neglect* 6: 285–293.

Association for Advanced Training in the Behavioral Sciences. 1986. *Preparatory Course for the Marriage, Family, and Child Counseling Licensing Examination*. Los Angeles: Association for Advanced Training in the Behavioral Sciences.

Avery-Clark, C., J. A. O'Neil, and D. A. Laws. 1981. "A Comparison of Intrafamilial Sexual and Physical Child Abuse." In *Adult Sexual Interest in Children*, edited by M. Cook and H. Kevin, 3–39. London: Academic Press.

Axline, V. 1969. *Play Therapy*. New York: Ballantine Books.

Bagley, C., and R. Ramsay. 1985–1986. "Disrupted Childhood and Vulnerability to Sexual Assault: Long-Term Sequels with Implications for Counseling." *Journal of Social Work and Human Sexuality* 4(1–2): 33–48.

Bandura, A. 1977. "Self-Efficacy: Toward a Unifying Theory of Behavioral Change." *Psychological Review* 84: 191–215.

Barrett, C. L., I. E. Hampe, and L. C. Miller. 1978. "Research on Child Psychotherapy." In *Handbook of Psychotherapy and Behavior Change: An Empirical Analysis*, edited by S. L. Garfield and A. E. Bergin, 411–435. 2d ed. New York: Wiley.

Battle, J. 1981. *Culture-Free SEI: Self-Esteem Inventories for Children and Adults*. Seattle: Special Child Publications.

Belsky, J. 1980. "Child Maltreatment: An Ecological Integration." *American Psychologist* 35: 320–355.

Berne, E. 1961. *Transactional Analysis in Psychotherapy*. New York: Grove Press.

Bixler, R. H. 1981. "The Incest Controversy." *Psychological Reports* 49: 267–283.

Blanck, G., and R. Blanck. 1974. *Ego Psychology: Theory and Practice*. New York: Columbia University Press.

Brickman, J. 1984. "Feminist, Nonsexist, and Traditional Models of Therapy: Implications for Working with Incest." *Women and Therapy* 3(1): 49–67.

Brière, J. 1984. "The Long-Term Effects of Childhood Sexual Abuse: Defining a

Post–Sexual-Abuse Syndrome." Paper presented at the Third National Conference on Sexual Victimization of Children, Washington, D.C., April.

Brissett, D. 1972. "Toward a Clarification of Self-Esteem." *Psychiatry* 35: 255–263.

Bronfenbrenner, U. 1979. *The Ecology of Human Development.* Cambridge, Mass.: Harvard University Press.

Burgess, R. 1978. "Child Abuse: A Behavioral Analysis." In *Advances in Child Clinical Psychology,* edited by B. Lakey and A. Kazdin, 88–101. New York: Plenum.

Burgess, R. L., and J. Garbarino. 1986. "Doing What Comes Naturally? An Evolutionary Perspective on Child Abuse." In *The Dark Side of Families: Current Family Violence Research,* edited by D. Finkelhor, R. J. Gelles, G. T. Hotaling, and M. A. Straus, 35–54. Beverly Hills, Calif.: Sage.

Burke, P. J. 1980. "The Self: Measurement Requirements from an Interactionist Perspective." *Social Psychological Quarterly* 43: 18–29.

Butler, S. 1978. *Conspiracy of Silence: The Trauma of Incest.* New York: New Glide Publications.

Calam, R., and C. Franchi. 1987. *Child Abuse and Its Consequences: Observational Approaches.* Cambridge: Cambridge University Press.

Child Welfare League of America. 1973. *Standards for Child Protective Services.* New York: Child Welfare League of America.

Cohen, H., and G. Weil. 1971. *Tasks of Emotional Development Test.* Lexington, Mass.: D. C. Heath.

Cooley, C. H. 1902. *Human Nature and the Social Order.* New York: Scribner.

Coopersmith, S. 1967. *The Antecedents of Self-Esteem.* San Francisco: Freeman.

———. 1975. *Coopersmith Self-Esteem Inventory.* Palo Alto, Calif.: Consulting Psychologists Press.

Courtois, C. 1979. "The Incest Experience and Its Aftermath." *Victimology: An International Journal* 4: 337–347.

Covitz, J. 1986. *Emotional Child Abuse: The Family Curse.* Boston: Sigo.

Daro, D. 1987. Personal communication to author. March.

DeFrancis, V. 1969. *Protecting the Child Victim of Sex Crimes Committed by Adults.* Denver: American Humane Association.

DeMause, L. 1974. *The History of Childhood.* New York: Psychohistory Press.

Dembo, R., M. Dertke, L. La Voie, S. Borders, M. Washburn, and J. Schmeidler. 1987. "Physical Abuse, Sexual Victimization, and Illicit Drug Use: A Structural Analysis Among High-Risk Adolescents." *Journal of Adolescence* 10: 13–33.

Dietz, C., and J. Craft. 1980. "Family Dynamics of Incest: A New Perspective." *Social Casework* 61: 421–426.

Dinkmeyer, D. C., W. L. Pew, and D. C. Dinkmeyer, Jr. 1979. *Adlerian Counseling and Psychotherapy.* Monterey, Calif.: Brooks/Cole.

Dreikurs, R. 1957. *Psychology in the Classroom.* New York: Harper & Row.

Ellis, A. 1962. *Reason and Emotion in Psychotherapy.* New York: Lyle Stuart.

Elmer, E. A. 1977. "A Follow-Up Study of Traumatized Children." *Pediatrics* 59: 273–279.

Encyclopedia of Social Work. 1987. 18th ed. Silver Spring, Md.: National Association of Social Work.

Epstein, S. 1973. "The Self-Concept Revisited, or, A Theory of a Theory." *American Psychologist* 28:404–416.

Evans, A. L. 1980. "Personality Characteristics and Disciplinary Attitudes of Child-Abusing Mothers." *Child Abuse and Neglect* 4:179–187.

Family Welfare Research Group. 1986. "Community-Based Child Abuse Prevention and Treatment Programs." Typescript.

Famularo, R., R. Barnum, and K. Stone. 1986. "Court-Ordered Removal in Severe Child Maltreatment: An Association to Parental Major Affective Disorder." *Child Abuse and Neglect* 10:487–492.

Feshbach, S. 1980. "Child Abuse and the Dynamics of Human Aggression and Violence." In *Child Abuse: An Agenda for Action,* edited by G. Gerbner, C. J. Ross, and E. Zigler, 48–62. New York: Oxford University Press.

Festinger, L. 1954. *A Theory of Social Comparison Processes.* New York: Human Relations Press.

Finkelhor, D. 1986. "Designing New Studies." In *A Sourcebook on Child Sexual Abuse,* edited by D. Finkelhor, S. Araja, L. Baron, A. Brown, S. D. Peters, and G. E. Wyatt, 199–223. Beverly Hills, Calif.: Sage.

Fitts, W. 1965. *Manual for the Tennessee Self-Concept Scale.* Nashville, Tenn.: Counselor Recordings and Tests.

Franks, D. D., and J. Marolla. 1976. "Efficacious Action and Social Approval as Interacting Dimensions of Self-Esteem: A Tentative Formulation Through Construct Validation." *Sociometry* 39:41–58.

Freedman, A. M., I. Kaplan, and B. J. Sadock. 1980. *Modern Synopsis of Comprehensive Textbook of Psychiatry/II.* 2d ed. Baltimore: Williams & Wilkins.

Freud, S. 1932. *New Introductory Lectures.* Vol. 22 of *The Complete Psychological Works of Sigmund Freud,* standard ed., edited by James Strachey. London: Hogarth Press.

———. 1963a. *Civilization and Its Discontents.* New York: Norton.

———. 1963b. *An Outline of Psychoanalysis.* New York: Norton.

Fryer, G. E., S. K. Krazier, and T. Miyoshi. 1987. "Measuring Actual Reduction of Risk to Child Abuse: A New Approach." *Child Abuse and Neglect* 11:173–179.

Gambrill, E. 1981. "The Use of Behavioural Procedures in Cases of Child Abuse and Neglect." *International Journal of Behavioural Social Work and Abstracts* 1(1): 3–26.

Garbarino, J. 1987. "Background, Identification, Contextual Issues of Emotional Maltreatment." Paper presented at conference on Adolescent Emotional Maltreatment: Therapeutic Strategies, Alameda, Calif.

Garbarino, J., and G. Gilliam. 1980. *Understanding Abusive Families.* Lexington, Mass.: D. C. Heath.

Garfield, S. L., and A. E. Bergin, eds. 1978. *Handbook of Psychotherapy and Behavior Change: An Empirical Analysis.* 2d ed. New York: Wiley.

Gecas, V. 1971. "Parental Behavior and Dimensions of Adolescent Self-Evaluation." *Sociometry* 35:332–345.

————. 1982. "The Self-Concept." *Annual Review of Sociology* 8:1–33.
Gelles, R. J., and C. P. Cornell. 1983. "International Perspectives on Child Abuse." *Child Abuse and Neglect* 7:375–386.
Gelles, R. J., and J. B. Lancaster. 1987. *Child Abuse and Neglect.* New York: Aldine de Gruyter.
Giaretto, H. 1982. *Integrated Treatment of Child Sexual Abuse: A Treatment and Training Manual.* Palo Alto, Calif.: Science and Behavior Books.
Gil, D. 1976. *The Challenge of Social Equality.* Cambridge, Mass.: Harvard University Press.
————. 1978. "Societal Violence in Families." In *Family Violence: An International and Interdisciplinary Study,* edited by J. M. Eekelaar and K. N. Sanfor, 79–91. Toronto: Butterworth.
————. 1987. "Maltreatment as a Function of the Structure of Social Systems." In *Psychological Maltreatment of Children and Youth,* edited by M. R. Brassard, R. Germain, and S. N. Hart, 157–170. New York: Pergamon Press.
Giovannoni, J. M., and R. M. Becerra. 1979. *Defining Child Abuse.* New York: Free Press.
Glass, C. V., and M. L. Smith. 1976. "Meta-Analysis of Psychotherapy Outcome Studies." Paper presented at the meeting of the Society for Psychotherapy Research, San Diego, Calif., June.
Green, A. H. 1978. "Psychopathology of the Abused Child." *Journal of the American Academy of Child Psychiatry* 17:92–103.
Green, A. H., R. W. Gaines, and A. Sandgrund. 1974. "Child Abuse: Pathological Syndrome of Family Interaction." *American Journal of Psychiatry* 131:882–886.
Green, A. H., E. Power, B. Stembook, and R. Gaines. 1981. "Factors Associated with Successful and Unsuccessful Intervention with Child-Abusive Families." *Child Abuse and Neglect* 5:45–52.
Groth, N. A. 1982. Workshop on Child Sexual Abuse. Presented at a conference of the California Consortium of Child Abuse Councils, Los Angeles, February.
Groth, N. A., R. E. Longo, and B. J. McFaddin. 1982. "Undetected Recidivism Among Rapists and Child Molesters." *Crime and Delinquency* 18(3): 450–458.
Hart, S. N., and M. R. Brassard. 1987. "Psychological Maltreatment: Integration and Summary." In *Psychological Maltreatment of Children and Youth,* edited by M. R. Brassard, R. Germain, and S. N. Hart, 254–266. New York: Pergamon Press.
Helfer, R. E. 1982. "A Review of the Literature on the Prevention of Child Abuse and Neglect." *Child Abuse and Neglect* 6:251–261.
Herman, J. 1981. *Father-Daughter Incest.* Cambridge, Mass.: Harvard University Press.
Hudson, W. 1982. *The Hudson Clinical Package.* Homewood, Ill.: Dorsey.
Hughes, H. 1984. "Measures of Self-Concept and Self-Esteem for Children Ages 3–12 Years: A Review and Recommendations." *Clinical Psychology Review* 4:657–692.

James, B., and M. Nasjleti. 1983. *Treating Sexually Abused Children and Their Families*. Palo Alto, Calif.: Consulting Psychologists Press.

James, W. 1890. *The Principles of Psychology*. New York: Dover.

Jersild, A. T. 1969. *In Search of Self*. New York: Columbia University, Teachers College Press.

Jung, C. G. 1954. *The Collected Works of Carl Jung*. Vol. 17. Princeton, N.J.: Princeton University Press.

Justice, B., and R. Justice. 1976. *The Abusing Family*. New York: Human Sciences Press.

———. 1979. *The Broken Taboo: Sex in the Family*. New York: Human Sciences Press.

Katzen, W. G., and A. J. Stenner. 1975. *Administrative Manual: Self-Observation Scales*. Durham, N.C.: NTS Research Corp.

Kaufman, D. 1986. Untitled paper presented at Child Guidance Clinic in-service training session, Children's Hospital, San Diego, Calif., September.

Kempe, C. H., and R. E. Helfer, eds. 1977. *Helping the Battered Child and His Family*. Philadelphia: Lippincott.

Kempe, R. S., and C. H. Kempe. 1984. *The Common Secret: Sexual Abuse of Children and Adolescents*. San Francisco: Freeman.

Kinard, E. M. 1980a. "Emotional Development in Physically Abused Children." *American Journal of Orthopsychiatry* 50:686–696.

———. 1980b. "Mental Health Needs of Abused Children." *Child Welfare* 59:451–462.

———. 1982. "Experiencing Child Abuse: Effects on Emotional Adjustment." *American Journal of Orthopsychiatry* 52:82–91.

Knapp, J. 1973. *A Selection of Self-Concept Measures*. Princeton, N.J.: Center for Statewide Educational Assessment.

Korbin, J. 1981. *Child Abuse and Neglect: Cross-Cultural Perspectives*. Berkeley and Los Angeles: University of California Press.

Lieber, L., and J. M. Baker. 1977. "Parents Anonymous: Self-Help Treatment for Child-Abusing Parents." *Child Abuse and Neglect* 1:133–148.

McGuire, W. J., and A. Padawer-Singer. 1976. "Trait Salience in the Spontaneous Self-Concept." *Journal of Personality and Social Psychology* 33:743–754.

McNeil, J. S., and M. L. McBride. 1979. "Group Therapy with Abusive Parents." *Social Casework* 60:36–42.

Malan, D. H. 1976. *Toward the Validation of Dynamic Psychotherapy: A Replication*. New York: Plenum.

Martin, B. 1972. "Parent-Child Relations." In *Application of Behavior Modification*, edited by T. Thompson and W. S. Dockens, 121–133. New York: Academic Press.

Martin, H. P., and P. Beezley. 1976. "Personality of Abused Children." In *The Abused Child: A Multidisciplinary Approach to Developmental Issues and Treatment. Behavioral Observations on Abused Children*, edited by H. P. Martin, 226–237. Cambridge, Mass.: Ballinger.

Martinek, T. J., and L. D. Zaichkowsky. 1977. *Manual for the Martinek-*

Zaichkowsky Self-Concept Scale for Children. Jacksonville, Ill.: Psychologists and Educators, Inc.

Maslow, A. H. 1971. *The Further Reaches of Human Nature.* New York: Viking Press.

Mead, G. H. 1934. *Mind, Self, and Society.* Chicago: University of Chicago Press.

Melnick, B., and J. R. Hurley. 1969. "Distinctive Personality Attributes of Child-Abusing Mothers." *Journal of Consulting and Clinical Psychology* 33:746–749.

Morris, M., R. Gould, and J. Matthews. 1964. "Toward Prevention of Child Abuse." *Children* 2:55–60.

Morris, S. B., C. W. Turner, and S. A. Szykula. 1988. "Psychotherapy Outcome Research: An Application of a New Method for Evaluating Research Methodology." *Psychotherapy* 25 (Spring): 18–26.

Moustakas, C. 1969. *Psychotherapy with Children.* New York: Ballantine Books.

Nagi, S. Z. 1977. *Child Maltreatment in the United States.* New York: Columbia University Press.

Navarre, E. L. 1987. "Psychological Maltreatment: The Core Component of Child Abuse." In *Psychological Maltreatment of Children and Youth,* edited by M. R. Brassard, R. Germain, and S. N. Hart, 45–58. New York: Pergamon Press.

Oates, R. K., and D. Forrest. 1985. "Self-Esteem and Early Background of Abusive Mothers." *Child Abuse and Neglect* 9:38–92.

Oates, R. K., D. Forrest, and A. Peacock. 1985. "Self-Esteem of Abused Children." *Child Abuse and Neglect* 9:159–163.

Office of the Attorney General. 1985. *Child Abuse Prevention Handbook.* Sacramento, Calif.: Office of the Attorney General.

O'Toole P., P. Turbett, and C. Nalepka. 1986. "Theories, Professional Knowledge, and Diagnosis of Child Abuse." In *The Dark Side of Families: Current Family Violence Research,* edited by D. Finkelhor, R. J. Gelles, G. T. Hotaling, and M. A. Straus, 349–362. Beverly Hills, Calif.: Sage.

Parton, N. 1979. "The Natural History of Child Abuse: A Study in Social Problem Definition." *British Journal of Social Work* 9:427–451.

Patterson, C. H. 1973. *Theories of Counseling and Psychotherapy.* New York: Harper & Row.

Perls, F. S. 1969. *Gestalt Therapy Verbatim.* Moab, Utah: Real People Press.

Phelan, P. 1987. "Incest: Socialization with a Treatment Program." *American Journal of Orthopsychiatry* 57:84–92.

Piers, E. V. 1969. *Manual for the Piers-Harris Children's Self-Concept Scale.* Nashville, Tenn.: Counselor Recordings and Tests.

Polansky, N. A., J. M. Gaudin, P. W. Ammons, and K. B. Davis. 1985. "The Psychological Ecology of the Neglectful Mother." *Child Abuse and Neglect* 9:265–275.

Polster, E., and M. Polster. 1973. *Gestalt Therapy Integrated: Counters of Theory and Practice.* New York: Random House.

Polster, R. A., and R. F. Dangel. 1984. "Behavioral Parent Training: Where It

Came From and Where It's At." In *Parent Training*, edited by R. A. Polster and R. F. Dangel, 1–12. New York: Guilford.

Porter, F. S., L. C. Blick, and S. M. Sgroi. 1982. "Treatment of the Sexually Abused Child." In *Handbook of Clinical Intervention in Child Sexual Abuse*, edited by S. M. Sgroi, 109–146. Lexington, Mass.: D. C. Heath.

Prodgers, A. 1984. "Psychopathology of the Physically Abusing Parent: A Comparison with Borderline Syndrome." *Child Abuse and Neglect* 8: 411–424.

Purkey, W., and J. C. Schmidt. 1987. *The Inviting Relationship: An Expanded Perspective for Professional Counseling*. Englewood Cliffs, N.J.: Prentice-Hall.

Rogers, C. R. 1965. *Client-Centered Therapy*. Boston: Houghton Mifflin.

Rohner, R. 1984. "Foundations of Parental Acceptance-Rejection Theory." Mimeo.

Rosenberg, M. 1965. *Society and the Adolescent Self-Image*. Princeton, N.J.: Princeton University Press.

———. 1979. *Conceiving the Self*. New York: Basic Books.

———. 1981. "The Self-Concept: Social Product and Social Force." In *Social Psychology: Sociological Perspectives*, edited by M. Rosenberg and R. H. Turner, 593–624. New York: Basic Books.

Rosenberg, M., and L. C. Pearlin. 1978. "Social Class and Self-Esteem Among Children and Adults." *American Journal of Sociology* 84: 53–77.

Rosenberg, M. S. 1987. "New Directions for Research on the Psychological Maltreatment of Children." *American Psychologist* 42: 166–171.

Rosenfeld, A. A., C. C. Nadelson, and M. Krieger. 1979. "Fantasy and Reality in Patients' Reports of Incest." *Journal of Clinical Psychiatry* 40: 159–164.

Rush, A. J., A. T. Beck, J. Kovacs, and S. Hollon. 1977. "Comparative Efficacy of Cognitive Therapy and Pharmacotherapy in the Treatment of Depressed Outpatients." *Cognitive Therapy and Research* 1: 17–37.

Rush, F. 1980. *The Best-Kept Secret: Sexual Abuse of Children*. Englewood Cliffs, N.J.: Prentice-Hall.

Russell, D. E. H. 1984. "The Prevalence and Seriousness of Incestuous Abuse: Stepfathers vs. Biological Fathers." *Child Abuse and Neglect* 8: 15–22.

———. 1986. *The Secret Trauma: Incest in the Lives of Girls and Women*. New York: Basic Books.

Ryan, T. S. 1986. "Problems, Errors, and Opportunities in the Treatment of Father-Daughter Incest." *Journal of Interpersonal Violence* 1(1): 113–124.

Schmitt, B. D. 1980. "The Prevention of Child Abuse and Neglect: A Review of the Literature with Recommendations for Application." *Child Abuse and Neglect* 4: 171–178.

Schneider, C., J. K. Hoffmeister, and R. Helfer. 1976. "A Predictive Screening Questionnaire for Potential Problems in Mother-Child Interaction." In *Child Abuse and Neglect: The Family and the Community*, edited by R. Helfer and C. Kempe, 393–407. Cambridge, Mass.: Ballinger.

Sgroi, S. M., ed. 1982. *Handbook of Clinical Intervention in Child Sexual Abuse*. Lexington, Mass.: D. C. Heath.

Sgroi, S. M., and N. T. Dana. 1982. "Individual and Group Treatment of Mothers of Incest Victims." In *Handbook of Clinical Intervention in Child Sexual Abuse*, edited by S. M. Sgroi, 191–214. Lexington, Mass.: D. C. Heath.

Shorkey, C. T. 1979. "A Review of Methods Used in the Treatment of Abusing Parents." *Social Casework* 60:360–367.

———. 1980. "Sense of Personal Worth, Self-Esteem, and Anomia of Child-Abusing Mothers and Controls." *Journal of Clinical Psychology* 36: 817–820.

Sloan, M. P., and J. H. Meier. 1983. "Typology for Parents of Abused Children." *Child Abuse and Neglect* 7:443–450.

Sloane, R. B., F. R. Staples, A. H. Cristol, N. J. Yorkston, and K. Whipple. 1975. *Short-Term Analytically Oriented Psychotherapy vs. Behaviour Therapy*. Cambridge, Mass.: Harvard University Press.

Smith, S. 1986. *Child Welfare in the United States: Fifty-State Survey Report*. Denver: National Conference of State Legislatures.

Solomon, B. B. 1976. *Black Empowerment*. New York: Columbia University Press.

Spearly, J. L., and M. Lauderdale. 1983. "Community Characteristics and Ethnicity in the Prediction of Child Maltreatment Rates." *Child Abuse and Neglect* 7:91–105.

Steele, B. F. 1980. "Psychodynamic Factors in Child Abuse." In *The Battered Child*, edited by C. H. Kempe and R. E. Helfer, 49–85. Chicago: University of Chicago Press.

Steele, B. F., and C. B. Pollock. 1974. "A Psychiatric Study of Parents Who Abuse Infants and Small Children." In *The Battered Child*, edited by C. H. Kempe and R. E. Helfer, 89–133. Chicago: University of Chicago Press.

Straus, M. A., R. J. Gelles, and S. K. Steinmetz. 1980. *Behind Closed Doors: Violence in the American Family*. Garden City, N.Y.: Anchor/Doubleday.

Stryker, S. 1977. "Developments in Two Social Psychologies: Toward an Appreciation of Mutual Relevance." *Sociometry* 40:145–160.

Sturkie, K., and J. P. Flanzer. 1987. "Depression and Self-Esteem in the Families of Maltreated Adolescents." *Social Work* 33:491–496.

Summit, R. 1983. "The Child Sexual Abuse Accommodation Syndrome." *Child Abuse and Neglect* 7:177–193.

Thorpe, L. P., W. W. Clark, and E. W. Tiegs. 1953. *Manual for the California Test of Personality*. Los Angeles: California Test Bureau.

Tracy, F., H. Donnelly, L. Morgenbesser, and D. Macdonald. 1983. "Program Evaluation: Recidivism Research Involving Sex Offenders." In *The Sexual Aggressor: Current Perspectives on Treatment*, edited by J. Green and I. Stuart, 198–213. New York: Van Nostrand Reinhold.

Tsai, M., and N. Wagner. 1978. "Therapy Groups for Women Sexually Molested as Children." *Archives of Sexual Behaviour* 75:417–427.

Westat Development and Associates. 1981. "National Study of the Incidence and Severity of Child Abuse and Neglect." Prepared for the National Center on Child Abuse and Neglect under contract no. 105–76–1137, Washington, D.C., September.

Wodarski, J. S. 1981. "Treatment of Parents Who Abuse Their Children: A

Literature Review and Implications for Professionals." *Child Abuse and Neglect* 5:351–361.

Wylie, R. C. 1979. *The Self-Concept*. Vol. 2, *Theory and Research on Selected Topics*. Rev. ed. Lincoln: University of Nebraska Press.

Yalom, I. D. 1975. *The Theory and Practice of Group Psychotherapy*. 2d ed. New York: Basic Books.

Yates, A., J. W. Hull, and R. B. Huebner. 1983. "Predicting the Abusive Parent's Response to Intervention." *Child Abuse and Neglect* 7:37–44.

Zigler, E. F. 1983. "Understanding Child Abuse: A Dilemma for Policy Development." In *Children, Families, and Government: Perspectives in America*, edited by E. F. Zigler, S. L. Kagan, and E. Klugman, 189–206. Cambridge: Cambridge University Press.

Self-Esteem and Failure in School: Analysis and Policy Implications

Martin V. Covington

Introduction

The failure to learn can be catastrophic for an individual and eventually staggering in its costs to society. A few statistics may present the broad dimensions of the problem. For example, an estimated 25 percent of the students who enter first grade in the United States each year drop out before high school graduation, and in some ghetto schools 30 percent of the students never complete eighth grade. In California, three out of ten students entering the ninth grade do not graduate from high school. Moreover, among those students who do graduate, average reading proficiency is below the ninth-grade level.

These statistics are shocking enough in themselves. But what is even more sobering is the larger implication of lives blighted, talent unused, and minds wasted. These losses are most clearly manifest in human terms as a paralysis of the will both to learn and to continue to learn as future circumstances change. In effect, a substantial number of our students face an unknown world utterly unprepared. Ultimately it is this failure of will that should concern us most—not solely the failure to read, to write, or to calculate, but the inability to adapt and cope, especially in a society where change is the only constant. For instance, Americans who enter the permanent work force in the year 2010 (those children beginning kindergarten in the next several years) will change careers—not just jobs, but careers—an average of five times before they retire. Without the capacity to learn from such change, and from occasional upheaval, individuals will become crippled, confused, and then eventually overwhelmed by a vastly changed future society in which they will no longer know how to participate. To what extent is the will to learn and the quality of one's academic preparation controlled and influenced by an individual's perceptions of self?

The main burden of this chapter is to summarize the case for a causal link between self-esteem and the widespread failure of students to learn. Assuming that such a case can be made, a second purpose is to identify the conditions of classroom learning and those teacher/student relationships that are thought to promote self-esteem and those believed to inhibit it. The basic reasoning behind this two-step analysis assumes that if low self-esteem interferes with learning—and positive self-esteem promotes learning—then educational failure should be lessened to the extent that we promote those conditions known to enhance self-esteem.

A third and final aim is to consider various recommendations for change in current educational policy and practice. We will place several restrictions on the kind and scope of proposals to be offered here. First, we will limit ourselves to recommendations that follow uniquely from a perspective that focuses on self-esteem. There are various economic and political interpretations of school failure that not only are plausible but also likely contain a portion of the truth (e.g., Bowles and Gintis 1976; Jencks et al. 1972). Our analysis here, however, is limited by the mandate of the task force to a consideration of self-esteem. In effect, we will ask if there is any unique contribution that a perspective focused on self-esteem can make to our understanding of the complex phenomena of learning and failure in schools. Second, we will restrict ourselves to recommendations that are eminently practical and possible to implement within a relatively short time, say, within three to five years. Moreover, there must be a reasonable prospect that such improvements in the educational climate can influence the current generation of students, that their effects will not be delayed until some distant, future time.

But does the "self-esteem perspective" admit to any such possibilities, even in theory? And what is the hope for any practical success, especially given that student indifference, truancy, and poor achievement often go hand in hand with classroom violence, drug dealing in the schoolyard, and various forms of child abuse and exploitation? It seems obvious that academic failure is as much, if not more, the result of the inevitable pressures and risks of growing up as it is the fault of any improper educational policy. Perhaps, after all, schools can do little to reverse the statistics of failure cited earlier. We must also be prepared to consider that low self-esteem is the result of the accumulation of various social ills and, as a consequence, may itself play little if any role in academic failure. But to abandon the search for esteem-related solutions because divisive factors are operating beyond the control of schools is to admit defeat before exploring all our options. Basically, we will argue that even if schools were drug-free, uncompromised by hatred and fear, and not a dumping ground for the rebellious or the unwanted, certain aspects of schooling would still be a threat to self-esteem and to the will to learn. These dangers—no matter how modest they may be, given the larger circle of threat—are what will drive our recommendations for educational change.

The assumption that self-esteem influences behavior has long been a guiding theme in the social sciences, as has the proposition that increasing a person's feelings of self-worth will promote more constructive, socially valued behaviors. The significance of self as a scientific construct is apparent not only in sociological and educational circles but also in the field of psychotherapy, where a changed self-image and increased self-understanding are often emphasized as major criteria for judging the effectiveness of therapy. Moreover, the presumed importance of perceptions of self and of positive self-change is widely accepted by the lay public, in many quarters as a fundamental article of faith. Whether or not this faith is justified on scientific grounds is a major focus of this chapter.

Before we turn to our review and analysis, we would do well to consider several issues briefly.

Evidence for Causation

The first issue concerns the question of what counts as scientific evidence in favor of the proposition that self-esteem influences, or causes, school achievement. Most empirical studies bearing on this proposition are correlational in nature. As a statistical index, correlation coefficients reflect the strength of an association between two variables, say, between a measure of self-esteem and school test scores. Most correlational studies report a positive association between achievement and indices of self-esteem: as the level of self-esteem increases, so do achievement scores; and as self-esteem decreases, so does achievement.

This simple relationship in itself does not prove causality, however. Certainly, such data establish the plausibility of the argument that self-esteem influences achievement. But other interpretations of this association are equally plausible, including the reverse argument that it is high achievement that causes self-confidence and poor performance that spawns self-deprecation. And, of course, both positions could be correct: self-esteem may be both a cause *and* a result of achievement. Simple correlational analyses by themselves are not especially helpful in disentangling these complex relationships.

The association between self-esteem and school performance may also be spurious, that is, the correspondence may be caused by some third factor—in this instance, perhaps intellectual capacity. Bright students typically hold themselves in higher regard and perform better than do students who are less bright. Thus, self-esteem might be simply a by-product of ability status and may exert little influence on school performance. To complete the example, it may be differences in ability, not in self-esteem, that cause variations in achievement. Again, simple correlational data do little to further our understanding of the intricate dynamics implied by this example. And, most important, they are not as helpful as other data or procedures in determining if there is any truth in our hypothesis.

Only a true experimental design can provide evidence to prove causality. Evidence of causality involves demonstrating that changes in a dependent variable—say, levels of reading achievement—respond in lawful ways to changes in an independent factor. For us, the independent factor of greatest interest is some index of self-esteem. The tricky part of such experiments is to manipulate artificially the degree of self-esteem (or confidence) experienced by subjects, and to do so in ways that are convincing.

Such manipulations are relatively infrequent in the research literature, but they can be accomplished successfully, as illustrated by the research of Weiner and Sierad (1975). These investigators, working with college subjects classified by high and low levels of self-confidence, administered a drug (actually a placebo) to the subjects immediately before assigning them a learning task. The drug was alleged to interfere with hand-eye coordination. Armed with some explanation for a potentially poor performance other than their own inability, the subjects with low self-confidence were expected to perform better than usual. In contrast, the more self-confident subjects were expected to perform worse than usual, owing to the presumed interference of the drug. These predictions were borne out. This experiment neatly demonstrates the causal influence on performance of cognitions (or thoughts) associated with self-esteem. For all their definitiveness and precision, however, true experiments typically involve a considerable trade-off, namely, that proof is provided only in the context of highly artificial circumstances, in laboratory settings far removed from the realities of life. Nonetheless, such experiments are important because they help us isolate the basic underlying mechanisms of behavior that might otherwise go undetected if we limited ourselves to simple correlational procedures.

A third technique, multiple-correlation (or prediction) analysis, retains much of the ecological validity lost in the true experimental design. It is also a decided improvement over the simple, two-variable correlational study. Multiple-prediction analysis employs many predictors of school performance, which often include but are not limited to self-esteem variables. Predictor variables might include indices of the quality of study habits or the degree to which anxiety interferes with test taking, as well as measures of the reasons students themselves give for their successes and failures. This analysis allows us to investigate the relative importance of self-esteem variables in school performance, compared to the rival influence of other factors. Moreover, under a multiple-prediction design, data are often gathered for the same students in real-life settings at different times, say, over the course of several classroom tests, allowing a longitudinal perspective. By tracking individuals over time, we can, for example, determine if the factors associated with an initially satisfactory performance are the same as, or different from, those factors associated with later performances.

As for establishing causation, multiple predictors are usually selected in advance of the actual research, on the basis of some theoretical model. These models prescribe the presumed causal pathways that link the various predictors, one with another, and their individual relationship to academic performance. Because it seems natural to speak of causal relationships as pathways of influence, we will use the generic term *path analysis* to describe these multiple-prediction techniques (Anderson and Evans 1974; Pedhazur 1982).

For all the sophistication of path analysis, proof is still a relative matter. Perhaps it is fairest to say, and for us to remember, that path analysis is not a method for demonstrating causality. Rather, it is a method for comparing *observed* relationships among variables with those relationships *expected* if we assume causality. From the perspective of the lay public, such distinctions may be considered unnecessary, if not bordering on sophistry. Nonetheless, such reasoning provides a conservative test for the assumption of causality. Whenever stakes are high, especially regarding matters of social policy, it is always best to adopt a stringent criterion for what counts as evidence of causation.

Gaps in Knowledge

Evidence regarding causality in the social sciences is typically incomplete. After all the data have been winnowed, sifted, and analyzed, there will remain inconsistent findings, counterintuitive outcomes, and downright gaps in our knowledge. It is in this sense that the case for self-esteem as a prerequisite for effective learning is incomplete. But being incomplete is not the same as being implausible. In fact, the case for self-esteem is not only plausible but, some would argue, compelling. Such an opinion is reasonable, even in the face of imperfect evidence. First, the case is strengthened immeasurably by the use of a variety of research methodologies. Whenever different research methods—correlational, observational, clinical, and experimental—lead to similar findings, we can be more secure about the appropriateness of any causal arguments. Second, as already noted, whenever empirical findings conform to theoretical predictions, the validity of one's causal argument is further strengthened. This is especially true when the predictions are basically counterintuitive, that is, when the theory accounts for puzzling phenomena that cannot be as easily explained by alternative models, or when the theory leads us to explore directions that we might otherwise overlook. In both regards, we will find that several psychological theories inspired by notions of self-esteem have considerable heuristic value: they explain much that is otherwise mysterious, and they lead us to ask new, potentially provocative questions.

Various Models of the Self

The case for the centrality of self-esteem will also depend in an important way on how the notion of *self* is conceptualized. There are, of course, many definitions and approaches to the psychology of self. Some researchers focus on self as a convenient way to catalogue both positive and negative characteristics of the individual (Backman and Secord 1968). Other investigators stress self as an evaluative process (Epstein 1973). Still others emphasize the affective, or emotional, component of self (Rosenberg and Simmons 1973). Additionally, there is a tradition rich in research and clinical application that emphasizes a distinction between actual-self and ideal-self (Davids and Hainsworth 1967); for instance, numerous studies have revealed discrepancies between actual- and ideal-selves among underachievers, with the actual-self falling far short of the ideal (Birney, Burdick, and Teevan 1969). It is this discrepancy that often leads underachievers to punish themselves for failing to attain the perfection they can never reach.

There is no shortage of conceptual models when it comes to describing the relationship between different versions of self and academic performance. Typically, these different models are compatible. Occasionally, however, they represent rival conceptions that are difficult to reconcile. When this happens, they tend to complicate rather than clarify and may cause the public to become impatient and frustrated with what it perceives as "technicalities." Largely for this reason, the field of research on self-concept is seen by some to be in disarray, without a general, unifying theoretical perspective (see Gergen 1971; Wylie 1968, 1974, 1979).

Not all approaches to the concept of self are equally helpful in understanding the processes involved in academic failure and in self-change as a means to improve school achievement (Scheirer and Kraut 1979). Although it is important to recognize the many different and valid approaches to the study of self, it is also important that we do not permit such eclecticism to lead us into chaos. One of our main tasks will be to establish a serviceable, unifying theoretical framework and, in the process, to develop a concept of self that is compatible with the rigors and demands of school life. Fortunately, much of this work has been done for us within the past decade or two. To anticipate briefly, we will view the self, within the context of school, as a monitoring system in which the individual allocates personal resources to achievement tasks, where resources refer to ability, time, effort, and energy level.

A Review

The literature on self-esteem and self-concept is enormous. Few topics in the social sciences and education have sustained interest for so long among both popular and scholarly audiences, or promoted such vast amounts of research and almost unending speculation. However, amid this flood of findings and material, at least one important regularity emerges, one we have already mentioned. A large number of studies over the past seventy-five years have demonstrated a positive association between self-esteem variables and academic achievement. (For comprehensive reviews, see Purkey 1970; Walberg and Uguroglu 1980; Wylie 1979.) As a group, these studies have sampled students of widely different ages and learning characteristics—from the gifted to the retarded—and have also employed many different measures of self-esteem, as well as a variety of achievement indices, including grade point average, standard achievement test scores, and even performance on teacher-made tests. Thus the generality of this finding is not in dispute. But most of these studies are correlational, and as such are of little more than circumstantial value in making a case for causation or for the direction of any causal relationship.

Apart from their lack of conclusiveness about causation, the most disquieting feature of these studies is the generally low magnitude of association found between self-esteem and achievement. For instance, Hansford and Hattie (1982) reported in their review of twenty studies, representing some forty-eight thousand subjects, that the average correlation between measures of achievement and indices of self-description was .16. If we assume a causal interpretation of this statistic, only 4 percent of the variation in school achievement is accounted for by variation in self-concept. Likewise, a review by West, Fish, and Stevens (1980) of some three hundred studies revealed correlations ranging between .11 and .50, with the average being .18. Finally, Sandige (1976) added a measure of self-esteem to a multiple-prediction of school achievement that already included factors such as social class and intelligence. The self-esteem measure accounted for only an additional 3 percent of the explained variation in academic performance. This means that most of the variation in achievement we observe in classrooms—97 percent of it, according to Sandige's study—can be explained by influences other than those traditionally associated with the notion of self-concept.

These findings present us with a dilemma. If feelings of self-esteem are so important to achievement, then why is the demonstrated relationship between self-esteem and academic performance so uniformly low? On the face of this evidence alone, would we be better advised to concentrate our limited educational resources on potentially more effective and immediate ways to offset educational failure, such as teaching improved study habits or increasing the amount of time students spend on a task?

The situation is scarcely improved when we consider the research that has attempted to demonstrate experimentally that changes in self-concept lead to improved performance. Here, as we have seen, investigators manipulate levels of self-esteem, on the assumption that

these changes will induce students to perform differently (Aronson and
Mettee 1968; Silverman 1964; Stotland and Zander 1958; Webster and
Sobieszek 1974). Unfortunately, the results of these studies tend to be
somewhat contradictory and the effects of the manipulation are typically short-lived (Steele 1975).

Another source of evidence about the role of self-esteem comes from
the appraisal of special compensatory education programs aimed at
creating changes in self-concept in order to enhance academic performance. These programs include Head Start for preschoolers, Follow
Through in the primary grades, and Upward Bound for high school students. (For a review, see Scheirer and Kraut 1979.) The basic rationale
behind many of these programs is that high self-esteem is a necessary
condition for achievement (Gray and Klaus 1970). Put in terms of path
analysis, self-concept is treated as a mediator that is positioned between
instructional variables, on the one hand, and achievement outcomes, on
the other, implying that for changes in instruction to influence achievement they must first change the student's self-concept. This reasoning is
implicit in what have been identified as *student-centered* models of
achievement (Covington 1985b).

Student-Centered View

A schematic of the student-centered model is presented in Figure 3.1
(Model A). The arrows imply causality and indicate the presumed direction of causal influence. Some of the relevant studies attempt to
encourage environments of trust in the classroom (e.g., Reckless and
Dinitz 1972); others provide instructional options that allow students a
choice of workload (Jacoby and Covington 1973). Still other researchers
have introduced curricula that permit nongraded academic experiences
(Lawson 1974). These attempts to encourage learning through self-
change have been generally disappointing. Some studies show little or
no change in measured self-concept as a result of intervention, even
though indices of academic achievement increased (e.g., Grant 1973;
Lawson 1974; Stallings and Kaskowitz 1974). In other instances, although changes in measures of self-regard occurred, no parallel changes
in achievement were observed (Hunt and Hardt 1969; Logsdon and
Ewert 1973). Neither outcome is consistent with the assumption that
positive self-regard is a necessary and sufficient precondition for productivity in the schools.

Figure 3.1.   Causal Models of School Achievement

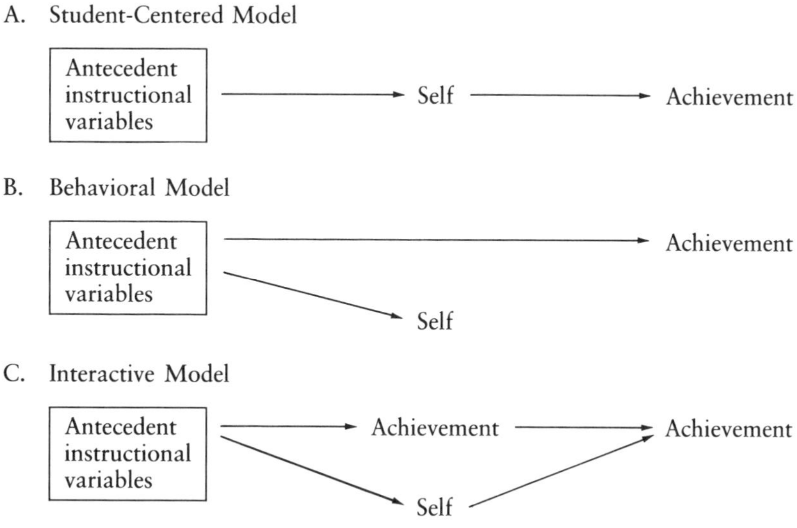

A. Student-Centered Model

    Antecedent instructional variables ⟶ Self ⟶ Achievement

B. Behavioral Model

    Antecedent instructional variables ⟶ Achievement
    ↘ Self

C. Interactive Model

    Antecedent instructional variables ⟶ Achievement ⟶ Achievement
    ↘ Self ↗

Behavioral View

A second, rival view of the role of self in the achievement process follows from a behavioral perspective. According to this tradition, the concept of self—like notions of motivation, emotion, and other "internal," subjective states—is of little value in understanding the dynamics of learning and performance. Behaviorists neither deny the reality of a subjective inner life nor reject the existence of emotions associated with success (pride) and failure (shame). But they do doubt that such general and diffused states of arousal could in themselves guide and direct human behavior in subtle ways.

Rather, they argue, it is the "external" features of instruction that control those actions traditionally associated with concepts such as motivation and self-esteem. These "motivated" behaviors include *choice* of learning task and *intensity* of study effort. According to many behaviorists, the main controlling factor is the schedule of reinforcements that teachers set up, in the form of grades, praise, and other rewards. Although psychologists still debate a number of subtle theoretical issues associated with such concepts as reward and reinforcement, it is nonetheless abundantly clear that on a practical, everyday level we tend to do those things that are rewarding and to avoid what is punishing or threatening. Other things being equal, students will typically do whatever they must to attain the highest grade possible. Indeed, many observational studies suggest that the teacher's grading policy controls almost everything about the student's academic work, including choice of task, intensity of effort, and duration of involvement in the task (Carter and Doyle 1982; King 1980). This is precisely why grading practices have come under such intense and increasing criticism in recent years. For many students, grades have become more important than learning itself.

For good or ill, grading policies control the quality and amount of student achievement to a remarkable degree, and so do a host of other instructional factors, including the amount of time spent studying, the quality of study (Rohwer 1984), and the quality and timing of feedback concerning performance. With respect to feedback, numerous demonstrations support the claim that a fundamental component of effective instruction is the degree to which learners have a clear picture of what is expected of them, as well as clear information about their progress toward these goals. (A review can be found in Doyle 1983.) For instance, students who do not receive information about how well or how poorly they are doing may subsequently perform less well than if they have been given consistently negative feedback (Butler and Nisan 1986).

From this perspective, it is unnecessary to introduce concepts such as "self" to explain the difference between good, poor, and mediocre performers in school. The essence of the behavioral model is that if and when positive changes in self-concept occur, they are most likely the result of successful performance rather than its cause, and that in turn such changes will exert little influence on the quality of future performance. In effect, the notion of self is simply an unnecessary explanatory complication. This view is depicted in Figure 3.1 (Model B). Interestingly, we would find it difficult to refute this rather stark proposition using the literature generated from the student-centered model.

Interactive View

The interactive model combines elements of both the behavioral and the student-centered views. It is portrayed in Figure 3.1 (Model C). Moving from left to right, we see that an increase in academic skills—say, learning to diagram sentences—triggers gains simultaneously both in self-esteem (as in the student-centered model) and in achievement (as in the behavioral model) and that enhanced self-esteem in turn favors further academic improvements. In short, by improving the student's scholastic skills we initiate a recursive, upward cycle of emotionally driven successes—hence the term *interactive*.

But can we ever expect to demonstrate such complex pathways empirically, especially in light of previous failures under the far simpler student-centered model? The answer is yes, albeit a cautious affirmation. But what has changed? The interactive model itself is not a recent introduction; actually, in one form or another, it has long been implicated in arguments favoring the view that self-esteem affects achievement. What *has* changed, however, is the greater precision with which this model is now being evaluated and the increased number of variables being considered by researchers. Above all, we are now beginning to conceptualize the notion of self in new ways. A novel, unifying view of self as applied to educational achievement is rapidly emerging, born out of recent advances in attribution theory, research on fear-of-failure dynamics, and self-defensive motivation. We now turn to these developments.

Puzzles Involving Self-Esteem

Until recently, self-esteem has been too poorly defined and imperfectly measured to provide much assistance in understanding the causes of academic success and failure. Many definitions of self-esteem can be reduced to statements about how individuals perceive themselves along various value-laden dimensions including good and bad, worthy and unworthy. Although these labels are a powerful part of our selfhood, they are not always related to achievement in any direct or obvious way. For example, we know that some people who hold themselves in low esteem are nonetheless highly creative members of society (Ghiselin 1955). It is as if these individuals are trying to convince themselves that they are acceptable by achieving in extraordinary ways (Coopersmith 1967). But can the absence of self-esteem really stimulate true competency, let alone greatness?

And there are other questions and puzzles. First, if high self-esteem favors achievement, and if noteworthy accomplishments increase esteem even more, then why should there be so little relationship between a sense of personal satisfaction in school and grade point average? One might assume that if high grades are a potential source of status and prestige—which they clearly are—then an outstanding academic record should lead to feelings of pride and worthiness; but apparently this is not always the case. Second, why do many students with low self-esteem perform at their best when the odds against succeeding are at their worst? Shouldn't a hopeless cause make them feel even more inadequate? Third, why should failure—which is known to elicit shame, guilt, and lowered self-esteem—actually mobilize some students to greater effort? Fourth, if success is so attractive and sought-after, then why should students with low self-esteem frequently reject success when it occurs? Fifth, if high self-regard is the product of numerous, accumulated past successes—as we generally assume—then why should some students' sense of confidence be devastated after only *one* failure? Shouldn't past successes count for something, compared to a single failure? Once again, these examples illustrate that the relationship between self-esteem and performance is complex and at times counterintuitive. When it comes to self-esteem, more is not always better where performance is concerned; and less is not always a liability.

Can we integrate these contrary observations into the simple models represented by the student-centered and the behavioral approaches? The answer is no. We can decipher these puzzles only in the context of an expanded version of the interactive model and in light of an alternative conception of self. One of the most fruitful ways to think about self as an instrument of achievement is to consider it as a complex set of personal resources. Those psychological resources most important to accomplishment include self-perception of ability, beliefs about the nature of the achievement process, and personal estimates of time and energy level. Notice that these are not actual resources objectively defined, say, by scores on standardized intelligence tests or physical indices of metabolic rate. Rather, they make up the subjective reality of each individual: one's sense of competency, personal aspirations, intentions, and desires.

Accumulated research over the past two decades indicates that such perceived resources are decisive in determining the quality of academic performance. These perceptions often enter into the process of achievement in the form of causal attributions (Weiner 1972, 1974, 1979). Most simply put, how individuals explain their successes and failures controls much of their achievement. The main perceived causes of achievement are said to be ability, effort, luck, and task difficulty (Heider 1958). For example, individuals who ascribe their successes to their own ability are likely to undertake similar tasks in the future because they anticipate doing well. In contrast, individuals will be less likely to try again if they believe their past successes were caused by external factors such as luck or chance, or if they believe that they are

Figure 3.2.   Revised Interactive Model

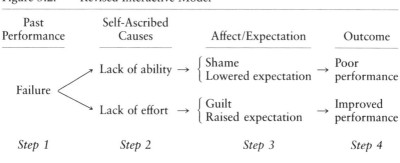

Past Performance	Self-Ascribed Causes	Affect/Expectation	Outcome
Failure	Lack of ability →	Shame / Lowered expectation →	Poor performance
	Lack of effort →	Guilt / Raised expectation →	Improved performance
Step 1	*Step 2*	*Step 3*	*Step 4*

SOURCE: Adapted from material found in Weiner 1985.

powerless to succeed again owing to insufficient ability. These perceived causes are thought to control not only the choice of the task undertaken and the quality of persistence but also the individual's emotional reactions to success (pride) and to failure (shame). Some observers argue persuasively that these self-referent attributions (or cognitions) and the emotions associated with them constitute a central part of self and self-consciousness (Brown and Weiner 1984; Kelley 1971; Weiner 1985; Weiner, Russell, and Lerman 1978, 1979). If we accept this view, the interactive model makes considerable sense, especially if it is recast in the slightly elaborated form presented in Figure 3.2.

This model suggests that students who interpret a disappointing performance as the result of insufficient ability are likely to suffer shame (low ability → shame) as well as to experience lowered expectations for future success (low ability → pessimism). Pessimism about the future may result because ability is perceived—at least by older students—as an internal, stable factor that is fixed by nature and also because ability is seen as the preemptive, overriding cause of achievement (Harari and Covington 1981; Weiner et al. 1971). In other words, if you are not smart, you can do only so well. In contrast, individuals who interpret the same failure as caused by insufficient or improper effort react with feelings of guilt, an emotion known to mobilize future effort (low effort → guilt → improved performance). By this reckoning, guilt is an effort-linked emotion (Covington and Omelich 1984a). And, because level of effort is seen as modifiable, expectations for future success remain high (Weiner et al. 1972; Weiner and Kukla 1970; Weiner and Potepan 1970). It is interesting to note that these attributional dynamics apply in essentially the same ways to a variety of learners, including the retarded and the learning disabled as well as students within the superior range of intelligence. (For a review, see Covington 1987.)

The psychological drama portrayed in Figure 3.2 involves a complex serial linkage: past performance → self-ascription of causes → affect/ expectations → future performance. This temporal sequence not only is interactive but is recursive as well. The process repeats itself from one achievement event to another, and for this reason its effects are also cumulative.

This model is appealing because it places notions of self, with both cognitive and emotional aspects, on a common footing with classroom achievement events, largely through the unifying principles of attribution theory. It also allows us to account for at least two of the puzzles mentioned above. First, it is not so much the occurrence of failure— even successful people occasionally fail—or the frequency of failure that disrupts future performance. Rather, the meaning the individual attaches to failure is the critical element. For those who see failure as the result of improper effort, failure presents a challenge. But for those who interpret it as evidence of inability or a lack of worth, it can be devastating. Depending on its meaning, then, failure can mobilize some students to greater effort and drive others to despair. Second, this attributional interpretation also helps us understand why some students reject success even though they may have desperately sought it. If success is seen as caused by forces beyond one's control, then it is meaningless; in addition, a student who embraces it may be expected to succeed in the future—something that he or she may doubt is possible.

Researchers have focused considerable attention on testing the general model portrayed in Figure 3.2 and on verifying the many implied causal pathways. Although some linkages have been investigated more intensively than others, the resulting literature generally supports the causal interpretations we have provided here. (For a comprehensive review, see Covington, in press.) Let us now briefly consider these confirming data, organized around the main self-referent resources of ability and effort.

Perceptions of Ability

Of the various self-perceived causes of achievement, ability is seen as the most significant influence on academic performance. For instance, of all the traditional dimensions of self-concept, the one that bears the highest consistent relationship to achievement is perception of one's ability. As part of the same meta-analysis cited earlier, Hansford and Hattie (1982) reported an average correlation of .42 between various achievement measures and self-perception of ability scales. In contrast, as already noted, the average composite correlations for other, more generalized measures of self, including feelings of worthiness and self-sentiment, was .16.

Actually, perceptions of ability bear a much more precise relationship to performance than is reflected in these simple correlations. For example, Covington and Omelich (1979a) conducted a path-analytic study to test all the sequential links in Figure 3.2 simultaneously. Self-perception of ability was the only attributional factor that linked the entire model, starting with self-cognitions and ending with actual test performance (ability perceptions → emotions → performance). Those students who ascribed an earlier failure to lack of ability experienced shame, which in turn inhibited subsequent performance. As to other aspects of the model, attributing one's performance to one's ability has been demonstrated to mediate pride in success (Covington and Omelich 1979c), shame and anxiety in failure (Covington and Omelich 1979b, 1981), and future expectations for success (Weiner, Nierenberg, and Goldstein 1976).

The importance of ability to students as a source of status and prestige is unrivaled even by the virtues of hard work. Students prefer to attribute their achievements to brilliance, not to effort (Brown and Weiner 1984). Moreover, ability is the most significant contributor to feelings of self-regard among students (Brown and Weiner 1984, Experiment I; Covington and Omelich 1984a). It seems fair to say that perceptions of ability profoundly influence virtually all aspects of the achievement process as it unfolds in the classroom.

Perceptions of Effort

Student perceptions of the intensity and effort put into study have also proven to be powerful determinants of the quality of future achievement. For example, one group of studies indicates that the more students study in a losing cause, the less sanguine they are about succeeding in the future (Fontaine 1974; McMahan 1973; Rosenbaum 1972; Valle 1974; Weiner et al. 1971). And we know that in turn subjective estimates of future success are highly influential in controlling actual performance (high expectations → improved performance) (Covington and Omelich 1979a, 1984b, 1984d). Also, intense effort increases pride in success (Brown and Weiner 1984; Covington and Omelich 1979c,

1981; Weiner et al. 1971), and pride in turn is known to influence future performance in a favorable direction (Covington and Omelich 1984b).

Other studies have helped to disentangle the relationship between attributions of ability and effort and their respective emotional components (Covington and Omelich 1984a). Failures that are attributed to inability elicit shame and humiliation, whereas explanations that focus on lack of effort trigger feelings of guilt. Conversely, trying hard reduces feelings of guilt. Yet, at the same time, failing despite intense effort implies lack of ability, which, we have noted, leads to shame (high effort → low ability → shame). Herein lies a cruel dilemma for many students. To try hard and fail anyway leads to shame and feelings of worthlessness (through a link with perception of ability); but not trying leads to feelings of guilt (Covington, Spratt, and Omelich 1980). In short, many students are caught between two rival sources of self-esteem—competency versus hard work—and they must sacrifice one to aggrandize the other.

Self-Worth Theory

One other significant theoretical development regarding the nature of self rivals in importance the attributional formulations just described. It involves the motivational aspects of self-process. Most simply put, motivational theorists are concerned with the question of *why*, rather than *how*, students learn. The reasons individuals learn are as important to the quality of achievement as are the attributions of cause these individuals make, and, in an important sense, motives actually determine the character and form of the attributions.

The evidence is steadily mounting that one main, even preeminent, reason that students achieve in school is to protect a sense of worth, especially in competitive situations. The self-worth theory of achievement motivation (Covington 1984a, in press; Covington and Beery 1976) holds that academic achievement is best understood in terms of students attempting to maintain a positive image of their own ability, especially when risking failure. This proposition is based on two widely held assumptions: first, that our society generally tends to equate the ability to achieve with human value (Gardner 1961); and second, that self-aggrandizement is a primary motivator of human behavior (Epstein 1973). In effect, whenever possible, individuals will act to maximize success, which reflects well on their ability, and to avoid failure, which casts doubts on their competency.

Given the extraordinary value accorded ability as a source of status, protecting one's sense of competency is of the highest priority—sometimes even a higher priority than achievement itself. For example, individuals may handicap themselves by striving for unattainable goals that invite failure—but such a failure would not reflect significantly on their ability, because almost no one could be expected to succeed. A variety of strategies for avoiding failure have been identified and experimentally documented by Birney, Burdick, and Teevan (1969) and by others (e.g., Berglas and Jones 1978; Sigall and Gould 1977). These strategies include academic cheating, as well as setting goals so easily attained that no risk of failure is involved. Another popular strategy involves procrastination. Handicapping themselves by studying only at the last moment, procrastinators can hardly be blamed for failure; and if they should do well, they will appear highly able, because they have succeeded with so little effort.

These strategies are often employed even though they eventually lead to the very failures that students are attempting to avoid. But at least the individual can obscure the cause of the failures for a time. When little or no effort is expended, estimates of one's ability remain uncertain, since a low level of effort is a sufficient explanation for failure (Kelley 1971). Consider the underachievers. By not trying, these students provide no information about their actual ability and as a result experience relatively little shame when they fail (Bricklin and Bricklin 1967). Moreover, through failure, underachievers can punish their parents, who often expect them to perform in near-perfect ways.

The central, activating principle behind such self-defeating tactics is that effort represents a potential threat to the student's sense of worth and self-esteem, because a combination of intense effort and failure implies lack of ability (Kun and Weiner 1973). This general line of reasoning leads to insights of special relevance regarding the causes of educational failure and the role played by self-process factors. For instance, according to the self-worth position, inadequate effort and indifference to learning are not always the products of insufficient motivation. Such behavior can in fact be highly motivated, but for the wrong reasons. Students who express apathy may be attempting to avoid failure; if they do fail, at least they can avoid the implications—that they lack ability and hence are unworthy. Moreover, by assuming that a struggle for self-regard is at the center of achievement dynamics, we are able to account for the remainder of the puzzles mentioned earlier.

First, the fact that a sense of personal satisfaction in school and grade

Figure 3.3. Stages of Academic Achievement

1. Anticipation of the Test	2. Preparation for the Test		3. Taking the Test		4. Reaction to the Test	
	Challenge vs.	*Threat*	*Success-Oriented* vs.	*Failure-Oriented*	*Success* vs.	*Failure*
Assessment of difficulty	Persistence	Irrational goal-setting	Confidence	Worry	Happiness	Disappointment
Grade goals	Optimism	Altering importance	Calmness	Tension	Relief	Shame
Importance of task	Task orientation	of the task		Bodily upset	Pride	Guilt
Personal resources		Procrastinating				Anxiety

point average are not necessarily correlated is now understandable. Some students, especially those we will later characterize as *overstrivers*, may accomplish extraordinary feats, but, again, for the wrong reasons (Beery 1975). These students are driven to succeed simply to avoid failure. But their successes, no matter how extraordinary, are unlikely to provide much satisfaction, for these students must prove themselves over and over against increasingly difficult odds. Such individuals demonstrate that high grade point average is no guarantee of personal fulfillment.

Second, fear-driven successes of the kind just described rarely convince individuals that they are worthy. It may appear that overstrivers possess great self-confidence, as a result of an unbroken string of successes. But given their underlying self-doubt, it may take only a few failures to convince them of what they have suspected all along: that they are really not bright enough to be worthy.

Third, what about the puzzling fact that some students with low self-esteem perform better when they know they will fail because the odds are heavily against them (Feather 1961, 1963; Karabenick and Youssef 1968; Sarason 1961)? Simply put, these students have been "allowed" to fail and now have the freedom to work up to their capacities; that is, failure will not necessarily reflect on their ability, because the task is impossible for almost everyone. Under the circumstances, effort is no longer a threat. Moreover, these failures provide positive benefits: we all admire the individual who struggles stoically and courageously for a worthy purpose against overwhelming odds.

Interactive View Revisited

This rapport among the cognitive, motivational, and affective aspects of self-process provides a broader, more complete appreciation of the achievement dynamic in schools. This perspective is best portrayed through one final elaboration on the interactive model, as shown in Figure 3.3. This second-generation model allows us to specify the temporal dimensions of the achievement process in far more detail.

The most common achievement event in schools, test taking, involves a time-ordered cycle with several stages. In the first stage, following the announcement of an upcoming test, students assess the likelihood of succeeding or failing. This complex judgment depends on the joint consideration of many factors, including one's past experience with similar tests and how realistic one's grade goals are. Of particular importance is the student's subjective estimate of resources. As already mentioned, these resources include the individual's perception of his or her own *ability*, typically reflected as a pattern of academic strengths and weaknesses; the amount of *effort* the individual plans to expend; and the actual *time* available for preparation.

In the second stage, students begin preparing for the test, a task that may involve a few minutes, a few hours, or perhaps even weeks. According to our interactive perspective, this preparation takes place in the context of various feelings, cognitions, and expectations regarding the wisdom or the futility of studying. For those individuals who judge their ability to be sufficient, the task represents a challenge; for those who believe they are inadequate to the task, school work becomes a threat. Individuals in this latter group are likely to engage in some of the defensive behaviors already described (e.g., procrastination) as a way of hedging their bets for a disaster that is now all the more likely.

In the test-taking stage, failure-oriented students experience tension, unpleasant physical arousal, and worry, all of which distract them and interfere with test performance. In the final, feedback stage, students react with various global emotions, including happiness or disappointment, depending on whether they judged their performance as a success or a failure, respectively. Other, more specific, emotions, such as pride or relief in the case of success, or shame and guilt in the event of failure, are also elicited. As we have seen, these emotions depend largely on the particular causes to which one attributes success or failure (Weiner 1985).

The available evidence suggests that as a student moves from one stage to another, psychological events within each stage are elicited by prior events and, in turn, act as triggers for successive events. Consider just one strand. The belief that one is able (stage 1) acts to discourage defensive thoughts and actions during study (stage 2) that would otherwise interfere with performance (feeling competent → reduced defensiveness → good performance). A number of studies using path analysis have also "mapped" other potential linkages based on Figure 3.3, establishing a complex network of cause-and-effect relationships that form the microscopic structure of academic achievement. (For reviews, see Covington, in press; Covington and Omelich 1988a; Covington, Omelich, and Schwarzer 1986.)

Types of Students

One of the most important conclusions to be drawn from this research is that the same achievement dynamics do not apply to all individuals. Several different types of students have been identified by researchers. These differences depend largely on whether a student is success-oriented, failure-avoiding, or some combination of these two tendencies (Atkinson 1957, 1964; Atkinson and Feather 1966). *Success-oriented* students learn for reasons that include the intrinsic value of satisfying curiosity, learning for its own sake, and the mastery of one's environment. In contrast, as already noted, *failure-avoiding* individuals learn for precisely that reason—to avoid failure or at least the implications of failure.

Other students reflect different combinations of these approach and avoidance tendencies (Covington and Omelich 1988b). Consider the *overstriver*, who shows strong tendencies for both approach and avoidance. In terms of self-worth, such students attempt to succeed in order to avoid failure. For this reason, learning becomes a highly conflicted process, although it usually ends in success. Because of the stress and conflict, these students enter the anticipation stage of our model in Figure 3.3 with heightened anxiety. But because they possess excellent study strategies, anxiety acts to mobilize their resources, as reflected in meticulous, often compulsive, overpreparation. As tensions mount during the test-taking phase, however, anxiety may interfere with the recall of the well-rehearsed information. Such negative arousal also tends to disrupt higher-level thinking processes temporarily (Covington 1967). The failing student who complains, "I knew the material cold before the exam," is most likely an overstriver (Covington and Omelich 1987).

Those who experience a relative absence of both hope and fear have been characterized as *failure-accepting* (Covington and Omelich 1985). These students appear to have given up on the pursuit of academic rewards and have resigned themselves to academic failure as a way of life. In terms of Figure 3.3, these students are marked by desultory, indifferent study patterns and by a relative absence of achievement affect. They express little pride in their successes, but neither do they express much shame in the event of failure. As a result, these students perform poorly because they lack both the proper study skills and the motivation to apply themselves, which is reflected by their general lack of emotional arousal.

Success-oriented students are of special interest to us, because the factors included in Figure 3.3 do a relatively poor job of predicting variations in their test performances. Whatever factors describe the unique psychology of success-oriented individuals, they are apparently not well represented in this portrayal of the achievement process. Even the ability perceptions of this group are only marginally related to achievement.

The most likely explanation is that this model typifies classroom learning in a predominantly competitive mode. In competition, the goal is to win by outperforming others, thereby enhancing one's ability status. The goal of learning becomes a secondary objective. Those students who have linked their sense of worth and self-esteem to the competitive learning game are well described by this model. They include over-strivers, failure-avoiding, and failure-accepting students. But for success-oriented individuals, a competitive model clearly misses the mark. These individuals are more likely to pursue learning not out of any need to gain power or prestige, but to satisfy intrinsic goals and interests. Such students will tend to perform well in any achievement context, no matter what the stakes or incentives, because they are confident and comfortable with themselves and with their own thought processes. Obviously, this is not true of those students who operate out of self-doubt and fear of publicly disclosing their incompetence. It is this latter group that is at special risk when confronting competitive learning goals.

These observations raise the prospect that lack of involvement in school, indifference to learning, and apathy—to the extent that such behaviors reflect misguided attempts to protect a sense of self-esteem—may be ameliorated by changing the goals of achievement from winning out over others to learning. We will consider this possibility later as we offer recommendations.

Repeated Failures

Recently, researchers have become interested in the dynamics of achievement as they unfold over several study/test/feedback cycles. Such a perspective requires that we expand the model portrayed in Figure 3.3 in a cyclical fashion, through time. The dynamics of achievement change from one test to another, depending largely on whether the individual's initial performance was judged a success or a failure (Covington and Omelich 1988a). In the case of an initial failure, levels of anxiety are elevated throughout the second study/test cycle. There is an increased willingness to externalize blame (i.e., to create excuses for failure) and to indulge in defensive study patterns. Students may also lower their estimates of their own ability, a change that is greatest among failure-avoiding and failure-accepting students (Covington and Omelich 1981). As perceived ability status decreases, estimates of the importance of ability as a causal factor in success increase. This combination places failure-prone students in a kind of double jeopardy.

Learned Helplessness

These findings provide us with unique insights into the phenomenon of *learned helplessness,* which has been described as a state of inaction and depression arising from a realization that one's efforts are ineffectual in attaining one's goals (Abramson, Seligman, and Teasdale 1978). Learned helplessness was originally observed in animals. Seligman, Maier, and Geer (1968) subjected dogs to electrical shock from which there was no escape. Subsequently, these dogs were provided with a way to avoid the shock by learning a simple response. Under normal circumstances, this escape response would have been learned in only a few trials. But many of the punished dogs never did learn it. This ineptitude was thought to be the result of losing a sense of power over events, a loss incurred during the original punishment phase. It is tempting to seek an analogy among those students who give up, having learned that no matter how hard they try or what they do, they cannot succeed (Dweck 1975; Diener and Dweck 1978; Dweck and Bush 1976). From a self-worth perspective, such helplessness represents the final phase in the process of demoralization that characterizes many failure-accepting students. This interpretation is supported by the results of a study by Schwarzer, Jerusalem, and Schwarzer (1983) in which high school students were tracked over a two-year period. Among many of those students whose grades progressively deteriorated, there was a concomitant increase in feeling helpless to alter events and a decrease in anxiety, reflecting resignation.

Instructional Context

These self-process dynamics must be considered in the larger context of the teacher/student relationship. The evidence just reviewed underscores the central role of perception of ability in the dynamics of competitive achievement. Students value ability and a sense of competency more than they value the virtues of hard work. There is an equally persuasive literature, however, suggesting that teachers value student effort. Teachers reason that although not all students can be equally bright, everyone can at least try. Students who are perceived as having tried hard are rewarded more in success and punished less in failure than are those who do not try (Eswara 1972; Rest et al. 1973; Weiner 1972, 1974; Weiner and Kukla 1970). Teachers further assume that they can manipulate student effort by dispensing and withholding rewards in the form of praise or reprimand.

But if teachers systematically reinforce an achievement pattern that favors student effort, why do so many students fail to respond? The answer lies in a conflict of teacher/student values. Teachers reward success that is achieved through intense effort, whereas for many students expending such effort poses a threat, especially when they are risking failure. If students try hard and fail anyway, the explanation for failure inevitably becomes inability. It is for this reason that effort has been described as a "double-edged sword" (Covington 1984a). This point was confirmed by an experiment (Covington and Omelich 1979b) in which college students indicated the degree of shame they believed they would experience after failing a test for which they had either studied a great deal or studied very little. Excuses for the failure were also available. In the case where little effort had been exerted, the excuse was that the student had been ill. In the case where the effort had been great, the mitigating explanation for the failure was that the teacher had emphasized materials insufficiently studied by the student. As expected, students experienced the most shame after having studied hard and the least after having studied little. When the excuses were considered, feelings of shame diminished, no matter how much effort had been expended.

In this experiment, the same students also adopted the role of teacher and were asked to reprimand hypothetical students under the same failure conditions. As "teachers," the subjects now punished most the very failures that elicited the least shame from students (i.e., low effort). Conversely, they rewarded most the circumstance that led to the greatest degree of student shame (i.e., high effort). Ironically, the condition that led to both minimal teacher punishment and maximal relief for students was a low level of effort combined with an excuse. In effect, despite the best efforts of teachers, students are encouraged by self-worth dynamics to try, or at least appear to try, but with excuses readily available. Obviously, this formula is ill suited to the pursuit of personal excellence. Teachers and students alike are apparently caught in a mismatch of values that sets in motion potential conflict, disharmony, and inferior levels of academic achievement, a situation for which neither party is necessarily to blame.

A simple reinforcement (behavioral) view of classroom achievement would presume that because teachers value and reward effort, students would soon internalize a work ethic. We now know that, at least among older students, questions of self-esteem confound these expectations. For junior high and senior high school students, a teacher's reinforcement of effort may lead to less rather than to more student involvement (Harari and Covington 1981). In contrast, data collected with young children, starting in the early primary grades, indicate that these young-sters behave in ways consistent with reinforcement principles (Blumen-feld et al. 1981). For young children, a sense of worth appears to depend less on ability status and more on trying hard, behaving oneself, and complying with authority. They respond with greater effort when re-warded by teachers and are quick to try harder after being reprimanded. Here we see a match, not a mismatch, between teacher and student values.

Interestingly, young students also value ability. But for these children the level of effort expended has not yet become a cue for inability, so effort is not threatening. To the contrary, in the early primary years abil-ity status is seen as depending on the amount of effort expended. Exert-ing an effort indicates ability, or, as one first-grader put it, "Smart stu-dents study, stupid ones don't" (Harari and Covington 1981). Young children also view ability as something that increases through effort (Nicholls 1978; Stipek 1981); to quote a second-grader, "If you try hard, your brain will get bigger" (Harari and Covington 1981). In short, young children view ability as modifiable, in the same sense that trying hard and behaving oneself are under personal control. The belief that ability can be perfected and increased through experience and hard work has been described as an "incremental" view of intelligence (Dweck and Bempechat 1983). This notion may be contrasted to an "entity," or fixed, view of intelligence that is often held by older students and adults. Research suggests that an incremental belief is associated with optimism about future success and with a willingness to try harder after an initial failure.

Analysis: The Competitive Classroom

Conceiving of self as a resource to be managed has proven important to our understanding of the psychological dynamics of school achieve-ment. This concept neatly combines cognitive, motivational, and emo-tional dimensions of human experience in ways that allow us to predict achievement outcomes with some accuracy. It also helps to account for a number of otherwise inexplicable student behaviors, including the longstanding observation that the same failure can goad some students to greater action and yet demoralize others, and the fact that despite the attractiveness of success, some students reject teachers' praise even though they may deserve it. At times, lack of a sense of worth is a more powerful stimulant to achievement than self-confidence is, and, depending on its source, a sense of self-esteem may not always promote the continued will to learn. Clearly, the relationship between self-process and academic performance is complex, indirect, and often counterintuitive. Yet despite these complexities, at the heart of the achievement process we find a struggle that, when reduced to its essence, reflects the need to establish and maintain feelings of worth and dignity.

What aspects of school life are likely responsible for this struggle, for the quality of student coping, and for the pervasive, often destructive need to enhance one's ability status? Does something inherent in the process of learning itself create this kind of vulnerability? No, not likely. The available evidence is quite clear on this point. By all accounts, the act of learning is a natural, adaptive event. Rather, the culprit is the *institutionalizing* of learning, as reflected in the incentive systems under which students learn. The basic problem is the indiscriminate and often excessive use of competition as a means to motivate students to achieve (Gardner 1961; Kohn 1986). Competitive incentives tie feelings of worth to how well one performs relative to others. But winning in competition with others is a counterproductive reason for achieving. More specifically, if shame in failure and pride in success depend largely on students' perceptions of their own ability, then students will continue to learn for only as long as they can aggrandize ability. This reason for learning is eventually self-defeating, because it destroys any intrinsic interest in achievement. In effect, when failure begins to threaten one's sense of competency, one is likely to withdraw from learning.

Few teachers deliberately set out to induce competition in their classrooms. Instead, most recognize the destructive nature of competition as a goad to learning and attempt to discourage it (Covington and Beery 1976). Yet, despite teacher efforts, most classrooms reflect competitive dynamics to one degree or another (Ames and Archer 1987). Competition appears to be almost inevitable, generated in part by a minority of students who define their worth in competitive ways. Thus it is not enough simply to oppose classroom competition in the abstract. Rather, teachers must actively restructure classroom learning incentives to encourage other, more beneficial, reasons for learning. We will discuss this point later in more detail.

In the meantime, let us briefly summarize the large body of research concerning the nature of competition in schools and how it appears to compromise the will to learn. The dynamics of classroom learning have been likened to a complex game (Alschuler 1969, 1973). Like all games, the classroom learning game has several formal properties. First, there is the scoring system by which players (students) receive points (rewards). Second, there are obstacles to gaining points and a variety of ways to lose them. Third, there is the issue of who makes the rules and enforces them. This responsibility primarily falls to the teacher. In competitively oriented classrooms, the scoring system elicits a power struggle in which students compete among themselves for a fixed, inevitably insufficient supply of rewards, so that the likelihood of a given student achieving success is reduced by the presence of other students competing for the same success. The reader will recognize this situation as a zero-sum game: when one player wins, others must lose. These dynamics are typically induced by "grading on the curve," by grouping students according to ability, or by calling public attention to the successes of some and the defeats of others. Under these circumstances, the implicit goal becomes "winning," that is, outperforming fellow students, rather than learning (Ames 1978; Deutsch 1979). One can hope to win only by gaining superiority over others. Yet for most students, given the scarcity and unequal division of rewards, the only option becomes avoiding failure, or at least avoiding the implications of failure (a sense of incompetence).

Research conducted over the past decade provides a glimpse of the specific microdynamics involved in competitive, failure-prone classrooms. The basic finding, and the central dynamic from which all negative consequences flow, is that competition causes students to focus on ability as the dominant causal agent. In competition, causal explanations for one's successes and failures become strongly associated with one's sense of either high or low ability, respectively (Ames 1978; Ames, Ames, and Felker 1979). These attributional patterns are all the more devastating because competition also promotes a belief in ability as fixed or immutable (i.e., the entity theory). This added dimension creates a sense of hopelessness, because nothing in the situation is within the power of the failing student to correct. Conversely, the perceived importance of effort in success and the virtues of hard work are downgraded under competitive conditions (Ames and Ames 1981). Finally, ascribing success to good luck is a common reaction (Ames 1981). In effect, for many students, success in competition merits only faint self-praise, because they believe success is caused by forces beyond their control.

This combination of factors provides all the elements necessary to promote learned helplessness. Moreover, the attributional patterns aroused by competitive goals are almost exactly the same as those singled out by researchers to describe failure-avoiding students (Weiner et al. 1971). Given this accumulation of evidence, we can conclude that attempts to motivate students through competition, far from increasing productivity, are likely to destroy the will to learn for many students. And what of those who appear to do well in the competitive game? For many of the most successful competitors, the rewards of success are compromised by feelings of guilt for having denied others a chance to succeed (Kohn 1986).

But these self-defeating attributional patterns are not the only negative consequences of competitive goal-setting. Competitive goals can also stimulate a divisive, misplaced pride in success. Under competitive conditions, youngsters who win are likely to see themselves as smarter than their companions and, as a result, to believe themselves more deserving (Ames, Ames, and Felker 1979). Conversely, for the losers, the self-punishment that follows failure in competition is especially devastating. These students believe that failure is their fault, even when their "failing" performance may be judged by others as perfectly adequate. Finally, under competitive circumstances, success does little to compensate for past failures (Ames and Ames 1981). Success is often viewed as the result of good luck; thus success does little to foster confidence in one's resources or to enhance the resolve to try harder next time.

From a self-worth perspective, educational failure and the paralysis of the will to learn arise whenever the individual's sense of worth becomes equated with the ability to achieve competitively. This linkage is strengthened by competitive learning environments, which magnify the importance of ability and tend to limit the supply of meaningful rewards. Without sufficient incentives for success, many—if not most—students must struggle to avoid failure and its accompanying sense of worthlessness.

Recommendations

We can now consider various ways to affect the causes of educational failure, at least those causes that stand indicted through our analysis, which has focused on self-worth. Here we enter the arena of advocacy, involving the promulgation of social policy on the broadest scale. Our analysis points to the structure of classroom learning and the educational goals implied by a given incentive system as the factors that largely control the quality and durability of student learning. If the implicit goal of competition is to outperform others, then perhaps the frequency of academic failures caused by competition—and even the meaning of failure—can be changed by altering the goals of the learning game, from being competitive to being individualized and cooperative. But from our perspective, what guidelines should be followed for reshaping the learning game? Four broad suggestions emerge from our review.

First, we need to increase the number of meaningful rewards available to students, so that all can approach success without consigning some to the burdensome and self-defeating task of simply avoiding failure. We must break the scarcity cycle that dominates the competitive learning game. This can best be achieved by redefining the meaning of success and failure in terms of individual striving. Success must come to depend on the individual exceeding his or her own aspirations, so that failure becomes a matter of falling short of one's own goals, not falling short as a person. In this context, we might expect that it would be tempting to set one's goals so low that success is virtually assured. But the research literature suggests that this does not typically happen. When students are not competing directly with one another, they usually set moderate learning goals slightly beyond their current level of performance (Lewin et al. 1944).

Second, any shift in the meaning of success and failure must be accompanied by a reemphasis on effort as the preferred means to success and on lack of involvement as the likely explanation for failure. This focus on effort should allow alternative explanations for failure, such as improper planning or unrealistic expectations, rather than assuming that lack of success means lack of ability.

Third, we must arrange school incentive systems so that self-praise (pride) and self-criticism (shame) come to depend not simply on success or failure, respectively, but rather on how hard or how little the student has tried. To fall short of reasonable but challenging goals need not be a disgrace if one has honestly tried; conversely, pride in even the most noteworthy accomplishment can easily be misplaced if success results from mere brilliance.

Fourth, we must promote an incremental view of ability. The belief that intelligence is an ever-increasing, expanding process is likely to counteract pessimism about the future and to promote effort as the highest classroom value.

None of these objectives is furthered in a competitive model. Indeed, the goal of competition—learning as a means to enhance one's ability status—is directly antithetical to the spirit and substance of these four guidelines. Therefore, we must seek out and encourage alternative achievement goals. One such goal involves satisfying one's curiosity and propagating a sense of wonder. Another is that of helping others or, more broadly stated, committing oneself to solving society's problems (Nicholls 1987). A third alternative goal is mastery or self-improvement, that is, becoming the best that one can be. Recent research suggests that it is these goals, and not those concerned with besting others for the sake of personal aggrandizement, that are associated with greater satisfaction in school, better grades, and the intention to attend college (Nicholls, Patashnick, and Nolen 1985).

Equity Systems

These self-enhancing goals are most likely to be promoted by incentive systems that have been described collectively as *equity structures* (Covington 1984a). Equity structures are intended to provide all students with equally attractive incentives to pursue the goal of learning. This implies that one of the major responsibilities of schools should be to equalize student motivation—to encourage learning goals within the reach of each individual. This equality of opportunity, so to speak, will not lead to equal outcomes, however. By encouraging all students to do their best, we will doubtless increase the average level of performance, that is, reduce the frequency of academic failures. Yet we may also increase the diversity of performance; less able students will do better, but then so will brighter students. This must be what is meant when educators refer to the goal of schools as encouraging "excellence through diversity." But can such excellence be sustained when differences in talent and ability become even more obvious, given that all students are maximally motivated? Put in a less abstract, more compelling form:

> But what of the student who discovers he has relatively few, if any, strong points or finds to his dismay that his particular "strengths" are no greater than the "weaknesses" exhibited by the student across the aisle? Can he avoid unfavorable comparisons and content himself with working within his reach, knowing all the while that he is foreclosed from prestigious occupations and status in adulthood owing to his limited gifts? (Covington and Beery, 1976, 146)

In the search for answers to these difficult questions, equity structures appear to hold some promise. One type of equity paradigm involves cooperative learning. Under this arrangement, several individuals are rewarded based on their performance as a group; when one student achieves his or her goal, then all those with whom the individual is co-operating achieve their goals as well (Slavin 1978, 1983, 1984). A second type of equity paradigm features individual incentives. Here, any number of individuals can be successful by reaching or surpassing the prevailing standards of excellence. These standards can be established by either the student or the teacher, or by a joint agreement. One example of student self-regulated learning is contingency contracting (Homme 1970), in which students set their own learning goals in consultation with a teacher and specify what work is to be done, when it is due, and the payoffs that are expected at completion. In contrast, teacher-regulated standards apply when the teacher requires that a certain level of proficiency be demonstrated before students can proceed to the next learning step. The most common form of teacher-controlled incentives is mastery learning, or outcome-based education (Block 1977, 1984; Bloom 1976; Spady 1982). Mastery learning is based on the philosophy that most students can learn basic subject matter if they are provided clear criteria as to what counts as mastery (e.g., 90 percent correct on each of three spelling tests) and have sufficient time to attain these standards through extra study and practice, should they initially fail to master the material. In these cases, if competition is involved at all, it is redefined in terms of overcoming one's own limitations rather than perceiving others as the main obstacle to success.

A surprisingly large body of literature on equity structures has developed, with references now running into the hundreds, if not thousands. (For reviews, see Ames 1984; Ames and Ames 1984; Block and Burns 1976; Burns 1987; Johnson and Ruskin 1977; Kulik, Kulik, and Cohen 1979; and Slavin 1987.) This evidence includes both well-controlled, laboratory-based studies and experimental field studies whose purpose is to validate the basic laboratory findings in naturally occurring classroom settings. A third kind of evidence comes from demonstration studies that make little pretense at formal research; their purpose is simply to illustrate that equity paradigms work, rather than explaining why or how they work. To these applied ends, the typical evaluation involves anecdotal case studies, staff reviews, and informal teacher observations.

Although we still have much to discover about institutionalized learning incentives, most research suggests that equity paradigms tend to promote the four instructional guidelines proposed earlier. For example, individual mastery incentives have been shown to encourage elementary school children to perceive effort as the major cause of school performance, while minimizing the presumed role of luck (Ames and Ames 1981). They also minimize the perceived importance of ability in success. This has been demonstrated both among children (Ames, Ames, and Felker 1979) and among college-level students (Covington and Omelich 1984c). Interestingly, self-estimates of ability, which predominate as predictors of academic performance in competitive circumstances, no longer do so under conditions of mastery learning (Covington 1985a; Covington and Omelich 1984c).

As to the other guidelines, equity structures also appear to promote a linkage between pride and effort accompanying success, while minimizing the association between pride and perception of ability (Ames and Ames 1981). Likewise, emotions associated with failure, such as guilt and remorse, come to result more from a feeling that one has not tried hard enough or in the right ways. These latter findings seem to reflect the fact that equity structures provide well-defined standards of performance. They make clear what is expected of students, whereas under a competitive arrangement standards of excellence are more elusive, because they depend on the relative performance of others.

In summary, it is clear that different incentive systems draw out different reasons for learning, for good or ill, and that these reasons influence not only the quality of student performance but also the student's willingness to continue to learn. Yet, within the broad outline of the existing evidence, our perspective prompts additional questions. For instance, if we make rewards more plentiful, will the increased number cheapen their incentive value? The available evidence, limited as it is, suggests that under equity approaches the value of rewards comes to depend more on the degree of risk involved in succeeding and less on how many other students are also rewarded (Covington 1984a). Even with this reassurance, it is also clear that for some students competitiveness is a way of life. We all know individuals who will try to turn any achievement situation, no matter how playful or spontaneous, into a competitive game. How should we deal with such youngsters? By increasing the number of available rewards, will we undercut the very reason that many of these competitively oriented students do so well? Also, is it possible that by increasing rewards we may actually create among some students exaggerated or false estimates of their abilities?

Although we cannot fully answer these questions now, they appear to be the right questions to ask when considering larger issues of educational policy. Moreover, these inquiries arise out of a solid, scientific understanding of the nature of academic failure. This understanding leads us to urge that a recommendation to promote more equity structures in schools should be seriously considered.

Strategic Thinking

A second, interlocking recommendation also flows from our perspective focusing on self-worth. It involves the need to encourage self-management skills among students. Equity paradigms provide considerable freedom for students to set their own learning goals and to decide how best to achieve them. But students are often unprepared for such freedom. For many youngsters, the prospect of independent action creates anxiety. Failure-prone students need autonomy the most, but they are the least prepared to take advantage of it. To them, success is an unexpected event, caused—they believe—by luck or by chance; as a result, success is something they may be unable to accept, let alone plan for. These students not only need to alter their reasons for learning but also need systematic instruction in the thinking and planning skills implied by the concept of self as a resource to be managed.

Central to the concept of self as a resource is the notion of *strategic thinking* (Covington 1985c, 1986). Strategic thinking refers to the overall process of planning a course of action to achieve a desired goal. It involves an awareness of one's pattern of cognitive skills, including both strengths and weaknesses; the ability to reflect on the quality and progress of one's work; and the capacity to recognize when one has learned something well enough or when one needs to study more. Strategic thinking also involves a sensitivity to changes in the nature of the study task, for example, recognizing when learning strategies that worked well in the past are no longer appropriate or have even become counterproductive. In the context of academic achievement, strategic thinking involves managing personal resources in an orchestrated attack on a problem—preparing for an upcoming test, developing a term project, or coordinating a team of other students toward a common purpose.

Strategic thinking bridges the cognitive, self-worth, and motivational domains described earlier in at least three ways. First, if students can analyze a learning task, discover the reasons why some tasks are easy and others difficult, and develop a plan of action for solving problems, then explanations other than lack of ability are possible in the event of failure. These strategy-oriented interpretations rob failure of its noxious, shame-evoking implication for ability status. This is especially true for the most threatening kinds of failure, those in which students tried hard and failed anyway. Research done by McNabb (1986) provides crucial evidence on this point. When students are given strategy messages (e.g., "to solve problems like these, you will have to use good methods"), as compared to simply telling them to try harder, they become more involved with the task, enjoy their work more, persist longer, and increase their expectations for future success. McNabb's conclusion, consistent with self-worth formulations, is that strategy messages provide insecure students with plausible explanations, not linked to ability, for their performances, thus freeing them to work harder. Similar findings by other investigators lend further credence to this interpretation (Anderson and Jennings 1980).

Second, like equity procedures, strategic skill training has also been shown to enhance both academic problem solving and the will to learn. Much of the evidence comes from a twenty-year program of research concerning the nature and facilitation of problem-solving ability (Covington 1985c; Olton and Crutchfield 1969). The central focus of this work was the development and evaluation of the *Productive Thinking Program,* a course in learning to think for upper elementary and junior high school students (Covington et al. 1974). This semester-long program is designed to strengthen a broad set of strategic skills involved in effective resource management and problem formulation, including the ability to choose among various solution strategies in a timely fashion and to remain sensitive to gaps and inconsistencies in available knowledge. The results of some twenty evaluation studies using this program indicate a number of motivational benefits. (See Covington 1986 for a review.) Instruction in strategic thinking increases the likelihood that students will choose to work on challenging yet reasonable tasks for which success is uncertain but not improbable (Olton and Crutchfield 1969). Also, trained students are less likely than untrained students to abandon their own judgments simply because they differ from the majority of peer-group opinion (Allen and Levine 1967).

A number of other school-based curricula that promote general problem-solving skills also appear to have considerable potential for furthering motivational objectives. These include the *Purdue Creative Thinking Program* (Feldhusen, Treffinger, and Bahlke 1970; Feldhusen, Speedie, and Treffinger 1971) and the *Philosophy for Children Program* (Lipman 1976, 1985). Other promising curricular approaches focus more specifically on building self-esteem by providing students with practice in setting personally meaningful goals, evaluating their competencies objectively, and accepting and understanding their feelings (Canfield 1986; Reasoner 1986).

Third, many cognitive researchers today view ability as created and enhanced through the strategic self-management of one's problem-solving resources, a process that can compensate for the sense that one lacks ability (Resnick 1987). This compensatory nature of ability allocation doubtless forms the basis for the belief that ability is an incremental, ever-expanding process. Individuals who hold such an incremental view are more likely to focus on the learning task at hand, are less preoccupied with school performance as a test of their worth, and display greater intrinsic involvement in learning. The available evidence suggests that strategic skill training also enhances this belief. Drawing on research with the *Productive Thinking Program,* we note that trained students show a greater appreciation for the fact that making mistakes is a natural, even necessary, part of problem solving and that students increase their capacity to learn through such a trial-and-error process (Covington 1967).

Overall, the accumulated weight of evidence suggests that all those attributes we have associated with self as a resource—namely, one's characteristic explanations for success and failure, one's repertoire of thinking skills, and one's beliefs about the nature and function of ability—can be modified through direct instruction and that such instruction can lead to achievement gains as well as to an increased willingness to use one's mind in a productive fashion.

For all their promise and demonstrated effectiveness, however, school-based efforts to teach students *how* to think rather than *what* to think are still relatively rare, despite repeated calls over the years for the development of process-oriented curricula (Aschner and Bish 1965; Fair and Shaftel 1967; Olton and Crutchfield 1969; Torrance 1965). There are several reasons for this lag. First, several unanswered conceptual questions hamper efforts to develop new, more far-reaching generations of strategic skill intervention. Chief among these issues is the largely unknown character of the relationship between skill instruction and cognitive development. More particularly, which general thinking skills should be taught, and at what point in a child's life, in order to promote mature, adultlike thinking in later years? If it is true that only long-term, comprehensive cognitive instruction will help reduce massive educational failure, then the staging and timing of such instruction becomes critical. But at present we know relatively little about the early precursors of later, adultlike thinking and planning. (See Friedman, Scholnick, and Cocking 1986 for a review.)

Second, there is considerable resistance to strategic skill instruction within the schools. Human information processing as a topic is as yet only imperfectly understood by scientists, and as a result it remains even more of a mystery to teachers, who would be expected to implement the goals of strategic thinking. Nevertheless, as implied by our review, we know at least enough to start. Ultimately, we must introduce widespread, intensive teacher training and preservice instruction in how to teach thinking skills and promote the independence of thought that we all cherish as adult learners. The most difficult part of teacher training will be to translate definitions of thinking skills, which often appear to be little more than abstract platitudes (e.g., "look at problems in new ways"), into forms that are readily useful in a variety of specific content areas such as biology, English composition, chemistry, and history.

Conclusion

These twin recommendations, which involve altering the prevailing reasons for learning and encouraging directly the capacity for strategic thinking, may at first appear unduly modest, given the massive, unparalleled problems facing schools today. It is axiomatic that big problems require big solutions. But these proposals require no major dislocation of responsibility for educating our young—educators still remain in control. Nor is an unprecedented infusion of federal or state funds called for. Any appearance of modesty may be a result of our initial promise to limit recommendations to those that are practicable and those that might have relatively immediate impact.

But appearances can be deceptive. Actually, what we have proposed here is exceedingly immodest and highly ambitious. The real value of the self-esteem perspective is not that it will necessarily overturn our national priorities or even successfully challenge the natural reluctance of our citizens to commit more tax dollars to yet another urgent problem. The concept of self-esteem carries with it no inherent economic or political imperatives. But it does contribute something unique to any debate concerning the public good. It challenges us to be more fully human. In addition to being an object of scientific investigation, as well as an explanation for behavior, self-esteem is above all a metaphor, a symbol that can ignite visions of what we as a people might become.

Perhaps only for the sake of self-esteem would we be willing to carry out policy recommendations that seriously question two of our most cherished beliefs: the cult of achievement and the myth of competition.

The Cult of Achievement

To most Americans, achievement is everything; it is our badge, our national identity. As a people, we are known for our ability to get the job done, and done on time. We have always been more committed to the *product* than comfortable with the *process,* and when productivity suffers we become uneasy and troubled. But there is much more to educational achievement than a test score, a course grade, or a report card. As virtues, effort and accomplishment will flourish only to the extent that we consider the *reasons* that students strive. This is the essential message of the self-esteem perspective. When we fail to consider motives and feelings, individuals may strive successfully, but for the wrong reasons—with the consequence that the benefits of these successes are illusory. In effect, the continued will to learn depends more on *why* one learns in the first place than on *what* one learns or even on how *well* one learns it. We must first set right the matter of motives, or the reasons for learning, and then achievement will follow and likely thrive. But if we concentrate on academic failure as anything more than a symptom, then in the end both achievement and self-esteem will suffer. This reality is hard for Americans to accept, given our impatience with such intangibles as feelings and emotions and our vague discomfort with process. Herein lies the first challenge to those who would promote a self-esteem perspective as the basis for educational policy making.

The Myth of Competition

The second challenge concerns the uniquely American commitment to competition and its corollary that competition is the best, if not the only, remaining way to ensure at least a minimum level of competence among millions of apparently shiftless, unmotivated, and dispirited students. This beguiling but mistaken belief is enormously powerful because of its intuitive appeal to reason. After all, if a competitive edge has sustained America's unprecedented economic prosperity over the years, could not the same formula work in our schools? The answer, as we have seen, is probably not. The essential point is that encouraging individuals to outperform one another—or other nations—however valuable such a strategy might be from an economic perspective, is counter-productive when it comes to the goal of maximizing learning for all individuals. Competition in school forces too many players (students) to focus on simply avoiding failure. As a result, performance suffers, giving the lie to arguments that competition motivates individuals to do their best. Moreover, as we have seen, achievement under competitive adversity, far from building character, as some claim, actually destroys self-confidence and encourages cheating, sabotage, and cynicism.

But even if all the damning research evidence on competition were widely acknowledged, one fundamental reason for maintaining a competitive climate in schools remains. This reason has little to do with the immediate purposes of schooling but rather with the economic and social realities that there are too many students aspiring for too few prestigious, high-paying jobs. Some orderly way must be found to distribute individuals across the work force, given that some jobs are more attractive, lucrative, and more highly sought after than others. By using schools as a sorting and screening device, we have created such a mechanism. Adult occupational status depends heavily on the grades received by students throughout their academic careers (Deutsch 1979). In effect, the better a student's grades, the more likely he or she is to be picked out for further schooling; and it is higher education that forms the gateway to prestigious occupations. For this reason, schools are held hostage in the battle for future economic security and prestige. As Campbell observes, "The whole frantic, irrational scramble to beat others is essential for the kind of institutions that our schools are . . . [namely,] bargain-basement personnel screening agencies for business and government" (1974, 145–147).

A number of alternative proposals for how to allocate talent across the existing range of jobs have been suggested over the years and need to be taken more seriously. (For reviews, see Deutsch 1979; Wolff 1969.) As a group, these proposals require a reconsideration of the basic competitive mentality that has long dominated the American scene. Herein lies the second challenge to the self-esteem perspective.

Finally, there remains the question implied from the outset: Can we really hope to improve future educational prospects, given the overwhelming problems that assail our children from so many quarters? To be candid, there is probably little hope, unless school-based changes occur in coordination with other reforms that address wider concerns such as drug dependency, crime, violence, and abuse. In this, we can learn from action research in the area of public health (Hamburg 1986). Sus-

tained health benefits are most likely to result when the target group—
say, school-aged children in a particular community—is immersed in a
circle of positive, interlocking influences in the form of parental health
education programs, church-based outreach groups, and community
service organizations. Only by harnessing a number of preventive and
promotion strategies in pursuit of a single goal will we have much reason for optimism about solving the many chronic and costly social
problems that threaten the well-being of our citizens. And, in the last
analysis, perhaps the most unifying and worthy goal is the promotion of
feelings of individual and collective esteem.

Bibliography

Abramson, L. Y., and H. A. Sackeim. 1977. "A Paradox in Depression: Uncontrollability and Self-Blame." *Psychological Bulletin* 84:838–851.

Abramson, L. Y., M. E. P. Seligman, and J. D. Teasdale. 1978. "Learned Helplessness in Humans: Critique and Reformulation." *Journal of Abnormal Psychology* 87:49–74.

Allen, V. L., and J. M. Levine. 1967. "Creativity and Conformity." Technical Report no. 33. University of Wisconsin Research and Development Center for Cognitive Learning, Madison, Wis.

Alschuler, A. S. 1969. "The Effects of Classroom Structure on Achievement Motivation and Academic Performance." *Educational Technology* 9: 19–24.

———. 1973. *Developing Achievement Motivation in Adolescents*. Englewood Cliffs, N.J.: Educational Technology Publications.

Ames, C. 1978. "Children's Achievement Attributions and Self-Reinforcement: Effects of Self-Concept and Competitive Reward Structure." *Journal of Educational Psychology* 70:345–355.

———. 1981. "Competitive Versus Cooperative Reward Structures: The Influence of Individual and Group Performance Factors on Achievement Attributions and Affect." *American Educational Research Journal* 18:273–388.

———. 1984. "Achievement Attributions and Self-Instructions Under Competitive and Individualistic Goal Structures." *Journal of Educational Psychology* 76:478–487.

Ames, C., and R. Ames. 1981. "Competitive Versus Individualistic Goal Structure: The Salience of Past Performance Information for Causal Attributions and Affect." *Journal of Educational Psychology* 73:411–418.

———. 1984. "Systems of Student and Teacher Motivation: Toward a Qualitative Definition." *Journal of Educational Psychology* 76:535–556.

Ames, C., R. Ames, and D. Felker. 1979. "Effects of Self-Concept on Children's Causal Attributions and Self-Reinforcement." *Journal of Educational Psychology* 71:613–619.

Ames, C., and J. Archer. 1987. "Mothers' Beliefs About the Role of Ability and Effort in School Learning." *Journal of Educational Psychology* 79:409–414.

Anderson, C. A., and D. L. Jennings. 1980. "When Experiences of Failure Promote Expectations of Success: The Impact of Attributing Failure to Ineffective Strategies." *Journal of Personality* 48:393–405.

Anderson, J. G., and F. B. Evans. 1974. "Causal Models in Educational Research: Recursive Models." *American Educational Research Journal* 11: 29–39.

Arnold, M. B. 1960. *Emotion and Personality*. New York: Columbia University Press.

Aronoff, J., and G. H. Litwin. 1966. "Achievement Motivation Training and Executive Advancement." Harvard University. Typescript.

Aronson, E., and D. R. Mettee. 1968. "Dishonest Behavior as a Function of

Differential Levels of Induced Self-Esteem." *Journal of Personality and Social Psychology* 9:121–127.

Aschner, M. J., and C. F. Bish, eds. 1965. *Productive Thinking in Education.* Washington, D.C.: National Education Association.

Atkinson, J. W. 1957. "Motivational Determinants of Risk-Taking Behavior." *Psychological Review* 64:359–372.

———. 1964. *An Introduction to Motivation.* Princeton, N.J.: Van Nostrand.

———. 1981. "Studying Personality in the Context of an Advanced Motivational Psychology." *American Psychologist* 36:117–128.

Atkinson, J. W., and N. T. Feather, eds. 1966. *A Theory of Achievement Motivation.* New York: Wiley.

Atkinson, J. W., and G. H. Litwin. 1960. "Achievement Motive and Test Anxiety Conceived as Motive to Approach Success and Motive to Avoid Failure." *Journal of Abnormal and Social Psychology* 60:52–63.

Atkinson, J. W., and P. A. O'Connor. 1966. "Neglected Factors in Studies of Achievement-Oriented Performance: Social Approval as an Incentive and Performance Decrement." In *A Theory of Achievement Motivation,* edited by J. W. Atkinson and N. T. Feather, 299–325. New York: Wiley.

Atkinson, J. W., and J. O. Raynor. 1974. *Motivation and Achievement.* New York: Wiley.

Atkinson, J. W., and W. R. Reitman. 1958. "Performance as a Function of Motive Strength and Expectancy of Goal Attainment." *Journal of Abnormal and Social Psychology* 53:361–366.

Backman, C., and P. E. Secord. 1968. "The Self and Role Selection." In *The Self in Social Interaction,* edited by C. Gordon and K. Gergen. New York: Wiley.

Battle, E. S. 1965. "Motivational Determinants of Academic Task Persistence." *Journal of Personality and Social Psychology* 2:209–218.

———. 1966. "Motivational Determinants of Academic Competence." *Journal of Personality and Social Psychology* 4:634–642.

Beck, A. T. 1967. *Depression: Clinical, Experimental, and Theoretical Aspects.* New York: Harper & Row.

Beery, R. G. 1975. "Fear of Failure in the Student Experience." *Personnel and Guidance Journal* 54:190–203.

Berglas, S., and E. Jones. 1978. "Drug Choice as a Self-Handicapping Strategy in Response to Noncontingent Success." *Journal of Personality and Social Psychology* 36:405–417.

Birney, R. C., H. Burdick, and R. C. Teevan. 1969. *Fear of Failure.* New York: Van Nostrand.

Block, J., and K. Lanning. 1984. "Attribution Therapy Requestioned: A Secondary Analysis of the Wilson-Linville Study." *Journal of Personality and Social Psychology* 46:705–708.

Block, J. H. 1977. "Motivation, Evaluation, and Mastery Learning." *UCLA Educator* 12:31–37.

———. 1984. "Making School Learning Activities More Playlike: Flow and Mastery Learning." *Elementary School Journal* 85:65–75.

Block, J. H., and R. B. Burns. 1976. "Mastery Learning." In *Review of Research in Education,* edited by L. S. Shulman. Itasca, Ill.: Peacock.

Bloom, B. S. 1976. *Human Characteristics and School Learning.* New York: McGraw-Hill.

———. 1987. "A Response to Slavin's Mastery Learning Reconsidered." *Review of Educational Research* 57:507–508.

Blumenfeld, P. C., P. R. Pintrich, J. Meece, and K. Wessels. 1981. "The Influence of Instructional Practices on Children's Criteria for Judging Ability, Effort, and Conduct." Paper presented at the annual meeting of the American Educational Research Association, Los Angeles.

Bowles, S., and H. Gintis. 1976. *Schooling in Capitalist America: Educational Reform and the Contradictions of Economic Life.* New York: Basic Books.

Bricklin, B., and P. M. Bricklin. 1967. *Bright Child—Poor Grades.* New York: Dell.

Brown, J., and B. Weiner. 1984. "Affective Consequences of Ability Versus Effort Ascriptions: Controversies, Resolutions, and Quandaries." *Journal of Educational Psychology* 76:146–158.

Burns, R. 1987. *Models of Instructional Organization: A Casebook on Mastery Learning and Outcome-Based Education.* San Francisco: Far West Laboratory for Educational Research and Development.

Butler, R., and M. Nisan. 1986. "Effects of No Feedback, Task-Related Comments, and Grade on Intrinsic Instruction and Performance." *Journal of Educational Psychology* 78:210–216.

Campbell, D. N. 1974. "On Being Number One: Competition in Education." *Phi Delta Kappan,* October, 143–147.

Canfield, J. 1986. *Self-Esteem in the Classroom.* Pacific Palisades, Calif.: Self-Esteem Seminars. [Address inquiries to 17156 Palisades Circle, Pacific Palisades, Calif. 90272.]

Carter, K., and W. Doyle. 1982. "Variations in Academic Tasks in High and Average Ability Classes." Paper presented at the annual meeting of the American Educational Research Association, New York.

Carver, C. S., and M. F. Scheier. 1984. "Self-Focused Attention in Test Anxiety: A General Theory Applied to a Specific Phenomenon." In *Advances in Test Anxiety Research,* vol. 3, edited by H. M. van der Ploeg, R. Schwarzer, and C. D. Spielberger, 3–20. Hillsdale, N.J.: Erlbaum.

Chandler, T. A., C. J. Spies, and F. M. Wolf. 1982. "Change in Strategy: The Relationship of Attribution, Expectancy, and Satisfaction." *Contemporary Educational Psychology* 7:9–14.

Chapin, M., and D. G. Dyck. 1976. "Persistence in Children's Reading Behavior as a Function of N Length and Attribution Retraining." *Journal of Abnormal Psychology* 85:511–515.

Coopersmith, S. 1967. *The Antecedents of Self-Esteem.* San Francisco: Freeman.

Covington, M. V. 1967. "The Effects of Anxiety on Various Types of Ideational Output Measures in Complex Problem Solving." Paper presented at the annual meeting of the Western Psychological Association, San Francisco.

———. 1983. "Anatomy of Failure-Induced Anxiety: The Role of Cognitive Mediators." Department of Psychology, University of California, Berkeley. Typescript.

————. 1984a. "The Motive for Self-Worth." In *Research on Motivation in Education,* vol. 1, edited by R. Ames and C. Ames, 77–113. New York: Academic Press.

————. 1984b. "The Self-Worth Theory of Achievement Motivation: Findings and Implications." *Elementary School Journal* 85:5–20.

————. 1985a. "The Effects of Multiple-Testing Opportunities on Rote and Conceptual Learning and Retention." *Human Learning* 4:57–72.

————. 1985b. "The Role of Self-Processes in Applied Social Psychology." *Journal of the Theory of Social Behavior* 15:355–389.

————. 1985c. "Strategic Thinking and the Fear of Failure." In *Thinking and Learning Skills,* vol. 1: *Relating Instruction to Research,* edited by J. W. Segal, S. F. Chipman, and R. Glaser, 389–416. Hillsdale, N.J.: Erlbaum.

————. 1986. "Instruction in Problem Solving and Planning." In *Blueprints for Thinking: The Role of Planning in Cognitive Development,* edited by S. L. Friedman, E. K. Scholnick, and R. R. Cocking, 469–511. New York: Cambridge University Press.

————. 1987. "Achievement Motivation, Self-Attributions, and Exceptionality." In *Intelligence and Exceptionality,* edited by J. D. Day and J. G. Borkowski, 173–213. Norwood, N.J.: Ablex.

————. In press. *Achievement Motivation and the Educational Process.* Cambridge: Cambridge University Press.

Covington, M. V., and R. G. Beery. 1976. *Self-Worth and School Learning.* New York: Holt, Rinehart & Winston.

Covington, M. V., R. S. Crutchfield, L. B. Davies, and R. M. Olton. 1974. *The Productive Thinking Program: A Course in Learning to Think.* Columbus, Ohio: Charles E. Merrill. [Address inquiries to Prof. Martin Covington, Department of Psychology, University of California, Berkeley.]

Covington, M. V., and C. L. Omelich. 1979a. "Are Causal Attributions Causal? A Path Analysis of the Cognitive Model of Achievement Motivation." *Journal of Personality and Social Psychology* 37:1487–1504.

————. 1979b. "Effort: The Double-Edged Sword in School Achievement." *Journal of Educational Psychology* 71:169–182.

————. 1979c. "It's Best to Be Able and Virtuous Too: Student and Teacher Evaluative Responses to Successful Effort." *Journal of Educational Psychology* 71:688–700.

————. 1981. "As Failures Mount: Affective and Cognitive Consequences of Ability Demotion in the Classroom." *Journal of Educational Psychology* 73:796–808.

————. 1984a. "Controversies or Consistencies? A Reply to Brown and Weiner." *Journal of Educational Psychology* 76:159–168.

————. 1984b. "An Empirical Examination of Weiner's Critique of Attribution Research." *Journal of Educational Psychology* 76:1214–1225.

————. 1984c. "Task-Oriented Versus Competitive Learning Structures: Motivational and Performance Consequences." *Journal of Educational Psychology* 76:1038–1050.

————. 1984d. "The Trouble with Pitfalls: A Reply to Weiner's Critique of Attribution Research." *Journal of Educational Psychology* 76:1199–1213.

————. 1985. "Ability and Effort Valuation Among Failure-Avoiding and Failure-Accepting Students." *Journal of Educational Psychology* 77:446– 459.

————. 1987. "'I Knew It Cold Before the Exam': A Test of the Anxiety-Blockage Hypothesis." *Journal of Educational Psychology* 79:393–400.

————. 1988a. "Achievement Dynamics: The Interaction of Motives, Cognitions, and Emotions over Time." *Anxiety Journal* 1:165–184.

————. 1988b. "Need Achievement Revisited: Verification of Atkinson's Original 2×2 Model." Department of Psychology, University of California, Berkeley. Typescript.

Covington, M. V., C. L. Omelich, and R. Schwarzer. 1986. "Anxiety, Aspirations, and Self-Concept in the Achievement Process: A Longitudinal Model with Latent Variables." *Motivation and Emotion* 10:71–88.

Covington, M. V., M. F. Spratt, and C. L. Omelich. 1980. "Is Effort Enough, or Does Diligence Count Too? Student and Teacher Reactions to Effort Stability in Failure." *Journal of Educational Psychology* 72:717–729.

Davids, A., and P. K. Hainsworth. 1967. "Maternal Attitudes About Family Life and Child-Rearing as Avowed by Mothers and Perceived by Their Underachieving and High-Achieving Sons." *Journal of Consulting Psychology* 31:29–37.

Day, V. H. 1982. "Validity of an Attributional Model for a Specific Life Event." *Psychological Reports* 50:434.

DeCharms, R. 1968. *Personal Causation: The Internal Affective Determinants of Behavior.* New York: Academic Press.

————. 1972. "Personal Causation Training in the Schools." *Journal of Applied Social Psychology* 2:95–113.

DeCharms, R., and W. J. Bridgeman. 1961. "Leadership Compliance and Group Behavior." Technical Report no. 9. Washington University, St. Louis.

Deutsch, M. 1979. "Education and Distributive Justice." *American Psychologist* 34:391–401.

Diener, C. T., and C. S. Dweck. 1978. "An Analysis of Learned Helplessness: Continuous Changes in Performance, Strategy, and Achievement Cognitions Following Failure." *Journal of Personality and Social Psychology* 36:451–462.

————. 1980. "An Analysis of Learned Helplessness: II. The Processing of Success." *Journal of Personality and Social Psychology* 39:940–952.

Doyle, W. 1983. "Academic Work." *Review of Educational Research* 53:159–199.

Dweck, C. S. 1975. "The Role of Expectations and Attributions in the Alleviation of Learned Helplessness." *Journal of Personality and Social Psychology* 31:674–685.

Dweck, C. S., and J. Bempechat. 1983. "Children's Theories of Intelligence: Consequences for Learning." In *Learning and Motivation in the Classroom,* edited by S. G. Paris, G. M. Olson, and H. M. Stevenson, 239–256. Hillsdale, N.J.: Erlbaum.

Dweck, C. S., and E. S. Bush. 1976. "Sex Differences in Learned Helplessness. I: Differential Debilitation with Peer and Adult Evaluators." *Developmental Psychology* 12:147–156.

Dweck, C. S., and N. D. Reppucci. 1973. "Learned Helplessness and Reinforcement Responsibility in Children." *Journal of Personality and Social Psychology* 25:109–116.

Dweck, C. S., and C. B. Wortman. 1982. "Learned Helplessness, Anxiety, and Achievement Motivation: Neglected Parallels in Cognitive, Affective, and Coping Responses." In *Achievement, Stress, and Anxiety,* edited by H. W. Krohne and L. Laux, 93–125. Washington, D.C.: Hemisphere.

Edwards, W. 1953. "Probability Preferences in Gambling." *American Journal of Psychology* 66:349–364.

Epstein, S. 1973. "The Self-Concept Revisited, or, A Theory of a Theory." *American Psychologist* 28:404–416.

Eswara, H. S. 1972. "Administration of Reward and Punishment in Relation to Ability, Effort, and Performance." *Journal of Social Psychology* 87:137–140.

Fair, J., and F. R. Shaftel. 1967. *Effective Thinking in the Social Studies.* Washington, D.C.: National Council for the Social Studies.

Falbo, T., and R. C. Beck. 1979. "Naive Psychology and the Attributional Model of Achievement." *Journal of Personality* 47:185–195.

Feather, N. T. 1961. "The Relationship of Persistence at a Task to Expectation of Success and Achievement-Related Motives." *Journal of Abnormal and Social Psychology* 63:552–561.

———. 1963. "Persistence at a Difficult Task with an Alternative Task of Intermediate Difficulty." *Journal of Abnormal and Social Psychology* 66:604–609.

Feldhusen, J. F., S. M. Speedie, and D. J. Treffinger. 1971. "The Purdue Creative Thinking Program: Research and Evaluation." *NSPI Journal* 10(3): 5–9.

Feldhusen, J. F., D. J. Treffinger, and S. J. Bahlke. 1970. "Developing Creative Thinking: The Purdue Creativity Program." *Journal of Creative Behavior* 4:85–90.

Fontaine, G. 1974. "Social Comparison and Some Determinants of Expected Personal Control and Expected Performance in a Novel Task Situation." *Journal of Personality and Social Psychology* 29:487–496.

Friedman, S. L., E. K. Scholnick, and R. R. Cocking, eds. 1986. *Blueprints for Thinking: The Role of Planning in Cognitive Development.* New York: Cambridge University Press.

Gardner, J. W. 1961. *Excellence: Can We Be Equal and Excellent Too?* New York: Harper & Row.

Gatchel, R. J., P. B. Paulus, and C. W. Maples. 1975. "Learned Helplessness and Self-Reported Affect." *Journal of Abnormal Psychology* 84:732–734.

Gergen, K. J. 1971. *The Concept of Self.* New York: Holt, Rinehart & Winston.

Ghiselin, B., ed. 1955. *The Creative Process.* New York: Mentor.

Glass, D. C., and J. E. Singer. 1972. *Urban Stress: Experiments on Noise and Social Stressors*. New York: Academic Press.

Goldman, R., D. Hudson, and B. Daharsh. 1973. "Self-Estimated Task Persistence as a Nonlinear Predictor of College Success." *Journal of Educational Psychology* 65 : 216–221.

Graham, S. 1984. "Teacher Feelings and Student Thoughts: An Attributional Approach to Affect in the Classroom." *Elementary School Journal* 85 : 91–104.

Grant, C. A. 1973. "Black Studies Materials Do Make a Difference." *Journal of Educational Research* 66 : 400–404.

Gray, S. W., and R. A. Klaus. 1970. "The Early Training Project: A Seventh Year Report." *Child Development* 41 : 909–924.

Hamburg, D. 1986. "Toward Health Development in Childhood and Adolescence." Charles M. and Martha Hitchcock Foundation Lectures, University of California, Berkeley.

Hansford, B. C., and J. A. Hattie. 1982. "The Relationship Between Self and Achievement/Performance Measures." *Review of Educational Research* 52 : 123–142.

Harari, O., and M. V. Covington. 1981. "Reactions to Achievement Behavior from a Teacher and Student Perspective: A Developmental Analysis." *American Educational Research Journal* 18 : 15–28.

Heckhausen, H., H.-D. Schmalt, and K. Schneider. 1985. *Achievement Motivation in Perspective*. Translated by M. Woodruff and R. Wicklund. New York: Academic Press.

Heider, F. 1958. *The Psychology of Interpersonal Relations*. New York: Wiley.

Hoffman, M. L. 1982. "Development of Prosocial Motivation: Empathy and Guilt." In *Development of Prosocial Behavior*, edited by N. Eisenberg-Borg, 281–313. New York: Academic Press.

Homme, L. 1970. *How to Use Contingency Contracting in the Classroom*. Champaign, Ill.: Research Press.

Hunt, D. E., and R. H. Hardt. 1969. "The Effect of Upward Bound Programs on the Attitudes, Motivation, and Academic Achievement of Negro Students." *Journal of Social Issues* 25 : 117–129.

Jacoby, K. E., and M. V. Covington. 1973. "Productive Thinking in an Introductory Psychology Course as a Function of an Independence-Conformance Dimension." Paper presented at the annual meeting of the American Psychological Association, Montreal.

Jencks, C., M. Smith, H. Acland, M. J. Bane, D. Cohen, H. Gintis, B. Heyns, and S. Michelson. 1972. *Inequity*. New York: Harper & Row.

Johnson, K. R., and R. S. Ruskin. 1977. *Behavioral Instruction: An Evaluative Review*. Washington, D.C.: American Psychological Association.

Karabenick, S. A., and Z. Youssef. 1968. "Performance as a Function of Achievement Motive Level and Perceived Difficulty." *Journal of Personality and Social Psychology* 10 : 414–419.

Kelley, H. H. 1971. "Causal Schemata and the Attribution Process." In *Attribution: Perceiving the Causes of Behavior*, edited by E. E. Jones et al., 151–174. Morristown, N.J.: General Learning Press.

King, L. H. 1980. "Student Thought Processes and the Expectancy Effect." Research Report no. 80–1–8. Centre for Research in Teaching, University of Alberta, Edmonton.

Klein, D. C., E. Fencil-Morse, and M. E. P. Seligman. 1976. "Learned Helplessness, Depression, and the Attribution of Failure." *Journal of Personality and Social Psychology* 33:508–516.

Kohn, A. 1986. *No Contest: The Case Against Competition.* Boston: Houghton Mifflin.

Kukla, A. 1972. "Foundation of an Attributional Theory of Performance." *Psychological Review* 79:454–470.

Kulik, J. A., C. C. Kulik, and P. A. Cohen. 1979. "A Meta-Analysis of Outcome Studies of Keller's Personalized System of Instruction." *American Psychologist* 34:307–318.

Kun, A., and B. Weiner. 1973. "Necessary Versus Sufficient Causal Schemata for Success and Failure." *Journal of Research in Personality* 7:197–207.

Lawson, R. E. 1974. *A Comparison of the Development of Self-Concept and Achievement in Reading of Students in the First, Third, and Fifth Year of Attendance in Graded and Non-Graded Elementary Schools.* Ann Arbor, Mich.: University Microfilms.

Lazarus, R. S. 1960. *Psychological Stress and the Coping Process.* New York: McGraw-Hill.

Lens, W., and M. De Volder. 1980. "Achievement Motivation and Intelligence Test Scores: A Test of the Yerkes-Dodson Hypothesis." *Psychologia Belgica* 20:49–59.

Lewin, K. 1935. *A Dynamic Theory of Personality.* New York: McGraw-Hill.

Lewin, K., T. Dembo, L. Festinger, and P. Sears. 1944. "Level of Aspiration." In *Personality and the Behavior Disorders,* vol. 1, edited by J. McHunt, 333–378. New York: Ronald Press.

Lichtenberg, P. A. 1957. "A Definition and Analysis of Depression." *Archives of Neurology and Psychiatry* 77:519–527.

Lipman, M. 1976. "Philosophy for Children." *Metaphilosophy* 7:17–39.

———. 1985. "Thinking Skills Fostered by the Middle-School Philosophy for Children Program." In *Thinking and Learning Skills,* vol. 1: *Relating Instruction to Research,* edited by J. W. Segal, S. F. Chipman, and R. Glaser, 83–108. Hillsdale, N.J.: Erlbaum.

Litwin, G. H., and J. A. Ciarlo. 1961. "Achievement Motivation and Risk-Taking in a Business Setting." Technical report. General Electric Company, Behavioral Research Service, New York.

Logsdon, D. M., and B. Ewert. 1973. "Longitudinal Study of an Operational Model for Enhancing Central City Youths' Self-Concept, Academic Achievement, Attitude Toward School, Participation in School, and Socialization/Maturation." University of Wisconsin, Milwaukee.

McClelland, D. C. 1965. "Toward a Theory of Motive Acquisition." *American Psychologist* 20:321–333.

———. 1969. *Motivating Economic Achievement.* New York: Free Press.

———. 1972. "What Is the Effect of Achievement Motivation Training in the Schools?" *Teachers College Record* 74:129–145.

————. 1980. "Motive Dispositions: The Merits of Operant and Respondent Measures." In *Review of Personality and Social Psychology,* vol. 1, edited by L. Wheeler, 10–41. Beverly Hills, Calif.: Sage.

————. 1985. "How Motives, Skills, and Values Determine What People Do." *American Psychologist* 40:812–825.

McMahan, I. D. 1973. "Relationships Between Causal Attributions and Expectancy of Success." *Journal of Personality and Social Psychology* 28:108–114.

McNabb, T. 1986. "The Effects of Strategy and Effort Attribution Training on the Motivation of Subjects Differing in Perceived Math Competence and Attitude Toward Strategy and Effort." American College Testing Program, Iowa City, Iowa. Typescript.

Marecek, J., and D. R. Mettee. 1972. "Avoidance of Continued Success as a Function of Self-Esteem, Level of Esteem Certainty, and Responsibility for Success." *Journal of Personality and Social Psychology* 22:98–107.

Meyer, J. P. 1980. "Causal Attribution for Success and Failure: A Multivariate Investigation of Dimensionality, Formation and Consequences." *Journal of Personality and Social Psychology* 38:704–718.

Miller, I. W., III, and W. H. Norman. 1979. "Learned Helplessness in Humans: A Review and Attribution-Theory Model." *Psychological Bulletin* 86:93–118.

Moulton, R. W. 1965. "Effects of Success and Failure on Level of Aspiration as Related to Achievement Motives." *Journal of Personality and Social Psychology* 1:399–406.

Naveh-Benjamin, M. 1985. "A Comparison of Training Programs Intended for Different Types of Test-Anxious Students." Paper presented at the annual meeting of the American Psychological Association, "Information Processing and Motivation" symposium, Los Angeles.

Nicholls, J. G. 1978. "The Development of the Concepts of Effort and Ability, Perception of Academic Attainment, and the Understanding that Difficult Tasks Require More Ability." *Child Development* 49:800–814.

————. 1987. "Motivation, Values, and Education." Paper presented at the annual meeting of the American Educational Research Association, "Enhancing Motivation: Values, Goals, Cognitions" symposium, Washington, D.C.

Nicholls, J. G., M. Patashnick, and S. B. Nolen. 1985. "Adolescents' Theories of Education." *Journal of Educational Psychology* 77:683–692.

Olson, C. B. 1988. "Success and Failure Attributions: Issues in Theory and Research." Department of Psychology, University of California, Berkeley. Typescript.

Olton, R. M., and R. S. Crutchfield. 1969. "Developing the Skills of Productive Thinking." In *Trends and Issues in Developmental Psychology,* edited by P. Mussen, J. Langer, and M. V. Covington, 68–91. New York: Holt, Rinehart & Winston.

Pedhazur, E. J. 1982. *Multiple Regression in Behavioral Research: Explanation and Prediction.* 2d ed. New York: Holt, Rinehart & Winston.

Purkey, W. W. 1970. *Self-Concept and School Achievement.* Englewood Cliffs, N.J.: Prentice-Hall.

Reasoner, R. W. 1986. *Building Self-Esteem*. Palo Alto, Calif.: Consulting Psychologists Press.

Reckless, W. C., and S. Dinitz. 1972. *The Prevention of Juvenile Delinquency: An Experiment*. Columbus: Ohio State University Press.

Resnick, L. 1987. *Education and Learning to Think*. Washington, D.C.: National Academy Press.

Rest, S., R. Nierenberg, B. Weiner, and H. Heckhausen. 1973. "Further Evidence Concerning the Effects of Perceptions of Effort and Ability on Achievement Evaluation." *Journal of Personality and Social Psychology* 28:187–191.

Rohwer, W. D., Jr. 1984. "An Invitation to a Developmental Psychology of Studying." In *Advances in Applied Developmental Psychology*, vol. 1, edited by F. J. Morrison, C. A. Lord, and D. P. Keating, 75–114. New York: Academic Press.

Rosen, B. C., and R. D'Andrade. 1959. "The Psychosocial Origins of Achievement Motivation." *Sociometry* 22:185–218.

Rosenbaum, R. M. 1972. "A Dimensional Analysis of the Perceived Causes of Success and Failure." Ph.D. dissertation, University of California, Los Angeles.

Rosenberg, M., and R. G. Simmons. 1973. *Black and White Self-Esteem: The Urban School Child*. Washington, D.C.: American Sociological Association.

Ryals, K. R. 1969. "An Experimental Study of Achievement Motivation Training as a Function of the Moral Maturity of Trainees." Ph.D. dissertation, Washington University, St. Louis.

Sarason, I. G. 1961. "The Effects of Anxiety and Threat on the Solution of a Difficult Task." *Journal of Abnormal and Social Psychology* 62:165–168.

Scheirer, M. A., and R. E. Kraut. 1979. "Increasing Educational Achievement Via Self-Concept Change." *Review of Educational Research* 49:131–150.

Schwarzer, R., M. Jerusalem, and C. Schwarzer. 1983. "Self-Related and Situation-Related Cognitions in Test Anxiety and Helplessness: A Longitudinal Analysis with Structural Equations." In *Advances in Test Anxiety Research*, vol. 2, edited by R. Schwarzer, H. M. van der Ploeg, and C. D. Spielberger, 35–43. Hillsdale, N.J.: Erlbaum.

Seligman, M. E. P. 1975. *Helplessness: On Depression, Development, and Death*. San Francisco: Freeman.

Seligman, M. E. P., S. F. Maier, and J. Geer. 1968. "The Alleviation of Learned Helplessness in the Dog." *Journal of Abnormal Psychology* 73:256–262.

Seligman, M. E. P., S. F. Maier, and R. L. Solomon. 1971. "Unpredictable and Uncontrollable Aversive Events." In *Aversive Conditioning and Learning*, edited by F. R. Brush. New York: Academic Press.

Sigall, H., and R. Gould. 1977. "The Effects of Self-Esteem and Evaluator Demandingness of Effort Expenditure." *Journal of Personality and Social Psychology* 35:12–20.

Silverman, P. 1964. "Self-Esteem and Differential Responsiveness to Success and Failure." *Journal of Abnormal and Social Psychology* 68:115–119.

Slavin, R. E. 1978. "Student Teams and Comparison Among Equals: Effects on

Academic Performance and Student Attitudes." *Journal of Educational Psychology* 70:532–538.

———. 1983. "When Does Cooperative Learning Increase Student Achievement?" *Psychological Bulletin* 94:429–445.

———. 1984. "Students Motivating Students to Excel: Cooperative Incentives, Cooperative Tasks, and Student Achievement." *Elementary School Journal* 85:53–64.

———. 1987. "Mastery Learning Reconsidered." *Review of Educational Research* 57:175–213.

Smith, C. P. 1963. "Situational Determinants of the Expression of Achievement Motivation in Thematic Apperception." Ph.D. dissertation, University of Michigan, Ann Arbor.

Spady, W. G. 1982. "Outcome-Based Instructional Management: A Sociological Perspective." *Australian Journal of Education* 26:123–143.

Stallings, J. A., and D. H. Kaskowitz. 1974. *Follow Through Classroom Observation Evaluation: 1972–73*. Menlo Park, Calif.: Stanford Research Institute.

Stebbins, L. B., R. G. St. Pierre, E. C. Proper, R. B. Anderson, and T. R. Cerva. 1977. *Education as Experimentation: A Planned Variation Model*. Vol. 4-A, *An Evaluation of Follow Through*. Cambridge, Mass.: Abt.

Steele, C. M. 1975. "Name Calling and Compliance." *Journal of Personality and Social Psychology* 31:361–369.

Stern, P. 1983. "A Multimethod Analysis of Student Perceptions of Causal Dimensions." Ph.D. dissertation, University of California, Los Angeles.

Stipek, D. 1981. "Children's Perceptions of Their Own and Their Classmates' Ability." *Journal of Educational Psychology* 73:404–410.

———. 1988. *Motivation to Learn: From Theory to Practice*. Englewood Cliffs, N.J.: Prentice-Hall.

Stotland, E., and A. Zander. 1958. "Effects of Public and Private Failure on Self-Evaluation." *Journal of Abnormal Psychology* 56:223–229.

Taylor, J. A. 1953. "A Personality Scale of Manifest Anxiety." *Journal of Abnormal and Social Psychology* 48:285–290.

———. 1956. "Drive Theory and Manifest Anxiety." *Psychological Bulletin* 53:303–320.

Tennen, H., and S. J. Eller. 1977. "Attributional Components of Learned Helplessness and Facilitation." *Journal of Personality and Social Psychology* 35:265–271.

Tolman, E. C. 1932. *Purposive Behavior in Animals and Men*. New York: Appleton-Century-Crofts.

Torrance, E. P. 1965. *Rewarding Creative Behavior: Experiments in Classroom Creativity*. Englewood Cliffs, N.J.: Prentice-Hall.

Trope, Y. 1975. "Seeking Information About One's Own Ability as a Determinant of Choice Among Tasks." *Journal of Personality and Social Psychology* 32:1004–1013.

Valle, V. A. 1974. "Attributions of Stability as a Mediator in the Changing of Expectations." Ph.D. dissertation, University of Pittsburgh.

Walberg, H. J., and M. E. Uguroglu. 1980. "Motivation and Educational Productivity: Theories, Results, and Implications." In *Achievement Motivation: Recent Trends in Theory and Research,* edited by L. J. Fyans, Jr. New York: Plenum.

Webster, M., and B. Sobieszek. 1974. *Sources of Self-Evaluation: A Formal Theory of Significant Others and Social Influence.* New York: Wiley.

Weiner, B. 1972. *Theories of Motivation: From Mechanism to Cognition.* Chicago: Markham.

———. 1974. *Achievement Motivation and Attribution Theory.* Morristown, N.J.: General Learning Press.

———. 1977. "An Attributional Model for Educational Psychology." In *Review of Research in Education,* vol. 4, edited by L. Shulman, 179–209. Itasca, Ill.: Peacock.

———. 1979. "A Theory of Motivation for Some Classroom Experiences." *Journal of Educational Psychology* 71:3–25.

———. 1983. "Some Methodological Pitfalls in Attributional Research." *Journal of Educational Psychology* 75:530–543.

———. 1985. "An Attributional Theory of Achievement Motivation and Emotion." *Psychological Review* 92:548–573.

Weiner, B., L. Frieze, A. Kukla, L. Reed, S. Rest, and R. Rosenbaum. 1971. "Perceiving the Causes of Success and Failure." In *Attribution: Perceiving the Causes of Behavior,* edited by E. E. Jones et al. Morristown, N.J.: General Learning Press.

Weiner, B., H. Heckhausen, W. Meyer, and R. Cook. 1972. "Causal Ascriptions and Achievement Behavior: A Conceptual Analysis of Effect and Reanalysis of Locus of Control." *Journal of Personality and Social Psychology* 21:239–248.

Weiner, B., and A. Kukla. 1970. "An Attributional Analysis of Achievement Motivation." *Journal of Personality and Social Psychology* 15:1–20.

Weiner, B., R. Nierenberg, and M. Goldstein. 1976. "Social Learning (Locus of Control) Versus Attributional (Causal Stability) Interpretations of Expectancy of Success." *Journal of Personality* 44:52–68.

Weiner, B., and P. Potepan. 1970. "Personality Characteristics and Affective Reactions Toward Exams of Superior and Failing College Students." *Journal of Educational Psychology* 61:144–151.

Weiner, B., D. Russell, and D. Lerman. 1978. "Affective Consequences of Causal Ascriptions." In *New Directions in Attribution Research,* vol. 2, edited by J. H. Harvey, W. J. Ickes, and R. F. Kidd, 59–90. Hillsdale, N.J.: Erlbaum.

———. 1979. "The Cognitive-Emotion Process in Achievement-Related Contexts." *Journal of Personality and Social Psychology* 37:1211–1220.

Weiner, B., and J. Sierad. 1975. "Misattribution for Failure and Enhancement of Achievement Strivings." *Journal of Personality and Social Psychology* 31:415–421.

West, C. K., J. A. Fish, and R. J. Stevens. 1980. "General Self-Concept, Self-Concept of Academic Ability and School Achievement: Implications for

'Causes' of Self-Concept." *Australian Journal of Education* 24:194–213.

Wicker, F. W., G. C. Payne, and R. D. Morgan. 1983. "Participant Descriptions of Guilt and Shame." *Motivation and Emotion* 7:25–39.

Wimer, S., and H. H. Kelley. 1982. "An Investigation of the Dimensions of Causal Analysis." *Journal of Personality and Social Psychology* 43:1142–1162.

Wolff, R. P. 1969. *The Ideal of the University*. Boston: Beacon Press.

Wong, P. T. P., and B. Weiner. 1981. "When People Ask 'Why' Questions and the Heuristics of Attributional Search." *Journal of Personality and Social Psychology* 40:650–663.

Wylie, R. C. 1968. "The Present Status of Self-Theory." In *Handbook of Personality Theory and Research*, edited by E. F. Borgatta and W. W. Lambert, 728–787. Chicago: Rand McNally.

———. 1974. *The Self-Concept*. Vol. 1, *A Review of Methodological Considerations and Measuring Instruments*. Rev. ed. Lincoln: University of Nebraska Press.

———. 1979. *The Self-Concept*. Vol. 2, *Theory and Research on Selected Topics*. Rev. ed. Lincoln: University of Nebraska Press.

Self-Esteem and Teenage Pregnancy

Susan B. Crockenberg and Barbara A. Soby

Introduction

> I knew I could get pregnant, but I didn't think about it much. I was too embarrassed to go to a clinic and tell a bunch of strangers that I was having sex. I couldn't talk to my boyfriend about birth control, either—he would have made fun of me. My mother would have grounded me permanently if she ever found out I was taking the pill. Anyway, I thought that maybe getting pregnant wouldn't be so bad—what else did I have to do?
>
> —Fictitious pregnant teenager

This vignette illustrates why adolescents with low self-esteem may be more likely to become pregnant than their peers with higher self-esteem. In this chapter, we suggest that adolescents perform—perhaps without realizing it—a cost/benefit analysis in their decisions to engage in sexual intercourse and to forego contraception. Self-esteem is important because it may influence how those costs and benefits are perceived. This intriguing possibility has implications for reducing the number of adolescent pregnancies.

The results of research studies tell a story that is much less straightforward than the one suggested in the vignette above, however. We begin by considering the birth rate among adolescents in the 1980s.

The birth rate among teenagers has declined in the past twenty years (U.S. Congress, House Select Committee on Children, Youth, and Families 1986), as it has among the general population. In California in 1985,

The authors gratefully acknowledge the assistance of Sandra Walker in the preparation of this chapter.

125

there were 52.5 births per 1,000 girls aged fifteen to nineteen, down from 68.9 births per 1,000 in 1970 (Brindis and Jeremy 1988). This decline has been greater for blacks than for whites, declining 35 percent and 24 percent, respectively, at the national level.* Judging from these statistics, we might expect the concern with teen pregnancy to have diminished correspondingly. Instead, it has increased dramatically, as seen in the number of studies funded, articles published, and congressional hearings convened that have focused on teenage pregnancy and parenting.

Three changes in the nature of teenage pregnancies may account for this concern. First, although the overall birth rate among teenagers has decreased significantly, it has increased among the youngest teens. In California, the birth rate among girls ten to fourteen years old rose between 1970 and 1985, from 0.8 to 1.0 births per 1,000 girls in that age group. One percent of all births to whites occurred in this age group, whereas 3 percent of births to Hispanics and 6 percent of births to blacks were to these young teens (Brindis and Jeremy 1988). Thus, the teenagers whose lives may be most adversely affected by a birth and who are presumably least able to care for a child are somewhat more likely to bear children today than they were twenty years ago.

This trend in the birth rate for young teenagers is apparent despite the availability and use of abortion, suggesting that the pregnancy rate would reveal an even steeper increase over time. It is estimated that in 1981 more than half of the pregnant teenagers in California (Brindis and Jeremy 1988) and more than 40 percent of pregnant teens in the United States (Hayes 1987b) terminated their pregnancies through induced abortions. Despite comparable rates of sexual activity, the United States has the highest pregnancy, abortion, and birth rates among adolescents of any developed country, especially among females under the age of fifteen. The birth rate among American adolescents in this age group is five times higher than it is among such young girls in any other developed country (Hayes 1987b).

The second change concerns the circumstances surrounding births to teenagers. In the past, the majority of births occurred in the context of marriage, albeit a hastily arranged one; today, the mother is more likely to remain single. In 1984, for girls between the ages of fifteen and nineteen, 34 percent of births to non-Hispanic whites, 45 percent of births to Hispanics, and 87 percent of births to blacks occurred outside of

---

*No comparative data concerning Hispanics are available, because birth rates have been calculated separately for Hispanic and non-Hispanic whites only since 1978.

marriage (Hayes 1987b). In contrast, in 1950 only 12.6 percent of all births to teens, 5.1 percent of births to white teenagers, and 68.5 percent of births to nonwhite teenagers were out of wedlock (Campbell 1980).

Not only are more babies born outside of marriage, but also the adolescent mothers today are more likely to keep their children and less likely to give them up for adoption than they were in the past (Vinovskis 1981). This is a third reason for concern, because it indicates that unwed adolescents, some of them quite young, will be raising the babies they bring into the world.

A major concern about teenage childbearing is the impact of a birth on the unmarried teen mother, whose subsequent life is viewed as both predictable and constricted. It is feared she will drop out of school, be unable to support herself and her child, and either marry someone she would not have chosen otherwise and then divorce or else enter the ranks of those on welfare. In fact, despite recent evidence of variability in the outcomes of adolescent childbearing (Furstenberg, Brooks-Gunn, and Morgan 1987), there is considerable evidence that these concerns are well founded (Hofferth 1987b). Virtually every study that has controlled for initial differences between adolescent and older childbearers has reported that early births carry an additional impact. In the Furstenberg, Brooks-Gunn, and Morgan (1987) study, for example, significant differences remained seventeen years later between the women who had waited until after age twenty to bear children and the teenage mothers. Fewer of the early childbearers had completed high school or obtained a GED, fewer were employed, and those who were employed were more likely to be in low-paying positions. More early childbearers were on welfare, more were poor, and more had divorced or separated from spouses.

Evidence that women who bear children as adolescents utilize public services more than other women do focuses attention on the economic costs to society of the increase in unmarried teenage mothers. These costs are considerable, as indicated by information collected by the National Research Council on Adolescent Sexuality, Pregnancy, and Childbearing and reported by Hofferth (1987b). In 1975, half of the budget for Aid to Families with Dependent Children (AFDC)—roughly $5 billion—went to households in which the mother was a teenager at first birth. When food stamps and Medicaid benefits are added to the bill, it rises to $8.55 billion. A 1985 estimate indicated that total welfare-related expenditures associated with teenage childbearing had nearly doubled in the preceding ten years, to $16.6 billion. In California, tax-payers spend an additional $1.24 billion each year on the direct and administrative costs of AFDC, Medi-Cal, and food stamps for families that were started when the mother was a teenager (Brindis and Jeremy 1988).

From this perspective, pregnancy (and therefore parenthood) among unmarried teens cannot be viewed simply as a violation of tradition or of certain moral standards, nor can it be viewed solely as a limiting individual choice. To the extent that social costs are associated with it, single parenthood among teenagers is a problem that society has an investment in solving.

The review that follows is consistent with this perspective. Unlike most other efforts to understand the factors contributing to adolescent pregnancy, however, we will focus primarily on the link between self-esteem and teenage pregnancy. We begin with a brief introduction to self-esteem as a psychological construct, followed by an analysis of low self-esteem as a possible contributor to teen pregnancy. We then describe and evaluate research that has tested whether low self-esteem increases the risk of a teen pregnancy. In the final section, we consider the implications of this research for social policy.

Self-Esteem

Self-esteem plays a central role in a number of psychological theories, each of which offers its own definition of the term (Wells and Marwell 1976). In nearly all these definitions, self-esteem refers to feelings and attitudes toward the self. These are described and measured along continuums that range from high to low or positive to negative. We have adopted this sparse definition of self-esteem here because it makes the fewest assumptions about the structure of personality, allowing for a more comprehensive review of studies that have considered the association between self-esteem and adolescent pregnancy. Other terms cited (self-attitude, self-regard, self-acceptance—or its opposite, self-derogation) also share the core meaning of feelings toward the self.

In their review of the literature, Wells and Marwell (1976) identify two components of self-esteem: an evaluative component and an affective component. The evaluative component addresses the issue of competence—how competent or successful an individual thinks he or she is. The affective component addresses the issue of acceptance—subjectively, how individuals feel about themselves. These different, though related, aspects of self-esteem are thought to result from different forms of experience. The evaluation of competence is associated with success at a task. If students do well in school or in some other activity that they consider important, they will presumably judge themselves as competent. Feelings of acceptance are associated with affiliative experiences, the ways in which significant others respond to an individual. If those responses are positive—that is, if one feels loved and accepted, despite imperfections—then the individual's internalized feelings about himself or herself should reflect this.

Although it is possible to distinguish these aspects of self-esteem, the two often are integrated, as in the definitions and descriptions of self-esteem provided by Rosenberg (1965), Coopersmith (1967), and Kaplan (1975) and in the measures designed by these psychologists to reflect these definitions (see Appendix). Rosenberg emphasizes the affective aspect and refers to self-esteem as "a positive or negative attitude toward a particular object, namely, the self" (1965, 30); but he acknowledges that these feelings derive from the individual's evaluation of self in relation to criteria of excellence, derived in turn from what is valued by the society. Coopersmith's definition—"the extent to which the person believes himself to be capable, significant, successful, and worthy"—emphasizes the evaluative component of self-esteem, but touches on the affective by including the notion of worthiness. Kaplan defines self-esteem as self-attitudes or feelings that "refer to the emotional experiences of the subject upon perceiving and evaluating his own attributes and behaviors" (1975, 10–11).

In general—and this oversimplifies the association considerably—high self-esteem is expected to reflect and predict good adjustment and behaviors valued by the society. In contrast, we expect low self-esteem to be associated with deviant behavior. Again, different theorists explain the dynamics of this association in various ways. Kaplan (1975) presents one of the clearest, yet most complex, descriptions of the association between self-esteem and behavior; his analysis will therefore form part of our theoretical framework for reviewing the research on self-esteem and adolescent pregnancy.

According to Kaplan, individuals attempt to develop, maintain, and improve positive self-attitudes. If they have not yet adopted deviant behaviors, we may assume that their positive self-attitudes are derived from culturally sanctioned (normative) experiences—acceptance and love at home, achievement at school. Because these experiences are associated with emotionally gratifying self-attitudes, they are expected to become gratifying in their own right and to encourage behavior that fosters other such experiences. Individuals who have developed positive self-esteem in this manner thus would continue to engage in behaviors valued by the culture.

We may also assume that negative self-attitudes derive from normative experiences. In these cases, however, such experiences have been unpleasant, threatening, or devaluing. Because these experiences are associated with emotionally distressing (negative) self-attitudes, they become highly distressing in their own right. Therefore, individuals with normatively derived negative self-attitudes not only are likely to avoid the distress-producing experiences, but also are "motivated to deviate from normative patterns by virtue of their intrinsically distressing nature." In Kaplan's view, "deviant patterns would offer the only remaining promise for satisfying the self-esteem motive" (1975, 54).

Using this analysis, one would predict correlations between high self-esteem and low frequencies of deviant behavior and between low self-esteem and high frequencies of deviant behavior only when positive self-attitude derives from so-called normative experiences (being loved by parents, accepted by friends, appreciated by teachers). If an individual has engaged in deviant acts, however, positive self-attitude may have derived from these acts, rather than from normative experiences. In that case, we would expect to find little empirical association between self-esteem and deviant behavior. Knowing the origins of self-esteem is therefore critical for evaluating the causal link between self-esteem and teen pregnancy, as we will discuss.

Linking Self-Esteem and Teen Pregnancy

Several analyses of the determinants of pregnancy or of deviant behavior would lead us to expect a higher incidence of pregnancy among adolescents with low self-esteem. The first is Kaplan's (1975), linking self-esteem and deviant behavior. A second is Luker's (1975) cost/benefit analysis of contraception and pregnancy, and a third is a variant of Luker's thesis that emphasizes the biological basis of adolescent pregnancy.

Becoming pregnant as an unmarried adolescent is deviant because only a small minority of adolescents do so and because it is not approved by the society at large. Thus, an individual who is motivated to deviate from normative patterns because of their negative connotation may become pregnant as a way of bolstering self-esteem. The adolescent may expect motherhood to improve her status: as a mother, she will have an important task to perform. She may also expect the baby to love her and the baby's father to feel bound to her. Alternatively, pregnancy could be simply an unconsidered outcome of sexual intercourse, which may be viewed as self-enhancing because it signals a movement away from childhood, because it is associated with the feeling of being loved, and because it may validate the adolescent as an attractive person. In either case, we would anticipate that adolescents with low self-esteem would be more likely to become pregnant.

An alternative view is that adolescent pregnancy becomes more common when the costs of pregnancy are low, especially if the costs of contraception are high (Luker 1975). An adolescent with low self-esteem may be unconcerned about avoiding pregnancy, simply because there is little to lose if she becomes pregnant. If she is not doing well in school and does not expect to get a job that is either interesting or lucrative, early pregnancy and parenthood will not interfere with any important individual goals and will carry little personal "cost." We would predict that this individual is more likely to become pregnant than an adolescent with high self-esteem. In addition, as Luker points out, just as there are costs to a pregnancy, there are costs to prevention, which requires either sexual abstinence or effective contraception. The higher the potential cost of these actions, the greater the cost associated with pregnancy will have to be to ensure that the adolescent successfully avoids becoming pregnant. If this perspective is accurate, it may be essential to include the cost of prevention in our model of self-esteem and teen pregnancy.

Still another view is that early sexuality should be viewed as "expected behavior," because sexual activity has always closely followed sexual maturity, not only in other animal species but also in most human societies prior to the twentieth century (Lancaster 1986). If we assume that the biological changes accompanying sexual maturity prime the individual to engage in sexual behavior, it is the inhibition of this behavior rather than its expression that needs to be accounted for. One plausible explanation is that inhibition will occur to the extent that engaging in early sexual intercourse has negative consequences for the individual. In American society, many of those consequences have diminished in the past thirty years. It is possible not only to prevent conception but also to abort an unwanted pregnancy after conception. Nor does an adolescent pregnancy carry the same stigma as in the past, although this clearly varies among social groups. Pregnant adolescents were once sent away to "homes for unwed mothers"; now they remain at home and attend special school programs. Consequently, teenage pregnancy and parenthood today, much more so than in the past, are individual decisions affected by perceived costs to the individual. If those costs are few, then pregnancy and parenthood will be more likely than if the costs are many and high.

Each of these perspectives would lead to similar predictions concerning self-esteem and pregnancy. Low self-esteem, we believe, would be associated with a greater risk of adolescent pregnancy.

Confounding Factors and Research Design

Factors other than self-esteem affect the teen pregnancy rate, and these factors vary across studies, making it difficult to evaluate the association between self-esteem and adolescent pregnancy. One such factor is race or ethnicity; others are social class, age, cohort (referring to the historical period during which the adolescent reached childbearing age), and availability of contraceptives.

Race/Ethnicity

Racial or ethnic background may be seen as a composite variable that encompasses differences in economic status, the value placed on motherhood, the disapproval associated with pregnancy, educational success and failure, and possibly self-esteem as well. Any of these factors, and therefore race or ethnicity, could affect the pregnancy rate directly, could interact with other predictors to affect the rate, or could confound or mask the association between self-esteem and pregnancy. Thus, in a subcultural group that highly values the maternal role, for example, pregnancy and motherhood may be especially attractive to adolescents and may also be associated with less social disapproval than would be the case in the dominant culture. In such a group, individual differences in self-esteem may play little role in predicting teen pregnancy.

Alternatively, low self-esteem may be associated with a high incidence of teen pregnancy only under certain, culturally linked, conditions. Thus, where there is an extremely high degree of parental or religious control over sexual behavior, low self-esteem may show less association with pregnancy than in a cultural context where the social constraints are weaker. This argument illustrates the difficulty of drawing clear inferences about what psychosocial factors might contribute to teen pregnancy. The possibility of racial or ethnic differences in predictors of teen pregnancy also has implications for attempts to reduce the pregnancy rate during the teenage years, for if the conditions that lead to pregnancy differ across ethnic groups, attempts to alter the pregnancy rate also must differ.

Social Class

Like race and ethnicity, social class is a composite variable that includes differences in income, occupational status, and education. Any of these factors could be expected to influence the probability of an adolescent pregnancy, through association with the various costs and benefits of pregnancy or its prevention. An adolescent whose parents have relatively little education and hold low-status jobs may not see an early pregnancy in terms of an interrupted education, lost career opportunities, or other such costs.

In addition, self-esteem may be influenced by experiences of success and failure in school, which are likely to be class-related. Thus, social class may be associated with the risk of pregnancy during adolescence as an effect of class-related expectations or as an effect of class-related experiences that contribute to differences in self-esteem. It follows that differences in social class may confound—that is, account for—any observed association between self-esteem and adolescent pregnancy.

Age

The adolescent's age or, more accurately, the age-linked probability that the adolescent has engaged in deviant behavior may influence what accounts for a teenage pregnancy. If we assume that adolescents often adopt deviant behaviors as a way of bolstering their self-esteem, then the younger they are when self-esteem is measured, the more likely we are to obtain an accurate view of the feelings that may later lead to deviant behavior. Self-esteem assessed early in or prior to adolescence should be a better predictor of teenage pregnancy than self-esteem assessed later in adolescence; the high self-esteem some older adolescents report may have derived from their deviant behavior or from devaluing acceptable behavior.

Cohort

The adolescent's cohort may well affect whether self-esteem predicts teen pregnancy. The percentage of adolescent females who report engaging in premarital sex has increased markedly since the early 1960s.

Although the causes of that increase cannot be determined conclusively, because so many other changes occurred at the same time, it is unlikely that a large-scale decrease in self-esteem accounts for the increase in premarital sex. More reasonable explanations are the increasing availability of contraceptives and abortion and the associated changes in opportunity for and acceptability of teenage sexual activity. To the extent that more adolescent females with high self-esteem also engage in premarital sex and become pregnant, self-esteem is less likely to predict pregnancy among those reaching adolescence in the 1970s and 1980s than it may have been in previous decades.

Availability of Contraceptives

The extent to which self-esteem, or any other psychosocial variable, predicts pregnancy may depend on the accessibility of contraceptives and contraceptive information or on fears associated with using contraceptives. For example, an adolescent girl with relatively high self-esteem and a desire to attend college may be motivated to prevent pregnancy, though not to the extent of foregoing sexual intercourse with her boyfriend. If she can obtain access to birth control easily, that is, conveniently and privately, she is more likely to use it effectively and to prevent pregnancy than a peer with lower self-esteem and less motivation would be. The more difficult it is to obtain contraceptives, however, or to maintain her privacy in doing so, the greater the probability that she will forego contraception and increase the risk of pregnancy. Thus, to the extent that access to contraceptives varies among the samples of adolescents studied, that access will be a confounding factor in testing the association between self-esteem and pregnancy in adolescence.

Because of these possible confounding factors, we have approached this review of the research on self-esteem and teen pregnancy, first, by eliminating studies in which differences of race or social class confound the results in obvious ways. Thus, a study that compared pregnant adolescents, the large majority of whom were black, with nonpregnant adolescents, the majority of whom were white, was discarded. Second, for the studies included, we note the ethnic or racial composition, social class, and age distribution of the sample and consider the implications of these factors for understanding the results or for limiting our ability to generalize them.

Third, to reduce possible cohort effects, as well as to identify data most relevant to adolescent pregnancy in the late 1980s, we have relied almost entirely on studies of those who reached adolescence in the 1970s or 1980s. This cut-off was selected to correspond to the increase in premarital sexual activity discussed earlier. It does not control entirely for differences in the accessibility of legal abortion as a way to terminate an unwanted pregnancy, a factor that also affects the adolescent pregnancy and birth rates. None of the studies reviewed includes information on abortion. Nor, to our knowledge, has anyone studied the association between self-esteem and the adolescent's decision to abort. We are therefore unable to address this important issue in our review.

Fourth, availability of contraceptives is another confounding factor for which there is no good control. Most studies do not consider access to contraceptives as a predictor of pregnancy, much less as a factor that may confound or interact with self-esteem. Thus, for the most part, we must infer the possible effect of such access from other information presented about the sample. Because this information is usually incomplete, availability of contraceptives will remain a factor that confounds the interpretation of the results of most studies linking self-esteem and teen pregnancy.

Important as these considerations may be to interpreting the reviewed research, the most serious potential confounding factor is the pregnancy itself.

Causal Inferences

The issue in this review is not simply whether adolescents who become pregnant have low self-esteem, but, rather, whether low self-esteem leads in some way to an increased risk of pregnancy during adolescence. To support such an inference, the measure of self-esteem must be obtained before the pregnancy and, for the reasons presented earlier, preferably before premarital sexual intercourse begins. The reason for this is obvious: if self-esteem is measured after the pregnancy or birth, the association may reflect the impact of the pregnancy on self-esteem, rather than the reverse. A pregnancy during adolescence may elicit disapproval and result in a lowering of self-esteem or, alternatively, self-esteem may rise, for reasons suggested above.

From this analysis, we conclude that it will be very difficult indeed to identify a causal link between self-esteem and teenage pregnancy. To support an inference of causality between self-esteem and pregnancy, longitudinal studies are necessary, in which self-esteem is measured before pregnancy and the adolescents are followed over time to determine whether in fact they become pregnant. To reduce the possibility that high self-esteem might be based on deviant rather than normative behavior, these longitudinal studies should begin very early in adolescence, before deviant behaviors are adopted. Unfortunately, very few longitudinal studies have considered adolescent pregnancy as an outcome measure, and an even smaller number have included some measure of self-esteem as a predictor. Our conclusions about the probable role of self-esteem in the etiology of adolescent pregnancy will be based, therefore, on a very small number of studies.

Review of the Research

Adolescent pregnancy is the consequence of engaging in sexual intercourse without adequate contraceptive protection. Thus, to understand the possible effect of low self-esteem on becoming pregnant, we will consider, first, the association between self-esteem and teenage sexual intercourse; second, the association between self-esteem and contraceptive use; and third, the association between self-esteem and pregnancy.

Self-Esteem and Teenage Sexual Intercourse

Four studies have investigated the association between self-esteem and either attitudes toward or actual engagement in sexual intercourse during adolescence (Cvetkovich and Grote 1980; Jessor and Jessor 1975; Herold and Goodwin 1979; and Miller, Christensen, and Olson 1987). Only the Jessor and Jessor study includes longitudinal data. As shown in Table 4.1, no consistent pattern of findings with respect to self-esteem and sexual behavior or attitudes is apparent from these studies.

Only Miller, Christensen, and Olson report a significant correlation between low self-esteem and permissive sexual attitudes and premarital sexual experience. The sample, made up of more than 2,400 males and females between the ages of fourteen and nineteen, was predominantly conservative and Mormon. The association between self-esteem and sexual behavior and permissive attitudes was apparent only for those who attended church weekly. Even in this group, the association was low, indicating that an adolescent's self-esteem provides very little practical information about his or her sexual attitudes and practices. Moreover, because self-esteem measures and sexual information were collected concurrently, it is not possible to determine whether engaging

Table 4.1.   Studies Examining the Association Between Self-Esteem and
              Teenage Sexual Activity/Attitudes

	Sample	Self-Esteem Scale	Association[a]
Self-esteem related to sexual activity			
Herold and Goodwin 1979	486 white females; 13–20 years old	MacKinnon Self-Esteem Scale	Positive
Jessor and Jessor 1975 (longitudinal)	483 white subjects, males and females; grades 9–12	Authors' own ten-item scale	Positive, for males only
Miller, Christensen, and Olson 1987	1,599 females, 824 males; of these, 2,060 were white, 363 Hispanic; 14–19 years old	Rosenberg Self-Esteem Scale	Negative, for active Mormons only
Self-esteem not related to sexual activity			
Cvetkovich and Grote 1980	195 white males, 253 white females, 117 nonwhite males, 119 nonwhite females; 15–18 years old	Personal Characteristics Inventory	

[a] A positive association indicates that high self-esteem is associated with greater sexual permissiveness.

in sexual intercourse produced low self-esteem in this highly religious sample of adolescents, rather than the reverse.

In contrast, two other studies report that high self-esteem was associated either with permissive attitudes toward sexual intercourse or with loss of virginity. Herold and Goodwin (1979) investigated this association in a sample of 486 white females attending birth control clinics in Canada. The young women ranged in age from thirteen to twenty, and most were attending school and living at home. Self-esteem was assessed by the MacKinnon Self-Esteem Scale, a ten-item, five-point scale with good internal validity. High self-esteem correlated with rejection of sexual abstinence, lack of sexual guilt, and endorsement of premarital intercourse involving strong affection; but it did not correlate with approval of intercourse without affection or intercourse with many partners.

We do not know whether the young women who endorsed these views were in fact sexually active, and we cannot therefore rule out the possibility that both permissive attitudes and high self-esteem are the result of that behavior. Nevertheless, these data do confirm that the association between self-esteem and sexual attitudes and behavior may vary with the perceived acceptability of those attitudes and behaviors. If permissive sexual attitudes and behavior are approved in a particular social group, high self-esteem should be associated with those attitudes and behavior, either as a determinant, a consequence, or both.

Jessor and Jessor (1975) investigated the transition from virginity to nonvirginity in a sample of 483 middle-class, Anglo-American students who were tested in each of four years between 1969 and 1972, beginning when they were in junior high school. The authors' self-esteem scale included ten items related to self-evaluation in four areas: intellectual competence, social attractiveness, decision-making ability, and potential for self-development. The scale has good internal validity and moderately high stability over the course of a year. At the fourth testing, when students were in grades ten to thirteen, self-esteem was significantly higher for nonvirgin than for virgin males. Moreover, males who had initially been virgins but reported that they had engaged in sexual intercourse by the time of the fourth testing had higher self-esteem before the sexual experience. This finding is consistent with the interpretation that high rather than low self-esteem leads to sexual intercourse during adolescence, at least for males. The results may be less straightforward than they appear to be, however. The two groups of males differed in other ways that might have affected their sexual behavior (e.g., grades and expectations for achievement), and those who became sexually active admitted to a higher level of general deviance prior to that activity. Thus, the high self-esteem these males reported may have been based on nonnormative rather than normative experiences and would fail for that reason to disprove the expected association between low self-esteem and early sexual intercourse.

The fourth study, by Cvetkovich and Grote (1980), investigated the association between self-esteem and sexual intercourse in a sample of 684 white and nonwhite males and females ranging in age from fifteen to eighteen. Seven intercorrelated items from a thirty-four-item self-reported Personal Characteristics Inventory were combined to form a self-esteem cluster. Self-esteem was not associated with sexual activity for either males or females. Some sexually active females reported, however, that they were likely to become sexually involved because they couldn't say "no," because they wanted to please and satisfy a boyfriend, or because it seemed to be expected of them. No attempt was made to determine whether females who gave this reason for entering into a sexual relationship also had lower self-esteem.

In sum, these studies do not support an association between self-esteem and sexual intercourse during adolescence, perhaps because premarital sexual intercourse can no longer be considered a deviant activity in the culture at large. This is the strongest claim that can be made, although it can be argued that because of design flaws none of the studies can be considered a good test of the hypothesized association. Low self-esteem may account for the behavior of the female adolescents described above, but this is sheer speculation at this point.

Self-Esteem and Use of Contraceptives

Four of the five studies investigating the association between self-esteem and contraceptive use report similar findings: low self-esteem is associated with less frequent or less sustained use of contraceptives. As shown in Table 4.2, the effect is sometimes apparent only for males, or only for females, or only under certain conditions. Always, however, when an effect is present, it is in the same direction. No study demonstrates a link between low self-esteem and effective use of contraceptives.

Two Canadian studies, one by Herold, Goodwin, and Lero (1979) and the other by Hornick, Doran, and Crawford (1979), investigated self-esteem in relation to contraceptive use by females. The sample and the measure in the former study were the same as those used in Herold and Goodwin's (1979) study investigating predictors of sexual attitudes. Females with high self-esteem expressed more positive attitudes toward using birth control pills, were more likely to have used effective contraception at last intercourse, and were more consistent in their use of birth control than were females with low self-esteem. When two groups of "extremes" were compared (sixty-eight users of birth control pills who were renewing their pill prescriptions, and seventy-nine subjects who had never used the pill or an IUD and had come for pregnancy testing), the self-esteem scores of the effective contraceptors were significantly higher than those of the ineffective contraceptors. The researchers conclude that self-esteem influences both attitudes toward and the actual use of contraceptives. They suggest that women who have a low sense of self-esteem may fail to use effective contraceptive methods,

Table 4.2.   Studies Examining the Association Between Self-Esteem and
              Contraceptive Use

	Sample	Self-Esteem Scale	Association[a]
Self-esteem associated with contraceptive use			
Ager, Shea, and Agronow 1982 (longitudinal)	30 white females, 113 nonwhite females; 13–17 years old	Coopersmith Self-Esteem Inventory	Positive, interacting with risk taking
Cvetkovich and Grote 1980	195 white males, 253 white females, 117 nonwhite males, 119 nonwhite females; 15–18 years old	Personal Characteristics Inventory	Positive, for white males only
Herold, Goodwin, and Lero 1979	486 white females; 13–20 years old	MacKinnon Self-Esteem Scale	Positive
Hornick, Doran, and Crawford 1979	144 females, 100 males; high school and university students	Coopersmith Self-Esteem Inventory	Positive, for females only
Self-esteem not associated with contraceptive use			
Rogel and Zuehlke 1982	118 black females, 2 nonblack females; 12–19 years old	Rosenberg Self-Esteem Scale	

[a]A positive association indicates that high self-esteem is associated with more effective use of contraceptives.

first, because the necessary planning would require acknowledging their intention to engage in sexual behavior and, second, because they would be concerned about negative reactions to their use of contraception.

These data on self-esteem and contraceptive use are open, however, to the alternative explanation that adolescents who have not used contraceptives and who believe they may be pregnant may have low self-esteem for precisely that reason. In a follow-up report, Herold and Samson (1980) attempted to address this issue by analyzing the differences between 48 females who had not yet had intercourse and had come to a clinic to obtain birth control and 183 women who were already sexually experienced at the time they visited a birth control clinic. The young women who obtained birth control before initiating sexual activity were older at the time of first intercourse (17.4 years old, as opposed to 16 years old) and had higher educational aspirations than the sexually experienced women. Unfortunately, no statistical tests were reported, and the measure of self-esteem was not mentioned.

The Hornick, Doran, and Crawford (1979) study of contraceptive use among sexually active adolescents was based on responses from 144 female and 100 male high school and university students in south-central Ontario. (No other sample characteristics were given.) Contraception included the high-risk methods of withdrawal and rhythm, as well as the low-risk methods of the birth control pill and the IUD. The average age of the high school females was 17; the average age for males was 16.9. The mean age of the university students was greater, 19.3 years for females and 20.1 years for males. Because only some of the respondents were adolescents and the data were analyzed for the combined sample, we can draw only limited generalizations about adolescents from this study. Nonetheless, the subject's age did not emerge as a "best predictor" of contraceptive use for either males or females, and the results are consistent with those of Herold, Goodwin, and Lero (1979). Along with a number of other variables, high self-esteem, as measured by the Coopersmith Self-Esteem Inventory, was associated with greater contraceptive use by females; this was not the case for males.

Ager, Shea, and Agronow (1982) studied 143 clients of a Planned Parenthood teen clinic for eighteen months, from the time the clients first came to the clinic to obtain contraceptives. All the subjects were female, 79 percent were black, and most lived in Detroit. Their ages ranged from thirteen to seventeen; the median age was 16.1 years at the start of the study. Continuance or discontinuance of contraception was charted over time, and reasons for discontinuance were investigated. The most frequent reasons given for discontinuing use of the birth control pill were experiencing side effects (42 percent) and fearing side effects (17 percent). Eleven percent indicated that the distance to the clinic or its eventual closing contributed to their decision to discontinue contraception. Self-esteem, as measured by the Coopersmith Inventory, did not differentiate those who continued and those who discontinued using birth control pills.

When the risk-taking behavior of the adolescents was identified, however, those with low reported self-esteem or a high inclination to take risks were significantly more likely to discontinue using the pill upon experiencing side effects than were those with high self-esteem and a low risk-taking personality. That is, the impact of side effects on behavior depended on the adolescent's personal characteristics. If she had high self-esteem and was a low risk-taker, she continued using the pill despite the side effects. From these data, we may infer that although many factors influence an adolescent's decision to discontinue using a "more effective" method of birth control, having high self-esteem, perhaps in combination with other characteristics, may influence her to persevere in using such a method, despite the difficulties.

In the studies described above, high self-esteem was associated with some measure of contraceptive use for females. Only one of these studies included both males and females in the sample and, again, the association between self-esteem and contraception was apparent only for females.

This was not the case in the only other study to report results for both male and female adolescents (Cvetkovich and Grote 1980). The characteristics of the sample and the self-esteem measure have been described earlier. In this study, contraceptive use was defined as the frequency with which some effective form of contraception had been used by either partner during intercourse in the previous three months. For white males only, more effective contraceptors reported higher self-esteem and did not relegate the responsibility for birth control to their female partners. They also disagreed with items implying that it was sometimes all right to chance a pregnancy.

Only Rogel and Zuehlke's (1982) study of contraceptive behavior in adolescence failed to find an association between contraceptive use and self-esteem. The 120 females who participated in the study ranged in age from twelve to nineteen, were predominantly black (98 percent), and were recruited from three clinics at the Michael Reese Hospital in Chicago in 1979. The majority of the girls were sexually active, and 75 percent either were or had been pregnant at the time of the study. The median age of first pregnancy was 15.6 years, with 81 percent of the pregnancies occurring by age seventeen. Self-esteem, measured by the Rosenberg Self-Esteem Scale, tended to be unusually high for the entire sample: 46 percent scored high on the scale (30 or higher on a scale that ranges from a low of 10 to a high of 40), and no one scored below 25. The high level and narrow range of self-esteem scores may explain why self-esteem failed to distinguish those who began contraception early from those who began late and from those who never used birth control.

The range of self-esteem scores does not explain why self-esteem should have been so unusually high in this group of adolescents. It may have been the result, as Kaplan (1975) argues, of the sexual activity and the heterosexual relationships with which that activity is associated. The researchers suggest that girls may use sexual activity as a means of attaining intimacy and closeness with a valued person outside the family; they point out that most of the girls had infrequent sex with only one sexual partner, whom they had known for more than a year. Participation in the relationship may have bolstered self-esteem, resulting in a surprisingly high level of self-esteem in the sample and in the process obscuring any association that might have existed initially between low self-esteem and failure to use contraception. This interpretation, although speculative, is consistent with Kaplan's prediction that measures of self-esteem obtained after deviant behavior has been adopted may be the result rather than the cause of that behavior.

In sum, there is evidence linking high self-esteem to more effective use of contraception among sexually active adolescents. Because none of the studies controlled entirely for the possibility that pregnancy or guilt associated with not using contraception might account for the lower self-esteem reported by the less effective users, any causal inference must be tentative. Moreover, in the research available to date, high self-esteem has been associated with effective contraception primarily for white adolescents, thereby limiting the applicability of these findings to other groups. Nevertheless, there is sufficient correlational evidence to further consider a possible causal link between self-esteem and contraceptive use.

Self-Esteem and Teen Pregnancy

Although there have been numerous studies of the correlates of teenage pregnancy, we located only seven that both included a measure of self-esteem and met our review criteria. Four of the studies examined self-esteem only after the adolescents became pregnant (Barth, Schinke, and Maxwell 1983; Brunswick 1971; Streetman 1987; and Werner and Smith 1977). In two of these, there was no association between self-esteem and pregnancy status. In the other two, the self-esteem scores of pregnant girls were significantly lower than those of girls in the control groups.

Brunswick (1971) collected data on 483 low-income males and females between the ages of twelve and seventeen in 1969–1970. Because 86 percent of the subjects were black, most of the pregnant teenagers were black. The median age at first pregnancy was fifteen. The 16 adolescents who were pregnant or who had already carried a baby to term were compared with 180 others on a self-esteem measure composed of three items from Rosenberg's scale and a fourth that asked the adolescent how much she would want to change herself if she could. There were no differences between the two groups either on the self-esteem measure or in their general mood or feelings of happiness. The pregnant women did report greater feelings of powerlessness, but, as the author points out, this may have reflected an accurate assessment of their life situation at the time.

In a more recent study, Streetman (1987) compared non-Caucasian teenage females without children to a group of teenage mothers and reported similar results. The sample included 93 females between the ages of fourteen and nineteen. More than 75 percent had at least one child. There were no differences between the groups on either the Coopersmith Self-Esteem Inventory or the Rosenberg Self-Esteem Scale.

Barth, Schinke, and Maxwell (1983) used a more sophisticated design and a more diverse sample in their study of pregnant adolescents. Participants were 185 young women, ranging in age from eleven to twenty-one, from three programs for school-aged parents and the alternative public high schools in which these programs operated. The schools were located in urban, suburban, and rural areas. Also unlike the previously discussed studies, only 49 percent of the young women were black; the rest were predominantly Anglo, with small percentages of Native Americans, Asians, and Hispanics. There were 62 pregnant females, 63 adolescent parents, and a comparison group of 60 female adolescents who were neither pregnant nor parents. The three groups were compared on five measures of well-being, including the Rosenberg Self-Esteem Scale. The self-esteem scores of both the pregnant teenagers and the adolescent parents were lower than those of the comparison group. Moreover, these differences continued to be significant after controlling statistically for differences associated with the adolescent's age, social class, and social support. Race does not appear to have affected the results, but this is not entirely clear from the report. In contrast to the Brunswick and Streetman studies, Barth, Schinke, and Maxwell used a larger sample of pregnant adolescents, distinguished between pregnant adolescents and adolescent parents, and controlled for a number of potential confounding factors, suggesting that their results should be given more weight.

A longitudinal study by Werner and Smith (1977) provides additional evidence for a link between low self-esteem and teen pregnancy.

The authors studied all the children born on the island of Kauai in 1955. During the eighteen-year follow-up conducted in 1973, the twenty-eight females who had become pregnant were compared with all other females in the sample. The teens who had become pregnant before turning eighteen differed from the comparison group on a large number of dimensions, including self-esteem as measured by a subset of questions from the California Personality Inventory. As in the Barth, Schinke, and Maxwell study, the pregnant teenagers had significantly lower self-esteem.

Because Werner and Smith's research was longitudinal, it was possible to investigate whether there were any childhood signs that indicated the risk of an early pregnancy. Unlike the children who later were identified as delinquents, those who became pregnant had not been identified as having a disproportionate number of learning disabilities or mental health problems at the age of ten. The variables at this age that did differentiate those who would become pregnant as teenagers were the family's social-economic status, the provision of educational stimulation, and ethnic background. Girls most likely to become pregnant were from the poorest families, with the least educational stimulation, and were at least part native Hawaiian—a group the authors described as valuing a nurturant maternal role and prizing children highly. No measure of self-esteem was obtained at age ten, and the measure of emotional support—a possible contributor to self-esteem—failed to distinguish the pregnant and nonpregnant adolescents, although emotional support was somewhat more likely to be associated with subsequent pregnancy for the non-Hawaiians (Werner 1988). Only three of the twelve Hawaiians who were pregnant were identified as receiving little emotional support when they were ten years old, whereas nine of the sixteen pregnant non-Hawaiians were so identified. The small sample and the level of statistical significance ($p < .10$) preclude any definite conclusions, but this finding does suggest that different factors may be causally linked to adolescent pregnancy in different ethnic or racial groups.

In sum, although the cross-sectional studies of self-esteem and teenage pregnancy yield no consistent pattern of findings, the better-designed research links low self-esteem to adolescent pregnancy. Consistent with the studies on self-esteem and contraceptive use, no study shows self-esteem to be higher for pregnant than for nonpregnant adolescents. We must emphasize, however, that these results do not necessarily demonstrate that low self-esteem increases the risk of pregnancy during adolescence. An equally plausible inference is that an adolescent pregnancy lowers self-esteem.

Three longitudinal studies offer a better test of the hypothesis that low self-esteem increases the likelihood of a teenage pregnancy. All three measured self-esteem at one point and later obtained information on pregnancies that subsequently occurred. Two of the three, based on the same data set studied at different time intervals, reported an association between low self-esteem and subsequent pregnancy; the third study reported no association.

Kaplan, Smith, and Pokorny (1979) obtained their sample from a 1971 survey of seventh-graders in a large urban school system. The survey included the Self-Derogation Scale as a measure of self-esteem. More than one year after the administration of the baseline questionnaire (and before each subject's eighteenth birthday), the researchers identified eighty-two adolescents who had given birth to their first child. (Evidence of birth was obtained from a clinic that provided perinatal services to the indigent, pregnant adolescents of the county.) The authors contrasted the unwed mothers with two comparison groups: one in which each unwed mother was matched with two adolescents by race, mother's education, and school; and one consisting of random controls selected from the female respondents from the baseline survey in seventh grade. Racial makeup was the only significant demographic difference between the groups: 90 percent of the unwed mothers and the matched comparison group were black, whereas only 25 percent of the subjects in the random control group were black.

Before becoming pregnant, the adolescents who later became unwed mothers were significantly more likely to have reported self-devaluing experiences associated with family and school and were less likely to have perceived themselves as succeeding, either at the time or in the future, than were the adolescents in either control group. They were also more likely to have had higher self-derogation scores (low self-esteem). Thus, low self-esteem as a result of family and school experiences distinguished adolescents who had babies from those who did not. Moreover, the black adolescents who did not become mothers thought it was more important to obey their parents and teachers than did those who had children. Together, these findings support Kaplan's (1975) theory that if children have positive family and school experiences, they feel good about themselves. They will want to maintain the good will and respect of the people in these situations and will behave in ways that they believe will ensure this.

The second analysis of this 1971 data set is reported by Robbins, Kaplan, and Martin (1985). To obtain information on out of wedlock pregnancies, 2,158 young adults (both males and females) from the original sample were contacted again when they were twenty-one years old. Of this later group of subjects, 63 percent were white, 27 percent black, and 10 percent Hispanic, indicating that the original group of unwed adolescent mothers and their matched controls, both of which were predominantly black, were underrepresented in this follow-up. Six items from the Self-Derogation Scale were used as a measure of self-esteem (alpha = .79). The findings with respect to self-esteem were weaker than in the earlier report, as would be anticipated, given that the researchers obtained pregnancy data retrospectively from the adolescents themselves and that those identified as unwed mothers in the earlier study were underrepresented. Nonetheless, high self-derogation in seventh grade was significantly associated with a higher risk of pregnancy before age twenty-one for females. From additional analyses, it could be inferred that the association between self-derogation and pregnancy was limited to ages twelve to fifteen during the three years following the original testing, corresponding most closely to the period in the 1979 study by Kaplan, Smith, and Pokorny.

Additional findings indicate, however, that self-derogation may have different effects at different ages under different conditions. First, family stress was positively related to pregnancy when self-esteem (low self-derogation) was moderate or high for young women over eighteen. The authors suggest this may reflect a rejection of parental control in late adolescence by self-confident girls. Second, although the Hispanic girls in this study were significantly more likely than others to have high self-derogation scores, they were less likely than either whites or blacks to become pregnant out of wedlock during adolescence. This finding may indicate that other characteristics of Hispanic culture, such as religious affiliation or the degree of control exercised by the family over the adolescent's behavior, result in a lower adolescent pregnancy rate. This could occur, for example, if Hispanic parents encourage adolescents to marry at an earlier age than that favored by parents from different ethnic or racial backgrounds.

These two studies provide the clearest evidence that low self-esteem is causally associated with a subsequent teenage pregnancy. Another longitudinal study failed to confirm these findings, however. Vernon, Green, and Frothingham (1983) questioned 858 low-income females between the ages of thirteen and nineteen, predominantly black (86 per-

Table 4.3.   Studies Examining the Association Between Self-Esteem and
              Teenage Pregnancy

	Sample	Self-Esteem Scale	Association[a]
Self-esteem related to teenage pregnancy			
Barth, Schinke, and Maxwell 1983	117 nonwhite females, 68 white females; 11–21 years old	Rosenberg Self-Esteem Scale	Negative
Kaplan, Smith, and Pokorny 1979 (longitudinal)	410 females	Self-Derogation Scale	Negative
Robbins, Kaplan, and Martin 1985 (longitudinal)	2,158 males and females; white, black, and Hispanic	Self-Derogation Scale	Negative, for females only
Werner and Smith 1977 (longitudinal)	614 males and females; 18 years old	California Personality Inventory	Negative
Self-esteem not related to teenage pregnancy			
Brunswick 1971	196 black females; 12–17 years old	Rosenberg Self-Esteem Scale (subset)	
Streetman 1987	93 nonwhite females; 14–19 years old	Coopersmith Self-Esteem Inventory; Rosenberg Self-Esteem Scale	
Vernon, Green, and Frothingham 1983 (longitudinal)	745 black females, 22 other nonwhite females, 91 white females; 13–19 years old	Coopersmith Self-Esteem Inventory	

[a]A negative association indicates that low self-esteem is associated with a greater risk of becoming pregnant during adolescence.

cent), who were enrolled in the ninth, tenth, and eleventh grades during the fall of 1980. Ninety-five of the subjects later became pregnant. The researchers measured self-esteem (using the Coopersmith Inventory) at the initial testing, as well as pregnancy outcome during the following year using reports from local clinical and laboratory facilities that provided health services. They found no differences in pregnancy rates for young women who scored in the low, intermediate, or high self-esteem groups. The pregnancy rate was higher, however, among those girls for whom the costs of pregnancy might be assumed to be lower: those who had lower vocational expectations, who attended church less often, and who had indicated that they would like or not mind being pregnant and would expect that their families would feel similarly about a pregnancy.

Table 4.3 indicates that studies investigating the association between self-esteem and teen pregnancy report mixed results. Only four studies (and three data sets) corroborate the anticipated association between low self-esteem and teenage pregnancy.

The failure to replicate findings is often sufficient reason to discount or to treat cautiously the results of a particular investigation. In this instance, however, the contradictory findings can be explained and indeed would have been expected from Kaplan's (1975) theory of the way in which engaging in deviant behavior may improve self-esteem. Participants in the Vernon, Green, and Frothingham (1983) study were in the ninth through eleventh grades at the time self-esteem was initially assessed, in contrast to the subjects in the other longitudinal studies, who were in the seventh grade. It is reasonable to assume that many of the older subjects had already become sexually active or had engaged in deviant behavior that would have increased their self-esteem. In short, although the observed association between low self-esteem and teenage pregnancy has not been well replicated, the design of those studies that have demonstrated such an association increases our confidence in the validity of the association.

Summary of the Review

What can we reasonably conclude from this review? Given the disparate results and the differences in design of the studies, reasonable people could justifiably draw different inferences from the data. Our approach is to make the strongest case possible, given the research, for the existence of a causal link between self-esteem and teenage pregnancy.

We conclude, therefore, that low self-esteem does contribute to the risk of an adolescent pregnancy. Although it is likely to be valid, the association between low self-esteem and pregnancy· is not strong. This finding, combined with evidence that a number of characteristics, conditions, or circumstances lead to an increased risk of pregnancy during adolescence, suggests that our understanding of teen pregnancy must be multifaceted.

We conclude also that self-esteem is more likely to have an impact on teenage pregnancy through its effect on increasing contraceptive use than through any effect it might be expected to have on reducing pre-marital sexual intercourse. There simply is no compelling evidence on which to base a claim that increasing self-esteem will reduce the number of teenagers who engage in premarital sex. Even if some teenagers engage in sex out of esteem-related interests, we would not expect raising self-esteem to have a major impact on adolescent sexual behavior, because so many other factors influence decisions regarding sexual activity.

In contrast, we believe the data, though imperfect, are consistent with the expectation that raising normatively based self-esteem would increase contraceptive use by both *males* and females, thereby reducing adolescent pregnancy. Adolescents with higher normatively based self-esteem would be more likely to have goals that would be compromised by an early pregnancy; they would thus be more motivated to practice effective contraception. They would presumably also be more willing to deal with the potential embarrassment and inconvenience often associated with obtaining and using contraceptives.

We had hoped to comment on the applicability of the findings to different ethnic or racial groups, but the relatively few studies that include adolescents from more than one group or analyze the association between self-esteem and outcome separately by race or ethnicity preclude this. We recommend caution in generalizing findings, because different factors may be causally linked to adolescent pregnancy in different ethnic or racial groups. To illustrate: Adolescents belonging to a recent immigrant group, the Hmong from Laos, are considered young adults by the age of thirteen and traditionally bear children soon after (Chan 1981). This cultural expectation may account for the group's inflated adolescent birth rate and would have to be considered in any attempt to reduce teenage pregnancy within this group.

The relatively high incidence of births to black adolescents noted throughout the chapter raises another important question: Do differences in self-esteem contribute to racial differences in the birth rate among adolescents? We have no data directly relevant to this question, for the reasons noted earlier. Even if black children are no more likely than others to develop low self-esteem, however, the conditions that give rise to low self-esteem may be more impervious to change for black children. To the extent that the opportunities for achievement are more restricted for blacks than for whites, attempts to raise self-esteem by focusing on families, schools, and community organizations may be seriously undermined.

Implications for Reducing Adolescent Pregnancy

It is beyond the scope of this review to fully consider all the factors associated with adolescent pregnancy. Nonetheless, even a cursory review of the research literature reveals numerous correlates of adolescent pregnancy, at least some of which also affect the likelihood of becoming pregnant (Hayes 1987b). Thus, attempts to reduce the incidence of adolescent pregnancy are not likely to be effective without using a multifaceted approach. We must keep this in mind when considering the potential impact of raising self-esteem.

Building Self-Esteem

As noted earlier, positive self-esteem results from experiences in membership groups that convey the idea that the individual possesses positively valued attributes, performs positively valued behaviors, and is the object of positive attitudes expressed by highly valued others. To the extent that these experiences occur in so-called normative membership groups such as the family and school, family- and school-related achievements and participation will be valued. If achievements and participation in these groups are incompatible with a pregnancy, the individual would be motivated to avoid it. In Luker's (1975) terms, the cost of a pregnancy to the adolescent would be high.

Thus, to encourage high self-esteem, we must consider the experiences of children and adolescents in their everyday environments. Our intent is not to design programs to promote high self-esteem, but rather to identify the kinds of family, school, and community experiences that should lead to higher self-esteem in children and adolescents.

Families

In the sample used in the study by Kaplan, Smith, and Pokorny (1979), adolescents who later became unwed mothers received the highest scores on measures of subjectively perceived self-devaluing experiences associated with family, school, and peers, as well as the highest self-derogation (lowest self-esteem) scores. The nature of those experiences was not described, but from other measures of maternal rejection we may infer that such experiences generally have to do with the extent to which parents convey that they enjoy spending time with the child, recognize and appreciate the child's characteristics and achievements, and avoid harsh criticism when the child engages in disapproved behavior (Coopersmith 1967; Sears 1970). It is reasonable to argue that family experiences characterized by this sort of "positive communication" form the basis of a child's positive or high self-esteem. Attempts to build this type of communication should therefore be at the center of efforts to reduce adolescent pregnancy by building self-esteem. To our knowledge, no program designed to prevent or reduce adolescent pregnancy has adopted this approach.

Kaplan, Smith, and Pokorny also report that the parents of the girls who did not become pregnant, but who were otherwise matched with those who did, consistently exerted social control over their children— control that the girls perceived as legitimate. This finding suggests that attempts to control adolescent behavior that are not firmly rooted in the adolescent's willingness to accept the control may be ill fated. The adolescent's perception of social control as legitimate depends in part on how the control is exercised (positive communication) and also on how salient the parents have been as sources of the adolescent's esteem-bolstering experiences. We may conclude that the enterprise of building self-esteem must begin well before the onset of adolescence if it is to affect adolescent pregnancy.

The effective exercise of social control by parents may be facilitated by contact with other families. In the Kaplan, Smith, and Pokorny study, the families of the girls who were at risk but did not become pregnant were likely to have lived in the area for more than five years and to have known one another well. This contact between families may have played an important role in establishing the legitimacy of familial control. If one family establishes rules that are at odds with those established by the families of the adolescent's friends, the adolescent may perceive the action as unreasonable and as a personal statement about how the parents view him or her. The adolescent in such a family also may successfully undermine those rules by pressuring parents to be more lenient. Thus, a family's ability to promote self-esteem and to exercise control over adolescent behavior may be facilitated by supportive connections with other, like-minded families. Encouraging such connections where they do not already exist may be one facet of successful programs to prevent teenage pregnancy.

Of course, families cannot always provide the kind of experiences that seem to be important in building self-esteem and exercising legitimate control over teenagers' behavior. Families may be split, and one parent may have to assume all the responsibilities that are shared in two-parent families. If the family is intact, the parents may have personal problems, sometimes linked to conditions of poverty, that may make simple survival, rather than the well-being of any one family member, the primary focus of the family. For children in such families, high self-esteem may be better encouraged by someone other than the parents. Indeed, given the number of mothers who are employed outside the home today (49.3 percent of those with children under six in 1986 [U.S. Department of Labor 1986]), even children in well-functioning families may be spending as much time with other adults, including teachers, as they do with their own parents. And of course these other adults may play an important role in encouraging high self-esteem.

Support for the value of alternative adult contacts for adolescents comes from Vincent (1961; cited in Kaplan, Smith, and Pokorny 1979), who reported that the only major difference between pregnant girls who had been rejected or had withdrawn from their parents and similar nonpregnant girls was that the nonpregnant girls had identified with a teacher or some other adult in the community who offered acceptance and counseled against premarital sex. Schools and other community organizations may therefore be an important aspect of attempts to raise self-esteem and reduce teenage pregnancy.

Schools

If positive experiences in school contribute to positive self-esteem, then ways must be found to make school a positive experience for children—not just for some children, but for all the children who are required to be there.

Success in school is defined primarily as achieving good grades, or at least as "passing." Intervening with children who are doing poorly in their schoolwork is thus essential to any school-based attempt to raise self-esteem. What that intervention should be remains to be determined. We do know, however, that the quality of schools—as measured by staff training, availability of learning resources, and teacher/student ratios— affects achievement and school retention, especially among the poor and racial and ethnic minorities (Rutter 1983).

Even if such interventions are effective in reducing failure, substantial differences in achievement among children are likely to remain, and some children will experience these differences as failures. One implication of this reality is the need to design a range of acceptable academic goals, along with alternative educational strategies. This has taken place already at the secondary level, in the form of alternative schools that stress individualized learning, counseling, social supports, remedial education, and work-study arrangements. Programs such as these not only reduce some of the more invidious comparisons between students, because "high achievers" are elsewhere, but also incorporate opportunities for success through work. Although assessments indicate that alternative programs can be effective in keeping young people in school and in boosting achievement, there are no data on whether such programs lower pregnancy rates (Hofferth 1987a).

We have focused thus far on achievement as the basis for success, positive responses from others, and subsequent positive feelings toward the self. Kaplan (1975) also concluded that high self-esteem is based on the perception, derived from group membership, that one possesses positively valued attributes and is the object of positive attitudes from highly valued others. These positive experiences can occur even in the face of failure, through communication between students and teachers—what is communicated about the child or adolescent, and how it is communicated, conveys whether the student is liked, appreciated, and respected. This dimension of the school experience is incorporated as "social support" in the alternative-school approach. Its value is suggested by Rutter's (1983) finding that disadvantaged children achieved more in schools in which teachers made more positive comments to them. As suggested earlier, another consequence of what we have referred to as positive communication may be that the school becomes or remains a legitimate source of control over the adolescent's behavior.

Communities

To the extent that programs such as Girl Scouts, 4-H, church groups, and team sports provide experiences that build competence and encourage relationships that convey appreciation, self-esteem should be affected positively when children and teenagers participate in them. The character and quality of the experiences and relationships identified earlier as determinants of high self-esteem are the same for any context, and we will not repeat them here. The special value of community groups is that children and adolescents participate voluntarily, in contrast to their participation in family or school life, and for that reason they may be motivated to engage fully in the activities. Training in child development, and especially in positive communication, for adult volunteer leaders and coaches, and a screening process to identify adults who lack the necessary skills to build and maintain high self-esteem are important to ensure that children benefit from their experiences in community programs.

Summary

We have suggested that attempts to reduce the incidence of adolescent pregnancy by building self-esteem should focus on, but not be limited to, the school and the family. We have left unspecified, however, the effect that high self-esteem may have on adolescent behavior. One effect could be to increase the age at which teenagers engage in premarital sexual intercourse. Although there is no evidence that self-esteem directly affects sexual behavior, there is evidence that age of first intercourse tends to be earlier for adolescents with lower school achievement. Thus, raising achievement level might be expected to influence sexual behavior. Moreover, individuals with high self-esteem may decide to become sexually active for reasons different from those of individuals with low self-esteem. For example, an adolescent with high self-esteem may engage in sex because she is involved in a loving relationship, whereas an adolescent with low self-esteem may do so because she is afraid of being rejected.

We argued earlier that the stronger link between self-esteem and pregnancy appears to be mediated by contraceptive use: adolescents with high self-esteem are more likely to use effective contraception. From this, we may conclude that attempts to build self-esteem will have a stronger effect on the incidence of adolescent pregnancy if they are linked with encouraging both sexes to use contraception. If families encourage high self-esteem and at the same time convey the unacceptability of using contraceptives, they must focus their efforts on preventing sexual intercourse—a difficult task, if the available research is to be trusted. Moreover, if they are unsuccessful, they may be faced with a choice between an abortion, which may be even less acceptable to them than contraceptive use, or a birth to an adolescent mother, which carries its own negative consequences. Thus, it seems reasonable to suggest that reducing adolescent pregnancies through raising self-esteem will be considerably more successful if such efforts are accompanied by information about, access to, and permission to use contraceptives.

There is another twist in the association between self-esteem and contraceptive use. Luker (1975) argues that women weigh the perceived cost of a pregnancy against the cost of preventing the pregnancy. Thus, the higher the psychological cost of obtaining contraceptives, the less likely the adolescent will be to try to obtain them. This cost may be particularly high for adolescents with low self-esteem, who may lack the assurance and assertiveness required to obtain and fill prescriptions in a context that lacks privacy and invites criticism. Reducing that cost should increase the probability that contraceptives will be used. If we acknowledge that self-esteem is most likely to affect teenage pregnancy through its effect on contraceptive use, it would seem self-defeating not to simultaneously attempt to make it easier for adolescents to obtain contraceptives.

Needed Research

Research of two types is needed to further our understanding of self-esteem as it relates to adolescent pregnancy and to determine how the adolescent pregnancy rate might be reduced. First, we need longitudinal studies designed to identify the characteristics and conditions that put an adolescent at risk for a pregnancy. Available research linking low self-esteem with adolescent pregnancy is suggestive, rather than compelling; the better studies are twenty years old; and few data are available on pregnancy among different ethnic groups, most notably Hispanics. In California, where almost 15 percent of Hispanic births in 1985 were to teenagers, in contrast to 7.9 percent of non-Hispanic white, 4.2 percent of Asian, and 18.2 percent of black births (Brindis and Jeremy 1988), this knowledge is critical. Second, we need research investigating the effects of programs designed to enhance self-esteem and to reduce the adolescent pregnancy rate.

Longitudinal Studies

We can identify several criteria against which any proposal for research on self-esteem and adolescent pregnancy should be evaluated. First, the research should be conceptually based; decisions about measures and analyses should be guided by well-developed ideas of the factors that might explain the likelihood of an adolescent pregnancy.

Second, the research should focus on many variables, not just one or two. Low self-esteem may predict adolescent pregnancy only in combination with other characteristics of the adolescent or her environment. By including multiple variables, we will be better able to discern such complexities. Race/ethnicity is one such variable; social-economic status is another. To design effective prevention efforts, we need to know whether different factors explain the incidence of adolescent pregnancy in different ethnic groups that vary in degree of acculturation (Becerra and de Anda 1984).

Third, the study should begin prior to the onset of puberty. Using chronological age as a marker variable, the first phase of data collection should begin no later than the child's tenth birthday, to reduce the possibility that sexual activity has already contributed to high or low self-esteem.

Fourth, the research should consider both process and outcome in studying adolescent pregnancy. We need to know not simply that the adolescent has or has not become pregnant, but whether she has been sexually active, whether she has used effective contraception, and her reasons for doing or not doing so.

Research on Prevention

Another approach to research is to test the effectiveness of programs designed to reduce the number of teenage pregnancies by raising self-esteem. We know from past experience that experimental social programs will be short-lived unless their effectiveness in meeting stated goals can be demonstrated convincingly. Prevention studies must have control groups; control groups and experimental groups must be comparable before intervention (with respect to self-esteem, ethnicity, achievement, age, or any other variable that may affect the likelihood of a teenage pregnancy); and researchers must obtain outcome data on sexual behavior, contraceptive use, and pregnancy over a significant period of time.

Equally important, the prevention programs must have a reasonable chance of succeeding. Success will be more likely if the programs are appropriate to the group they are intended to serve and if individuals at risk for an adolescent pregnancy, or adults in contact with them, participate in the programs. Ensuring that this will happen is one of the primary challenges of prevention programs and prevention-oriented research.

Appendix: Measures of Self-Esteem

In measuring any psychological construct, we want to know that the instrument accurately reflects the theoretical construct on which it is based and truthfully assesses the individual's internal reality. The first issue can be addressed by the measure's "face validity"—the extent to which individuals familiar with the theoretical construct agree that the measure adequately represents the construct; its "internal validity"—the degree to which the items in the measure intercorrelate, indicating a degree of psychological unity; and its "convergent validity"—the extent to which the measure is associated with other measures of the same construct.

Three additional types of evidence are relevant to determining whether the measure accurately describes the individual. The first is test-retest reliability—the extent to which individuals achieve the same scores relative to others in the sample over a short period of time, typically a few days to a few weeks. High test-retest reliability is consistent with the interpretation that the measure reflects something relatively enduring about the individual, rather than a fleeting or momentary mood state. The other two types of evidence are concurrent and predictive validity—the extent to which scores on the measure correlate with some other relevant measures assessed either at the same time (concurrently) or over a longer period (predictively).

Information concerning the reliability and validity of the three measures of self-esteem used most frequently in the studies we review—the Rosenberg Self-Esteem Scale (1965), the Coopersmith Self-Esteem Inventory (1967), and the Self-Derogation Scale from Kaplan, Smith, and Pokorny (1979)—is included below. We provide information on other measures when describing the individual study.

Rosenberg Self-Esteem Scale

The Rosenberg Self-Esteem Scale consists of ten items (e.g., "On the whole, I am satisfied with myself"), with one of four responses possible for each item: respondents are asked to strongly agree, agree, disagree, or strongly disagree with each test item.

Three properties of the measure are worth noting. First, the scale is designed to measure the respondents' *global self-esteem*. The items do not specify particular areas of activity or qualities that individuals must take into consideration when judging themselves. The scale attempts to gauge a respondent's basic attitude toward his or her own worth by allowing individuals to invoke their own frame of reference. Second, the scale is designed to capture the respondent's enduring, longstanding self-estimate. The emphasis is not on one's immediate or momentary self-perception; rather, the scale stresses the more permanent, more stable components of the self-image. Finally, a high score on this scale does not mean that the respondent stands in awe of himself or herself, nor does it mean that a respondent expects such awe or deference from others. Rather, it reflects the feeling that one is "good enough"—a person of worth, who merits self-respect.

The psychometric properties of this scale have been summarized by Wylie (1974). She points out that the Rosenberg Scale's face validity appears to be good and that its convergence with other measures of self-esteem is acceptably high, ranging from .67 to .83. A two-week test-retest reliability coefficient is similarly high—.85 for twenty-eight college-age respondents. In addition, the scale appears to have the ability to predict and concur with behaviors, attitudes, and experiences to which self-esteem is theoretically expected to be related (e.g., depressive affect, anxiety and psychosomatic symptoms, interpersonal insecurity, participation in activities, leadership, and parental disinterest).

Regarding the scale's ability to provide an accurate assessment of the individual's internal reality, there remains, as there does for all self-concept measures, the possibility that respondents may distort reality in order to provide socially desirable answers. Researchers hope that if they are able to establish rapport and guarantee anonymity, respondents will answer truthfully.

Coopersmith Self-Esteem Inventory

The Coopersmith Self-Esteem Inventory (SEI) for children is a fifty-item questionnaire intended to measure the evaluation that children from ages eight to fifteen make and customarily maintain with regard to themselves. The questionnaire presents respondents with generally favorable or generally unfavorable statements about the self (e.g., "I am pretty sure of myself," "I'm easy to like"), which they designate as "like me" or "unlike me." Assuming that self-efficacy may vary across different areas of experience, Coopersmith includes questions from five different domains: peers, family, self, school, and general social activities.

The scores from these subscales are combined for a general self-esteem score. The scale is accompanied by an eight-item lie scale to assess defensiveness.

Coopersmith developed the measure with the assistance of several "self-esteem experts," and all the items in the final scale were agreed upon by five psychologists, supporting the scale's face validity. Coopersmith, like many self-esteem researchers, assumes that one's global self-esteem score consists of the sum of scores in five separate areas, as described above. Whether or not this assumption is valid is not known, for no item analyses or internal factor analyses have been performed. Wylie (1974) reports low to moderate convergence, ranging from .17 to .40, between scores on the Coopersmith SEI and other measures of self-esteem, as well as similarly moderate correlations with measures to which self-esteem is theoretically expected to be associated (e.g., the Iowa Achievement Tests, $r = .36$; and a sociometric rating of popularity, $r = .29$). Test-retest reliability is high: .88 over a five-week interval for fifth graders (Coopersmith 1967).

Coopersmith attempts to control for acquiescent responses by including an equal number of favorably and unfavorably worded items. Again, it is hoped that guaranteeing anonymity and establishing rapport with the respondents will cause them to answer truthfully rather than providing socially desirable answers.

Self-Derogation Scale

Kaplan's self-derogation scale consists of the seven items that make up the first factor derived from a factor analysis of the Rosenberg Scale (Kaplan and Pokorny 1969). The scale indexes a lack of pride and self-respect and feelings of personal failure and worthlessness. Thus a low score indicates high self-esteem. Because the scale is made up of items from the Rosenberg Self-Esteem Scale, we may presume it is equally valid on its face.

The inter-item correlations for the seven items making up the scale, as reported by Kaplan (1980), are not high but are statistically significant. The scale's internal consistency is estimated at .79 (Cronbach's alpha) (Robbins, Kaplan, and Martin 1985). Kaplan does not report the scale's convergence with other measures of self-esteem, but it may be presumed that its convergent validity does not differ appreciably from the Rosenberg Self-Esteem Scale, on which it is based.

Unlike Coopersmith, Kaplan does not expect high long-term test-retest reliability scores, especially for children with low self-esteem. Accordingly, test-retest correlations ranged from .55 (over one year) to .40 (over a two-year interval) during adolescence. In addition, Kaplan and Pokorny (1969) report that high scores on the self-derogation scale are associated with several measures of psychosocial adjustment, including self-reports of psychological symptoms, scores on a depressive affect scale, and use of psychiatric services during the preceding year.

Bibliography

Ager, J. W., F. P. Shea, and S. J. Agronow. 1982. "Method Discontinuance in Teenage Women: Implications for Teen Contraceptive Programs." In *Pregnancy in Adolescence: Needs, Problems, and Management,* edited by I. R. Stuart and C. F. Wells, 236–263. New York: Van Nostrand Reinhold.

Barth, R. P., S. P. Schinke, and J. S. Maxwell. 1983. "Psychological Correlates of Teenage Motherhood." *Journal of Youth and Adolescence* 12 (6): 471–481.

Becerra, R. M., and D. de Anda. 1984. "Pregnancy and Motherhood Among Mexican-American Adolescents." *Health and Social Work* 9 (2): 106–123.

Brindis, C. D., and R. J. Jeremy. 1988. *Adolescent Pregnancy and Parenting in California: Building a Strategic Plan for Action.* San Francisco: Institute for Health Policy Studies.

Brunswick, A. 1971. "Adolescent Health, Sex, and Fertility." *Adolescent Sexuality* 61 (4): 711–729.

Campbell, A. A. 1980. "Trends in Teenage Childbearing in the United States." In *Adolescent Pregnancy and Childbearing: Findings from Research,* edited by C. Chilman, 3–13. DHHS Publication no. 81–2077 (NIH). Washington, D.C.: U.S. Department of Health and Human Services.

Chan, I. 1981. *The Hmong in America—Their Cultural Continuities and Discontinuities.* St. Paul, Minn.: Bush Foundation.

Coopersmith, S. 1967. *The Antecedents of Self-Esteem.* San Francisco: Freeman.

Cvetkovich, G., and B. Grote. 1980. "Psychosocial Development and the Social Problem of Teenage Illegitimacy." In *Adolescent Pregnancy and Childbearing: Findings from Research,* edited by C. Chilman, 15–41. DHHS Publication no. 81–2077 (NIH). Washington, D.C.: U.S. Department of Health and Human Services.

Furstenberg, F. F., J. Brooks-Gunn, and P. S. Morgan. 1987. *Adolescent Mothers in Later Life.* New York: Cambridge University Press.

Hayes, C. D. 1987a. "Adolescent Pregnancy and Childbearing: An Emerging Research Focus." In *Risking the Future: Adolescent Sexuality, Pregnancy, and Childbearing,* vol. 2, edited by S. L. Hofferth and C. D. Hayes, 1–6. Washington, D.C.: National Academy Press.

———, ed. 1987b. *Risking the Future: Adolescent Sexuality, Pregnancy, and Childbearing.* Vol. 1. Washington D.C.: National Academy Press.

Herold, E. S., and M. S. Goodwin. 1979. "Self-Esteem and Sexual Permissiveness." *Journal of Clinical Psychology* 35 (4): 908–912.

Herold, E. S., M. S. Goodwin, and D. S. Lero. 1979. "Self-Esteem, Locus of Control, and Adolescent Contraception." *Journal of Psychology* 101 (January): 83–88.

Herold, E. S., and L. M. Samson. 1980. "Differences Between Women Who Begin Pill Use Before and After First Intercourse: Ontario, Canada." *Family Planning Perspectives* 12 (6): 304–305.

Hofferth, S. L. 1987a. "The Effects of Programs and Policies on Adolescent Pregnancy and Childbearing." In *Risking the Future: Adolescent Sexuality,*

Pregnancy, and Childbearing, vol. 2, edited by S. L. Hofferth and C. D. Hayes, 207–263. Washington, D.C.: National Academy Press.

———. 1987b. "Social and Economic Consequences of Teenage Childbearing." In *Risking the Future: Adolescent Sexuality, Pregnancy, and Childbearing,* vol. 2, edited by S. L. Hofferth and C. D. Hayes, 123–144. Washington, D.C.: National Academy Press.

Hornick, J. P., L. Doran, and S. H. Crawford. 1979. "Premarital Contraceptive Usage Among Male and Female Adolescents." *Family Coordinator* 11: 181–190.

Jessor, S. L., and R. Jessor. 1975. "Transition from Virginity to Nonvirginity Among Youth: A Social-Psychological Study over Time." *Developmental Psychology* 11 (4): 473–484.

Kaplan, H. B. 1975. *Self-Attitudes and Deviant Behavior.* Pacific Palisades, Calif.: Goodyear.

———. 1980. *Deviant Behavior in Defense of Self.* New York: Academic Press.

Kaplan, H. B., and A. D. Pokorny. 1969. "Self-Derogation and Psychosocial Adjustment." *Journal of Nervous and Mental Disease* 149 (5): 421–434.

Kaplan, H. B., P. B. Smith, and A. D. Pokorny. 1979. "Psychosocial Antecedents of Unwed Motherhood Among Indigent Adolescents." *Journal of Youth and Adolescence* 8 (2): 181–207.

Lancaster, J. B. 1986. "Human Adolescence and Reproduction: An Evolutionary Perspective." In *School-Age Pregnancy and Parenthood,* edited by J. B. Lancaster and B. A. Hamburg, 17–37. New York: Aldine de Gruyter.

Luker, K. 1975. *Taking Chances: Abortion and the Decision Not to Contracept.* Berkeley and Los Angeles: University of California Press.

Miller, B. S., R. B. Christensen, and T. D. Olson. 1987. "Adolescent Self-Esteem in Relation to Sexual Attitudes and Behavior." *Youth and Society* 19 (1): 93–111.

Robbins, C., H. B. Kaplan, and S. S. Martin. 1985. "Antecedents of Pregnancy Among Unmarried Adolescents." *Journal of Marriage and the Family* 42:567–583.

Rogel, M. J., and M. E. Zuehlke. 1982. "Adolescent Contraceptive Behavior: Influences and Implications." In *Pregnancy in Adolescence: Needs, Problems, and Management,* edited by I. R. Stuart and C. F. Wells, 194–216. New York: Van Nostrand Reinhold.

Rogel, M. J., M. E. Zuehlke, A. C. Petersen, M. Tobin-Richards, and M. Shelton. 1980. "Contraceptive Behavior in Adolescence: A Decision-Making Perspective." *Journal of Youth and Adolescence* 9 (6): 491–506.

Rosenberg, M. 1965. *Society and the Adolescent Self-Image.* Princeton, N.J.: Princeton University Press.

Rutter, M. 1983. "School Effects on Pupil Progress: Research Findings and Policy Implications." *Child Development* 54(1): 1–29.

Sears, R. R. 1970. "Relation of Early Socialization Experiences to Self-Concepts and Gender Role in Middle Childhood." *Child Development* 41(2): 267–287.

Streetman, L. G. 1987. "Contrasts in the Self-Esteem of Unwed Teenage Mothers." *Adolescence* 22(86): 459–464.

U.S. Congress. House. Select Committee on Children, Youth, and Families. 1986. *Teen Pregnancy: What Is Being Done? A State-by-State Look.* Committee Print. Washington, D.C.: Government Printing Office.

U.S. Department of Labor. 1986. *Employment and Earnings Characteristics of Families: Second Quarter 1986.* USDL 86–300. Washington, D.C.: Government Printing Office.

Vernon, M., J. A. Green, and T. E. Frothingham. 1983. "Teenage Pregnancy: A Prospective Study of Self-Esteem and Other Sociodemographic Factors." *Pediatrics* 72(5): 632–635.

Vincent, C. E. 1961. *Unmarried Mothers.* New York: Free Press.

Vinovskis, M. A. 1981. "An Epidemic of Adolescent Pregnancy? Some Historical Considerations." *Journal of Family History* 6(2): 205–230.

Wells, L. E., and G. Marwell. 1976. *Self-Esteem: Its Conceptualization and Measurement.* Beverly Hills, Calif.: Sage.

Werner, E. E. 1988. Personal communication to Susan Crockenberg. March.

Werner, E. E., and R. Smith. 1977. *Children of Kauai.* Honolulu: University of Hawaii Press.

Wylie, R. C. 1974. *The Self-Concept.* Vol. 1, *A Review of Methodological Considerations and Measuring Instruments.* Rev. ed. Lincoln: University of Nebraska Press.

Crime, Violence, and Self-Esteem: Review and Proposals

Thomas J. Scheff, Suzanne M. Retzinger, and Michael T. Ryan

The role played by self-esteem in precipitating, influencing, or preventing violent behavior is problematic. In this chapter, we will survey studies of the relation of self-esteem to crime and violence, propose a new approach, and make recommendations for public policy. The literature review will include both a survey of studies that have used quantitative methods and a selective review of studies of emotion and self-esteem in violent behavior.

The first half of our review is a broad survey. But we have narrowed the focus of the second half to the role of self-esteem in crimes of violence. We made this decision for two reasons. First, level of self-esteem may be crucial in crimes of violence, particularly violence toward intimates. Violence of this type often appears to involve intense emotion; it is sometimes referred to as a "crime of passion." As we suggest below, the kinds of passions involved in family violence may be related to self-esteem.

Second, in crimes against property and against the public order, the connection with self-esteem is not clear. This is not to say there is no connection; rather, studies simply do not provide a clear picture. Our discussion of quantitative studies criticizes weaknesses in the design and methods of existing research. Perhaps future, more adequate, studies may yet uncover such relationships. But most crimes against property (theft, for example) may be "economic" crimes, not crimes of passion, and therefore not related to self-esteem. Most prisoners in the American corrections system have been convicted for crimes against property. It is possible that economic, political, and cultural forces, rather than psychological ones, swell our prison populations. These are important issues, but they will not be our focus here.

Quantitative Studies

Explanations of deviant behavior have a long tradition in psychology and sociology. As the influence of interactionist social psychology grew in the 1950s, theorists began including the idea of a self-concept in such explanations (Wells 1978). These theorists assumed that behavior is influenced by thoughts and feelings about self. The self-concept was seen as a product of socialization and interaction with significant others, an approach that could form a bridge between psychology and sociology. More recently, low self-esteem has been proposed as a cause of criminal behavior. Empirical validation, however, has been slow in coming. Examining the relevant studies will help us to assess the current state of this research.

Crime and violence are concepts that encompass diverse forms of specific behavior. The relevant research represents a wide assortment of approaches and concerns, and it also interprets the idea of self-esteem in a number of ways. The most common conception is *global self-esteem,* attitudes and feelings held toward the whole self, that is, "the degree to which an individual feels that he is personally and socially adequate" (Rosenbaum and deCharms 1962, 291). Other studies, however, concern the behavioral effects of levels of self-esteem that are temporarily *induced* (by insult or praise) under specific experimental conditions. A few have studied the consequences of interaction between global and induced self-esteem.

The population samples used in these studies also vary widely. Many are limited to a particular age group (e.g., children or adolescents), gender, social class, or other subgroup such as delinquents, making comparisons of the findings difficult.

Various types of behavior relevant to crime and violence have been investigated. Experimental studies have sought to link levels of self-esteem (both global and induced) with aggression, as well as with other forms of antisocial behavior such as cheating or dishonesty. In such studies, researchers first administer a questionnaire designed to measure self-esteem and then apply treatments that are assumed to raise or lower self-esteem. Subjects' responses to one or more experimental conditions are then measured. Because self-esteem is measured or induced before observing how the subjects respond, these studies are better able to show the causative effects of self-esteem than are correlational studies, which simply show an association between the measured variables.

The rich diversity of experimental research in this area is impressive, and certainly much is owed to the investigators for their ingenuity and persistence. It is therefore especially disheartening that the experimental studies have tended to be inconclusive, often demonstrating effects that are weak, nonexistent, or sometimes contradictory. Although much has been learned, the parts still fail to add up to a recognizable whole. Furthermore, because these studies are conducted in laboratory settings, the extrapolation of results to real situations is uncertain. Such studies may lack what is called "ecological" validity.

Other studies have investigated the relationship of self-esteem to hostility and aggression, as well as to criminal behavior. But most research conducted outside the laboratory has attempted only to demonstrate correlations between levels of self-esteem and behavior, showing the possibility of a relationship without establishing causation. Even with such a limited goal, the correlations reported have been weak at best. Clearly, longitudinal studies are required to ascertain whether level of self-esteem plays a *causal* role in violent or criminal behavior. Very few such studies have been conducted, however, and these have focused principally on only one field, juvenile delinquency. Nevertheless, because of the care with which this research was done, we review it at some length below.

Many early studies of aggression focused on the "frustration-aggression" hypothesis (Dollard et al. 1939), which views aggression as a response to any stimulus that blocks "goal-directed" activity (i.e., the attempt to gain a valued reward such as money, food, or social approval). This line of research, popular into the 1960s (see, for example, Berkowitz 1962; Buss 1961), suggested that individuals differ in their predispositions to anger and aggression and therefore in their susceptibility to frustration. Such differences came to be seen as the product of the individual's self-concept or self-esteem.

Rosenbaum and deCharms (1962) conceptualized self-esteem as a "mediating response" that determines expectations of reward or punishment, success or failure, and so on. Persons with low self-esteem, having more negative expectations, should therefore be more sensitive to disapproval or rejection, and hence more easily "frustrated" and prone to aggression. At the same time, however, expectations of punishment and failure should be expected to inhibit the overt expression of aggressive impulses by such individuals. A series of experiments showed support for both hypotheses: subjects with low self-esteem appeared to be more angered by verbal attacks than were subjects with high self-esteem, yet the former group also seemed more inhibited in expressing aggression.

Though not conclusive, these results suggest why there have been so many weak or contradictory findings. Depending on which proposed effect of self-esteem is more strongly elicited or on how aggression is measured, self-esteem may be positively *or* negatively correlated with aggression; or the countervailing influences may simply cancel each other out. Kingsbury (1978), for example, found that subjects with low self-esteem who were insulted by a confederate "punished" the confederate in a bogus learning task with levels of electrical shock that were substantially higher than those administered by similar subjects who had not been insulted. Among subjects with high self-esteem, there was no significant difference between those who were insulted and those who were not, supporting the notion that persons with low self-esteem are more easily angered by insults. But subjects with low self-esteem also administered higher shock levels than subjects with high self-esteem did, both when insulted and when not insulted (though the latter difference was not statistically significant), contrary to the prediction that those with low self-esteem should be more inhibited in expressing such aggression.

In another experiment, however, Worchel (1958) allowed subjects to use a questionnaire to express aggressive feelings toward an instructor who had insulted them. Subjects with high self-esteem exhibited levels of aggression that were substantially greater than those expressed by subjects with low self-esteem, supporting the idea that individuals with low self-esteem are more inhibited. But the contingent conditions for inhibition are neither specified by the theory nor explicitly controlled for in such experiments, making it difficult to generalize their findings. Cohen (1959) found evidence that people with low self-esteem are more vulnerable to the exercise of power over them than are people with high self-esteem, suggesting that at least some of the effects observed among subjects with low self-esteem may be inadvertent results of the experimenter's or other influence, perhaps in anticipation of approval or punishment. These considerations imply that the notion of a single, linear relationship between self-esteem and behavior is overly simplistic.

Rosenbaum and deCharms (1962) also noted that it was not clear whether the differences they observed between the two sets of subjects could be generalized to task-oriented frustration. Epstein and Taylor found that when subjects competed in a "reaction time" test in which the winner administered a shock to the loser, the subjects used higher shock settings only when the opponent was also clearly aggressive, leading the researchers to conclude that "perception of the opponent's aggressive intent is a far more potent instigator to aggression than frustration in the form of defeat" (1967, 286). Geen (1968) similarly found personal insult to instigate aggression more effectively than did frustration per se. Feshbach, in an influential theoretical statement, concluded that "violations to self-esteem through insult, humiliation, or coercion are . . . probably the most important source of anger and aggressive drive in humans" (1971, 285). Feshbach's forceful statement is significant for the theory that will be proposed later in this chapter.

Concurrent with investigations of the frustration-aggression hypothesis were studies of environmental factors that lead to aggressive behavior. McCord, McCord, and Howard (1961) reanalyzed data from the Cambridge-Somerville Youth Study of the 1930s, in which the home lives of 650 nine-year-old boys had been observed over a five-year period. Half the sample, who were judged to be "maladjusted" and potentially delinquent, formed the control group. Subjects in the other, "normal" half were observed to fall into three categories: those who were consistently "aggressive," those who were merely "assertive" (occasionally aggressive), and those who were consistently "nonaggressive." Researchers found that the aggressive boys had experienced significantly higher levels of direct parental attacks (physical abuse, verbal threats of punishment or abandonment, derogation, and rejection) than the other boys had faced. As the authors observed: "These attitudes and actions are all, presumably, direct attacks on the child's sense of security; they all tend to undermine the boy's conception of himself as a person of worth and significance; and they all carry the implication that the world is a dangerous, hostile environment" (1961, 84).

Additionally, the aggressive boys were more likely to have experienced parental conflict in the home, as well as deficient (weak and inconsistent) parental controls, which, at least in current clinical opinion, might also be seen as contributing to low self-esteem. The authors noted that the aggressive boys displayed a greater tendency to reject their parents and the parents' values, more often choosing a "reference group" outside the home, such as a gang of delinquents or other group of neighborhood boys. (The relationship of this point to self-esteem will be seen more clearly in our discussion of Kaplan's theory of deviance, below.) Parents who typically responded with aggression to crises in and outside the home, however, did not seem to be more common among the aggressive group of boys, suggesting that the modeling of such behavior was less important than the emotional climate of the familial relationships.

These observations support the earlier findings of Glueck and Glueck (1950), who worked with a somewhat different sample of lower-class boys. They found that many delinquent boys came from homes similarly characterized by severe punitiveness, parental rejection, inconsistency, and parental discord. Delinquents were described as more insecure and anxious and less cooperative and trusting than their nondelinquent counterparts. Bandura and Walters (1959) also reported comparable findings in their extensive study of middle-class delinquents.

Toch (1969) interviewed sixty-nine prison inmates and parolees who had a history of violence. He concluded that there were ten characteristic approaches to interpersonal situations that promoted violence. The most common, "self-image compensating," involved aggression in defense of self-image (as retribution against an individual who may have cast aspersions on one's self-image) or to promote self-image (to demonstrate worth). In both cases, the need to resort to aggression was believed to stem from feelings of extremely low self-esteem.

These studies are correlational only, even though they provide far richer and much more detailed evidence than that available from laboratory studies. They convincingly show an association between the presumed antecedents of low self-esteem and aggressive or delinquent behavior, but they fail to demonstrate that the relationship is a causal one.

The most comprehensive theoretical elaboration of the relationship between self-esteem and criminal behavior—and the most convincing empirical investigation thus far—is based on Kaplan's (1975, 1980) "esteem-enhancement" model of deviance. Kaplan proposes that delinquent behavior serves to enhance self-esteem for individuals who have experienced failure and lowered self-esteem.

Fundamental to this theory is the assumption of a "self-esteem motive"—defined by Kaplan (1975) as "the personal need to maximize the experience of positive self-attitudes and to minimize the experience of negative self-attitudes"—which stems from the child's early dependence on adults. As Kaplan describes it, the need to behave in a way that evokes positive adult behavior sensitizes the child to adult reactions to his or her self. Over time, therefore, the role of others will be adopted as a guide to appropriate behavior, until a symbolic association is formed between the *imagined* responses of others and one's own responses to self.

When an individual's past experiences in a particular membership group have led to negative self-attitudes, according to the theory, the individual will associate that membership group with self-derogating experiences, ultimately losing the motivation to conform to normative expectations—and gaining the motivation to deviate from such expectations. Deviance becomes attractive to the extent that it represents opportunities for self-enhancing experiences. Whether deviant behavior is adopted and which type is chosen depend on circumstances—what kinds of deviant activity are visible and available, the perceived attractiveness of these opportunities, and so on. Whether the involvement is continued, says Kaplan, depends in turn on the extent to which the deviant activity is in fact felt to be self-enhancing or self-derogating.

To test this theory, Kaplan conducted a survey of seventh-grade students each year for three years. This age group (eleven to thirteen years old) was a compromise, likely to predict adult behavior, yet minimizing prior involvement in deviant activities. More than three thousand students were surveyed each year. Self-derogation and self-esteem were measured using seven items from Rosenberg's ten-question scale (those items Kaplan judged to measure "affective" components of self-esteem). Deviant behavior was measured by self-reports of twenty-eight "presumably deviant acts." Questions pertaining to other aspects of the theory (such as attitudes toward normative expectations) were also asked.

In the first analysis of the data (Kaplan 1980), several steps in the causal chain specified by the theory were investigated. Most relevant to our purposes here is the analysis of the effects of self-esteem on subsequent delinquency. Kaplan found that among subjects presumed not to have already adopted deviant behaviors, those with initially lower levels of self-esteem (and those with greater antecedent increases in self-rejecting attitudes) were more likely than others to subsequently adopt deviant patterns.

The effects of social class (defined in terms of the mother's education) and gender were also examined, for it was argued that deviance would be more normative for lower-class students than for middle-class students and less normative (i.e., more "deviant") for females than for males. The relationship of self-rejection to subsequent deviant behavior was shown to be stronger and more consistent for middle-class students, weaker and in many cases insignificant for lower-class subjects. In both classes, the association was stronger for females than for males.

Variables that might have intervened between self-esteem and deviance, such as the subjective association of negative self-attitudes with membership group experiences and the development of contra-normative attitudes, were also investigated.

Finally, the proposed increase in self-esteem following the adoption of deviant behavior was examined. Here, a clear relationship was not immediately found. Additional conditions were considered: (1) lack of defenses against or vulnerability to self-derogating experiences in normative settings (reflecting an inability to satisfy the self-esteem motive within normative membership groups); (2) the perceived self-enhancing potential of the normative environment (presumed to indicate the degree to which "deviant" acts were actually defined as such by the subjects); and (3) gender (taken as a rough estimate of the subjects' vulnerability to the self-derogating consequences of *deviant* behavior patterns, because females were expected to be more dependent than males on approval from—and hence less likely to reap the rewards of deviating from—the normative setting). In each case, the expected results were obtained, to varying degrees, although the authors acknowledge that their measures represented only coarse approximations of the conditions required by their theory.

Because of the piecemeal approach taken by this analysis, it fails to provide a convincing confirmation of the overall theory. Kaplan selectively points out only the significant effects that appear to support the esteem-enhancement model, based at least partially on "predictions" apparently formulated after the data were already in hand. Furthermore, because the twenty-eight different self-reported measures of deviance are analyzed separately, it is difficult to assess the strength of the relationships proposed. Multivariate analyses of other longitudinal data by Bynner, O'Malley, and Bachman (1981), Wells and Rankin (1983), and McCarthy and Hoge (1984) used path analysis techniques to simultaneously estimate the effects of the entire esteem-enhancement model. All three of these studies concluded that the direct effects of self-esteem on deviance were negligible or nonexistent, although two (excepting Wells and Rankin 1983) found support for the self-enhancing effects of delinquent behavior. These three studies assume considerable importance for our review, because they fail to support Kaplan's main findings.

Subsequent analysis of the Kaplan data by Kaplan, Martin, and Johnson (1986) posited three deficiencies in all of the earlier analyses.

First, the measurement of self-rejection or self-esteem had been inadequate, since the theory proposes that it is the combination of global feelings of inadequacy *and* the individual's association of such feelings with membership group experiences that disposes the person to deviance. Second, measures of deviance had most often been specified as a continuous variable covering specific kinds of behavior, whereas the theory asserts that it is "not the amount of deviance but rather the engagement in any of a range of functionally equivalent deviant behaviors that is predicted" (Kaplan, Martin, and Johnson 1986, 393). Third, and more fundamental, the earlier analyses had erred in focusing only on the *direct* relationship of self-esteem to deviance, whereas "self-rejection, theoretically, has direct effects on deviant dispositions, not on deviant behavior" (391). Thus, the disposition to deviance needed to be defined as an intervening variable in the model. The variables were respecified, using multiple indices. Strong support was found for the theoretical model. Estimated coefficients for the direct effect of self-rejection at time-1 on disposition to deviance at time-2 ($= .76$) and disposition to deviance at time-2 on deviance at time-3 ($= .52$) were both large and significant beyond the .001 level.

An elaboration of the model was provided by Kaplan, Johnson, and Bailey's (1986) addition of the latent construct "early involvement in deviant activities" (as reported at time-1) to the earlier analysis. Early deviance was expected to show a direct negative effect on self-esteem, by violating internalized norms and by evoking negative responses from the individual's social milieu. This effect was then expected to indirectly influence subsequent deviance both positively *and* negatively. That is, if self-rejection, or low self-esteem, increases the disposition to deviance, the likelihood of deviance should also increase. But low self-esteem was also expected to show a *negative* effect on deviant behavior in the new model, as a result of feelings of inefficacy and an increased need to conform to normative standards. (Negative self-feelings presume that the individual still desires positive regard from others and has internalized the norms that proscribe deviant behavior.)

Thus, as in Rosenbaum and deCharms's (1962) proposal regarding the countervailing effects of low self-esteem on aggression, self-rejection was hypothesized to motivate the person to further conform to membership group constraints, even as he or she becomes disposed to subsequently deviate from them. In addition, early deviance reported at time-1 was expected to have a direct positive effect on the disposition to deviance at time-2, as well as a direct positive effect on later deviance at time-3 through maintaining or increasing opportunities to learn deviant behaviors from others.

Inclusion of the new variable also permitted a test of whether the previously noted indirect influence of self-rejection on subsequent deviance was an independent causal effect, as predicted by the model, or was dependent on earlier deviance. The estimated coefficients indicated support for the model and were all found to be significant beyond the .001 level of probability:

effects of early deviance at time-1 on self-rejection at time-1 (.568), disposition to deviance at time-2 (.224), and deviance at time-3 (.340);

direct effects of self-rejection at time-1 on disposition to deviance at time-2 (.426) and deviance at time-3 (−.180);

and direct effects of disposition to deviance at time-2 on deviance at time-3 (.510).

In the most recent refinement of the model by Kaplan, Johnson, and Bailey (1987), yet another variable was added: "deviant peer association" at time-2, measured by self-reports of deviant behavior engaged in by friends and peers at school. It was predicted that such associations would positively affect subsequent deviant behavior, and this prediction was supported. The direct effect of deviant peer association at time-2 on deviance at time-3 was estimated to be .387.

The added variable changed the effect of disposition to deviance at time-2 on deviance at time-3 from .510 to .197, while the direct effect of disposition to deviance at time-2 on deviant peer association at time-2 was estimated to be a substantial .635. Interestingly, no opposite effect was found—apparently, deviant peer associations do not affect disposition to deviance, as some theorists have asserted (cf. Matsueda 1982). The picture that emerges is one in which the disposition to deviance most often led students to adopt associations with deviant peers; these associations, much more than the disposition to deviance itself, provided the strongest impetus to subsequent deviance.

Kaplan and his associates certainly deserve praise and encouragement for their efforts. Having provided a comprehensive longitudinal study, complete with extensive theoretical underpinnings, they continue to test and refine the model with painstaking diligence. The final verdict on this research may still be years away, however, and it must be pointed out that several unresolved issues remain. Most notably, the posited self-enhancing effects of deviant behavior, on which the theory is substantially based, have yet to be convincingly demonstrated. Nor has the possible bias from sample attrition been adequately addressed. Only 33.7 percent of the original sample completed all three tests; analyses of the initial questionnaires indicated that the most significant correlate of sample attrition was self-report of early deviance, a variable subsequently included in the structural equation model. Further, because it is impossible to know how the missing students may have differed from the final sample over time, the results cannot be generalized.

Similarly, students' self-reports of deviance may be unreliable. For more than half of the twenty-four items also reported on by school officials, for example, students reported fewer than 50 percent of the activities the officials "knew" had occurred. For three of the items, more than 60 percent of those who reported an act the first year subsequently denied it the next.

What does the esteem-enhancement model tell us about the relationship of self-esteem to crime and violence? In the end, the answer may be as equivocal as the one implied by Rosenbaum and deCharms (1962) more than a quarter century ago: "It depends." As more variables are added to the model, the practical utility of its insights may diminish, leaving us awash in a sea of conditional probabilities.

The implication of the numerous studies of self-esteem may be that the concept as it has been used so far is complex and contradictory, more indicative of propensities to particular kinds of influence and patterns of avoidance than of specific behaviors. Because such issues have not been resolved, quantitative studies have thus far been unable to significantly advance our practical understanding of the relationship between self-esteem and crime and violence.

The problem of defining the concept of self-esteem surfaces in all quantitative studies of the subject, not only those that seek to relate it to crime, violence, and aggression. Morris Rosenberg (1988), a pioneer in the quantitative study of self-esteem, estimates that approximately *ten thousand* such studies of the concept have been conducted. Each study has used a self-esteem scale, usually consisting of a small number of questions, most often ten to thirty. In the absence of a standard, agreed-upon conceptual definition of self-esteem, these scales have proliferated: there are now at least *two hundred* in use (Rosenberg 1988). These scales, for the most part, are not comparable. This lack of comparability alone would create chaos, a Tower of Babel, in any field of study.

Given the vast number of quantitative studies, there are surprisingly few overall assessments of their findings. We located only five general reviews of the entire field and one review of a very large subfield, adolescent self-esteem. Four of these six reviews are quite critical. Diggory does not mince words: he concludes his overview with a commentary on the "utter bankruptcy of it all" (1966, 62). Crandall's assessment is also harsh: "Despite the popularity of self-esteem, no standard or operational definition exists" (1973, 45). He also criticizes the lack of evidence for validity and the theoretical and conceptual confusion. (His review is extremely useful, for he lists at least several items from thirty of the most widely used scales.) In their review of studies of adolescent self-esteem, Savin-Williams and Demo join the critical chorus: "Despite 1,500 articles on adolescent self-esteem . . . we know relatively little of its correlates, determinants, or predictors" (1983, 121). The most recent general review is also the most critical:

> What has emerged . . . in the self-esteem literature is a confusion of results that defies interpretation. Hypotheses have been tested about the relationships between self-esteem and hundreds of other psychological variables. Many of these hypotheses have been formally supported, but most observed trends have been weak and insubstantial. There are few replications or systematic extensions, and it is difficult to know which findings are worth pursuing. Moreover, because different investigators begin with different assumptions, their findings stand in obscure relation to one another. (Jackson 1984, 2–3)

The two positive reviews, by Wells and Marwell (1976) and Wylie (1979), are more comprehensive than the negative ones. Both positive reviews report in detail the procedures used and the results found in the self-esteem studies. Both accentuate the positive: the authors sympathize with the systematic nature of the quantitative studies, and they praise the precision and reliability of the procedures. The optimistic and laudatory tone stands in stark contrast to the tone of the four critical reviews.

In one crucial respect, however, these two reviews are in complete agreement with the critics: *the absence of significant findings*. Wells and Marwell (1976, 72–73) go to great pains to document the contradictions among various studies. They report disagreement among twenty-nine studies on the direction of the relationship between self-esteem and seven variables, such as authoritarianism, admitting unflattering descriptions about oneself, persuasibility, and so on. Because of these contradictions, we are unable to interpret any of these relationships; that is, the findings have been nil. In the broadest and most careful of the re-

views, Wylie (1979, 690, 692) agrees, pointing to the "striking incidence" of findings that are weak, null, or contradictory.

Readers of the last two studies may conclude that these reviews represent the state of the field as healthy. But it is possible to construe them,
in concert with the four critical reviews, in a different way: *even re-
viewers who are completely sympathetic to the intentions of the quantitative studies acknowledge that these studies have produced no results.* In our opinion, the implication of all six of the general reviews is
not that the field is healthy but that it is in a state of crisis, and has been
for some time. This interpretation has been underlined since the publication of the two positive reviews (in 1976 and 1979). Several thousand quantitative studies later, there are still no results that are both
strong and replicated. How many inconclusive studies will be conducted before basic premises are examined?

It should be emphasized that the series of studies by Kaplan was not
referenced by the six general reviews. His findings seem to contradict
the conclusion we draw from the reviews, that the relationships reported between self-esteem and deviance have been weak or null. Some
of his correlations were substantial, and his work may thus seem to be
an exception. As already indicated, however, three subsequent studies
by other investigators failed to replicate his findings. For this reason,
our critique of the quantitative studies is not overturned by Kaplan's
work.

We do not claim that the quantitative studies have been useless. On
the contrary, we believe they were necessary. Their very lack of success
suggests the need for new directions in theory and method that might be
more suited to the problem at hand. The existing paradigm in the field is
a general one, treating self-esteem as an attitude that can be studied like
any other attitude. Perhaps what is needed is a new paradigm more
closely connected with the particular problem of self-esteem. If, as suggested below, self-esteem turns out to be a complex cognitive-emotional
structure, then a new paradigm might clear the path toward proving
causation.

A Theory of Self-Esteem

As we have indicated, the vast body of quantitative studies does not
establish level of self-esteem as a cause of crime and violence. Perhaps
much more exploratory research and theoretical work will be necessary
before valid quantitative studies can be designed. As a beginning step in

this direction, our focus now shifts to a theory of self-esteem and several studies that seem to support it. Like the quantitative research we have just criticized, these studies do not prove causation. None of them attempts such a task; they are all exploratory in design. We believe, however, that these studies, unlike the quantitative studies, may point toward a new direction in research and public policy.

Our purpose is to build a prima facie case for the importance of self-esteem in the causation of violent crimes. Public policy does not wait for final proof in other realms, and even a case that is merely plausible should provide grounds for debate and discussion of possible new law and policy in the area of corrections. We see no need to be defensive about advocating the importance of self-esteem, because the case that can be made for it is at least as good as the case that has been made for existing laws and policies.

Self-Esteem and Emotion

The theory and research to be discussed here suggest a new way to conceptualize self-esteem in terms of emotions, the basic emotions of pride and shame. The idea of connecting self-esteem to these emotions is not completely new, but it has only recently been made explicit. Our theory emphasizes what already seems to be understood in everyday usage, that self-esteem concerns how we usually *feel* about ourselves. High self-esteem means that we usually feel justified pride in ourselves, low self-esteem that we often and easily feel ashamed of ourselves or try to avoid feelings of shame. All of the correlates of self-esteem (perceptions, beliefs, and concepts regarding the self; attributions regarding others' perception of self; and behavior toward self and others) may derive from these self-feelings—whether we are usually proud or usually ashamed of ourselves.

In this view, level of self-esteem is a summary concept, representing how well one does overall in managing shame. For persons with high self-esteem, shame is painful but not overwhelming. Such persons have sufficient experiences of pride in their lives that they can usually manage the shame they experience.

Persons with low self-esteem appear to lack sufficient experiences of pride to be able to manage shame; for them, shame is a calamity, to be avoided at all costs. When it cannot be avoided, its effects are often disruptive or even catastrophic. What makes shame so problematic in our society is that, in adults, it is nearly always hidden. We have learned to be ashamed of being ashamed (Scheff 1988). Both laypeople and re-searchers often ignore pride and shame as causal agents, because these emotions usually have low visibility and because we have all been trained to ignore them.

In modern societies, it is taken for granted that shame is a rare emo-tion among adults. This belief is reflected in the anthropological divi-sion between shame and guilt cultures: supposedly, traditional societies rely on shame for social and self-control, modern societies on guilt. A similar premise is found in psychoanalytic theory, which places near-total emphasis on guilt as the adult emotion of self-control, with shame deemed "regressive," that is, childish. (For an early critique of both premises, see Piers and Singer 1953.)

There is also an opposing tradition in the scientific literature, how-ever, which maintains that shame is a primary emotion, generated by the constant monitoring of self from the point of view of others. Such monitoring, it is argued, is not rare but incessant, even in solitude. This thread can be found in Darwin (1872), MacDougall (1908), Cooley (1902), Lynd (1958), Goffman (1967), and Lewis (1971). Their argu-ments can be summarized by three propositions:

1. In adults, social monitoring of self is continuous. We are, as Cooley put it, "living in the minds of others without knowing it."

> We do not think much of [self-feeling] so long as it is moderately and regularly gratified. Many people of balanced mind and congenial ac-tivity scarcely know that they care what others think of them, and will deny, perhaps with indignation, that such care is an important factor in what they are and do. But this is illusion. If failure or disgrace arrives, if one suddenly finds that the faces of men show coldness or contempt in-stead of the kindliness and deference that he is used to, he will perceive from the shock, the fear, the sense of being outcast and helpless, that he was *living in the minds of others without knowing it*, just as we daily walk the solid ground without thinking how it bears us up. (Cooley 1902, 208; emphasis added)

2. Social monitoring always has an evaluative edge and gives rise, therefore, to either pride or shame.

These first two propositions, taken together, create a puzzle. If social monitoring is so incessant, and if it produces either pride or shame, why do we see so little of either emotion?

3. Adults are almost always in a state of pride or shame, but these emotions have such low visibility that we seldom notice them.

This review suggests that although pride and shame may determine behavior, they usually go unnoticed. Their lack of visibility involves both the stimulus and response sides. On the stimulus side, adults are careful to conceal their manifestations of pride and shame (Goffman 1967, 101–104). On the response side, these emotions are socially unacceptable, to the point that one is not supposed to discuss, express, or even feel them (Scheff 1984). We live in a shame-denying society, in that the denial and disguise of pride and shame are not only matters of individual propensity but also institutionalized patterns of collective behavior. Our very vocabulary denies shame, projecting it instead onto the outer world. We say, "It was an awkward moment for both of us," rather than leveling about emotions by saying, "We were both embarrassed."

Perhaps this institutionalized denial is the reason that self-esteem has never been adequately defined; it touches, after all, on the collective secret of pride and shame. For purposes of discussion, we will here define level of self-esteem as each person's *ratio of pride to shame states*. This definition is rudimentary, but it may help to stimulate further discussion and research. For example, even though the definition is crude, it could serve as a basis for classifying most of the thousands of items in the existing self-esteem scales. Showing that scale items are facets of either pride or shame, or perhaps are sources or consequences of these emotions, would be a first step toward making the scales comparable.

Because most states of pride and shame are carefully disguised, this definition concerns, for the most part, unacknowledged, low-visibility pride and shame. It parallels Satir's (1972) definition of what she calls "low pot": one is "low pot" when one experiences undesirable feelings but tries to behave as if the feelings weren't there. Her definition of self-esteem does not actually name what we now think is the specific emotion involved in "feeling low," shame. Rather, it follows the contemporary custom of not explicitly naming shame.

Recent developments in theory and method now provide a way of detecting low-visibility shame and demonstrating its role in behavior. The first step was taken by Gottschalk and Gleser, who developed reliable scales for inferring emotion from verbal statements. Although much of their focus is on detecting low-visibility anger and anxiety, they also furnish a scale for low-visibility shame (or "shame-anxiety," as they call it [Gottschalk, Winget, and Gleser 1969, 49–52]). Although compatible with Gottschalk and Gleser's approach, the approach taken by Lewis (1971), a psychoanalyst, is much broader. Her laborious, moment-by-moment analysis of the audiotapes of several hundred psychotherapy sessions provides the rationale for inferring low-visibility shame from observable external cues, both verbal and nonverbal (loudness, pitch, rate of speech, intonation, and so on). In her study, she demonstrates that, although neither patient nor therapist seemed aware of it, episodes of low-visibility shame occurred in every session.

Lewis divides unacknowledged shame into two basic types: *overt, undifferentiated* shame; and *bypassed* shame. Overt, undifferentiated shame involves painful feelings that are not identified as shame by the person experiencing them. Rather, they are labeled with a wide variety of terms that serve to disguise the experience of shame: having low self-esteem, feeling foolish, stupid, ridiculous, inadequate, defective, incompetent, awkward, exposed, vulnerable, insecure, helpless. Our culture provides a great many such codewords. Lewis classifies all the terms listed above as shame markers, because *they occurred only in a certain context and only in association with specific types of nonverbal markers.* The context always involved a perception of self as negatively evaluated, by either self or other—the basic context for shame. In this context, Lewis always found a change in the patient's manner, characterized by such nonverbal markers as speech disruption (stammers, repetition of words, speech static like "well" or "uhhh," long pauses), lowered or averted gaze, blushing, and, especially noticeable, a sharp drop in the loudness of speech, even to the point of inaudibility.

Both the verbal and nonverbal markers of overt shame can be characterized as forms of "hiding" behavior. The verbal terms hide shame under a disguising label, and the nonverbal forms suggest physical hiding: covering the face with the hands, averting or lowering one's gaze to escape the other's eyes, and using speech disruption or overly quiet speech to hide the content of one's speech and thoughts. At times, but not always, the ideation of the person undergoing overt shame may also involve hiding: "I wanted to disappear"; "I wished that the earth had opened and swallowed me."

Because Lewis's work was based on audiotapes, her markers for shame are limited to verbal and paralinguistic cues. In contrast, our study of the "moment of truth" in "Candid Camera" television shows was based on videotapes, and we found that very flagrant *gestural* markers of overt shame sometimes accompany verbal and paralinguistic cues or may occur alone (Scheff 1985; Scheff and Retzinger n.d.). When subjects learned they had been caught on camera in what they thought was a private moment, some of them showed extreme hiding behavior: they not only hid their face with both hands, but some also simultaneously turned away from the camera, and others even attempted to hide completely. (One man crawled beneath a desk.) We also observed gestures that we interpreted as hiding behavior, although they appeared in what Tomkins (1963) characterized as a "miniaturized" form. For example, at the moment of truth, many subjects began to bring one or both hands up to the face as if to cover it. Instead of covering it, however, they ended up only touching it.

Because the concept of hiding brings together many different types of ideational, verbal, and nonverbal markers, it is a significant aspect of overt shame. It is of considerable interest, therefore, that one of the markers, face touching, has been independently validated by a study with a very different methodology. Edelman (1989) surveyed five different European countries, focusing on the experience of embarrassment. Although the subjects also associated various other gestures with that emotion, face touching was mentioned in all five countries.

To summarize: overt, undifferentiated shame is marked by (1) a context in which self is perceived as negatively evaluated, by either self or other; (2) "hiding" behavior; and/or (3) the use of undifferentiated terms such as those listed above. In these instances, the negative evaluation of self appears to cause so much pain that it interferes with the fluent production of thought or speech, even though the pain is mislabeled.

Like the overt pattern, *bypassed* shame occurs in a context in which self is perceived as negatively evaluated. But unlike the markers of undifferentiated shame, which are often flagrant and overt, those of bypassed shame may be subtle and covert. Although thought and speech are not obviously disrupted, they take on a speeded-up but repetitive quality that Lewis refers to as "obsessive." Typically, her patients repeated a story or series of stories, talking rapidly and fluently, but not quite to the point. They appeared unable to make decisions, because of seemingly balanced pros and cons ("insoluble dilemmas"). They complained of endless internal replaying of a scene in which they felt criticized or in error. Often they reported that when they first realized the error, they winced or groaned and then immediately began to obsessively focus on the incident. In such situations, the mind seems to be so caught up with the unresolved scene that one feels unable to become directly involved in events in the present, even though there is no obvious disruption. One is somewhat distracted.

The two patterns of shame appear to involve opposite styles of response. In overt shame, the victim *feels* so much emotional pain that it obviously retards or disrupts thought and speech. In bypassed shame, the victim *avoids* the pain before it can be completely experienced, through hyperactive and rapid thought, speech, or actions.

Adler's (1956) theory of human development anticipated Lewis's discovery of the two basic types of unacknowledged shame. Although he did not use the term, Adler described a "feeling of inferiority," that is, shame, that played a central role in his theory. He argued that children's primary need is for love (for what Bowlby [1969] called a "secure attachment"). If love is not available at crucial points, the child can proceed along one of two paths. One path is to develop an "inferiority complex"—to become prone to overt, undifferentiated shame. The other is to compensate by seeking power—to avoid feeling shame by bypassing it, through what we have termed hyperactive and rapid thought, speech, or actions.

Although the two formulations are compatible, Lewis's work marks a significant advance over Adler's. His theory, true to the psychoanalytic genre, uses concepts that are static and highly abstract. For this reason, his propositions, though provocative, are virtually untestable. No one has envisioned the observable markers of feelings of inferiority, the inferiority complex, or the compensatory drive for power. Nor has the process implied by this theory been spelled out in sufficient detail to allow observations to evaluate its accuracy. Through what concrete steps does deprivation of love cause either an inferiority complex or the drive for power? Adler's theory is couched in concepts that are only "black boxes"; the wiring within and between these boxes is not specified. His "theory" is not testable as it stands.

In contrast, Lewis's formulations provide the foundation for a testable theory, because they describe or at least imply observable markers for the major concepts involved and for the events in the connecting causal chain. She also specifies the behavioral manifestations of Adler's structures, allowing their presence or absence to be detected in actual episodes of social interaction. To our knowledge, hers is the first general theory of human behavior with these desirable characteristics.

Although overt shame and bypassed shame appear to be very different in terms of behavior, the difference is one of outer style; the different appearances mask an underlying similarity. Both the slowed-down pattern of overt shame and the speeded-up pattern of bypassed shame are disruptive; both involve rigid and distorted reactions to reality. Both kinds of shame are equally invisible—one is misnamed, the other ignored. These two basic patterns explain how shame might be ubiquitous, yet usually escape notice.

A series of studies by Scheff (1986, 1987, 1989) has shown how Lewis's theory and method can be applied to audiotaped discourse to demonstrate the cycle of insult, humiliation, revenge, counterrevenge, and chronic resentment that characterizes interminable quarrels and silent impasses. Retzinger (1988) reports similar results with videotapes of marital quarrels, using standard methods for rating visual, as well as verbal and paralinguistic, cues. The analysis of audio and videotapes may provide a new path toward establishing a causal relationship involving self-esteem, emotion, and behavior.

The concept of low-visibility shame may give us a key to what has been a very important unsolved problem: the origins of destructive anger. The cause of angry violence, of anger that goes out of control, has always been something of a mystery. We know that anger alone does not usually result in violence, because most anger is of brief duration and relatively low intensity. What, then, is the additional ingredient that results in violence?

The additional ingredient, according to several theorists, is what Lewis (1971) calls *unacknowledged shame*. She argues that the combination of unacknowledged shame and anger causes a feeling trap, an alternation between shame and anger, taking the form of a chain reaction that can lead to explosive violence. She calls the result *humiliated fury*—feeling ashamed that one is angry, angry that one is ashamed, and so on, in a sequence that will not subside.

The psychoanalyst Heinz Kohut (1977) uses a somewhat different term, "narcissistic rage," for what seems to be the same state; he identifies it as a compound of shame and rage. A similar concept, which he called "impotent rage," can be found in Nietzsche. Interpreting the feeling of impotence as a variant or cognate for unacknowledged shame, Gottschalk, Winget, and Gleser (1969), Lewis (1971), and Wurmser (1981) all suggest that violence results from a mixture of shame and anger. Similar suggestions have already been mentioned above, particularly in the emphasis that Geen (1968) and Feshbach (1971) place on the role of insult and humiliation in causing aggression.

Lewis's discovery of unacknowledged shame and the affinity between shame and anger provides the basis for an explicit theory of the role of emotion in aggression and violence (Scheff 1987, 1988). According to this theory, pride and shame states almost always depend on the level of deference accorded a person: pride arises from deferential treatment by others ("respect"), and shame from lack of deference ("disrespect"). Gestures that imply respect or disrespect, together with the emotional response they generate, make up the *deference/emotion system,* which exerts a powerful influence on human behavior. Because both the level of deference being accorded and the person's emotional reactions are usually not acknowledged, this system has seldom been noticed, much less carefully studied. We will develop this analysis further in our discussion of the Attica prison riot, below.

The theory outlined here is supported by a series of exploratory studies, each study conducted independently, and independent of Lewis's work and the theory developed from it. Katz (1988) analyzed descriptions of several hundred criminal acts: vandalism, theft, robbery, and murder. In many of the cases, Katz found that the perpetrator felt humiliated and had committed the crime as an act of revenge. In some cases, the sense of humiliation was based on actual insults: "[A] typical technique [leading to murder] is for the victim to attack the spouse's deviations from the culturally approved sex role. . . . For example, a wife may accuse her husband of being a poor breadwinner or an incompetent lover . . . or the husband may accuse his wife of being 'bitchy,' 'frigid,' or promiscuous" (1988, 16).

In other cases, it was difficult to assess the degree to which the humiliations were real or imagined. Whatever the realities, Katz's findings support the model of the shame/rage feeling trap. In his analysis of the murder of intimates, he says: "The would-be killer must undergo a particular emotional process. He must transform what he initially senses as an eternally humiliating situation into a blinding rage" (1988, 19). Rather than acknowledging his or her shame, the killer masks it with anger, which is the first step into the abyss of shame/rage, ending in murder. Katz reports similar (though less dramatic) findings with respect to the other kinds of crimes he investigated. Because shame may be the key ingredient in a low level of self-esteem, Katz's study seems to implicate low self-esteem in the causation of criminal acts.

One issue not addressed by Katz's study concerns the conditions under which humiliation is transformed into rage. Because not all humiliation leads to blind rage, there must be some element not indicated in Katz's cases. Studies of family violence by Lansky strongly suggest what this extra element might be. In order to lead to blind rage, the shame component in the emotions that are aroused must be *unacknowledged.*

Lansky has published several studies of family violence. The first (1984) describes six cases, the second (1987) describes four. Another recent study (Lansky n.d.) analyzes a session with a single couple. In all eleven cases, Lansky reports similar emotional dynamics: violence resulted from the disrespectful and insulting manner that husbands and wives adopted toward each other. Although some insults were overt (cursing, open contempt and disgust), most were more covert (innuendo or double messages). Underhanded disrespect seemed to give rise to unacknowledged shame, which led in turn to anger and violence, as predicted by Lewis. It was difficult for participants to respond to innuendo and double messages; these forms of communication seemed to confuse them. Instead of admitting their upset and puzzlement, they answered in kind. The cycle involves disrespect, humiliation, revenge, counter-revenge, and so on, ending in violence.

Both spouses often seemed unaware of the intense shame their behavior generated, as Lansky described in one of the cases:

> A thirty-two-year-old man and his forty-six-year-old wife were seen in emergency conjoint consultation after he struck her. Both spouses were horrified, and the husband agreed that hospitalization might be the best way to start the lengthy treatment that he wanted. As he attempted to explain his view of his difficult marriage, his wife disorganized him with repeated humiliating comments about his inability to hold a job. These comments came at a time when he was talking about matters other than the job. When he did talk about work, she interrupted to say how immature he was compared to her previous husbands, then how strong and manly he was. The combination of building up and undercutting his sense of manliness was brought into focus. As the *therapist* commented on the process, the husband became more and more calm. . . . After the fourth session, he left his marriage and the hospital for another state and phoned the therapist for an appropriate referral for individual therapy. On follow-up some months later, he had followed through with treatment. (Lansky 1984, 34–35; emphasis added)

The wife's humiliation of the husband in this case was not disguised through innuendo; rather, her disparagement was overt. Her shaming tactics were disguised by her technique of first building him up by stating how "strong and manly" he was, then cutting him down. Perhaps she managed to confuse herself with this tactic as much as she confused him.

Lack of awareness of shame can be seen in Lansky's (n.d.) report of a conjoint session with a violent man and his wife. In this case, the wife dressed in a sexually provocative way, and her bearing and manner toward the interviewer were overtly seductive. Yet neither spouse acknowledged her activity, even when the interviewer asked them whether the wife was ever seductive toward other men. Although both answered affirmatively, their answers concerned only past events; there was an astonishing lack of comment on what was occurring at that very moment in the interview. It would seem that blind rage requires not only shaming and shame but also blindness toward these two elements.

Collective Violence

The studies by Katz and Lansky are only exploratory, but they may be used in reinterpreting earlier studies of collective violence, such as those concerned with the 1971 prison riot and killings at Attica State Prison in New York. It is not just the fact that the guards in the Attica prison were humiliated that may explain the riot; rather, their humiliation was unacknowledged and, for this reason, transformed into blind rage.

This general point is especially clear in Lansky's work. He argues that, before clinical intervention, unacknowledged shaming and shame lead to humiliation, rage, and violence. Then he shows that after an intervention in which the therapist comments on and helps the individuals acknowledge the shame process, the level of violence sharply drops. In the riots to be discussed here, this second step, the acknowledgment of shame, was of course absent. The details of the shame and anger process at the interpersonal level may help us understand causation at the level of organizations such as prisons and mental hospitals.

The studies by Katz and Lansky may also have implications for social policy. Lansky's work in particular—both the clinical studies already mentioned and his organizational studies, to be reviewed later—would seem to have policy implications. We will return to this issue at the end of this chapter.

Our analysis of the Attica riot implicates unacknowledged shame, and therefore level of self-esteem, as a causal agent in large-scale, collective violence. The extensive report by the McKay Commission (1972) and a study by Stotland suggest that the level of self-esteem of both prisoners and guards is a key issue in corrections policy. As Stotland describes it: "For both troopers and guards, sense of competence, violence, and self-esteem . . . are linked" (1976, 88). He further notes that "a person's self-esteem can be threatened by failure [and] insults" (86). Because we believe that these studies have both direct and indirect implications, we will devote considerable attention to them.

The analysis of self-esteem and aggression parallels more recent work on shame and humiliation leading to aggression (Katz 1988; Lansky 1987; Retzinger 1987, 1989). These studies suggest a powerful affinity between shame and rage. When a person is shamed, anger is quick to follow if shame is not acknowledged (Horowitz 1981; Katz 1988; Lan sky 1987; Lewis 1981; Retzinger 1987; Scheff 1987). These studies suggest two conditions in which unacknowledged shame leads to rage, one concerning *personality*, the other concerning *situational elements*. Persons who are prone to shame may respond quickly and violently to their perceptions of slights against the self. But even persons who are not especially prone to shame may also respond violently to insult and humiliation in certain situations—for example, if they perceive themselves as isolated from others, with no one to turn to in their anguish. The status of the social bonds the shamed person or group shares with others (Bowlby 1969) may be crucial. Strong bonds can facilitate the management of shame; weak or severed bonds can impair it.

Stotland's analysis of the role of self-esteem in riots can be expanded by reference to the theory and research reviewed here. Stotland describes frequent episodes of shame and humiliation, but he does not give these episodes the crucial causal role that we do. As suggested in our quotations from his articles, he notes shame and humiliation only in passing.

In our theory, rage is used as a defense against a threat to self, that is, feeling shame, a feeling of vulnerability of the whole self. Anger can be a protective measure to guard against shame, which is experienced as an attack on self. As humiliation increases, rage and hostility increase proportionally to defend against loss of self-esteem; there is a decrease in the ratio of pride to shame states.

Another case that can be reinterpreted in this way is the 1970 shooting of demonstrators by National Guardsmen at Kent State University in Ohio. In their interpretation of the violence at Kent State, Stotland and Martinez conclude:

> The events . . . leading up to the killings were a series of inept, ineffectual, almost *humiliating* moves by the Guardsmen against the "enemy." . . . The answer to these threats to their self-esteem, to their sense of competence, was violence. . . . Another aspect . . . which added to the threat to the self-esteem of the Guardsmen [was that] during their presence on . . . campus . . . the students insulted Guardsmen . . . [and the Guardsmen] were not in a position to answer back. Their relative silence was another *humiliation* for them. (1976, 12; emphasis added)

In these cases, hostility can be viewed as an attempt to ward off feelings of humiliation (shame) generated by inept, ineffectual moves, a sense of incompetence, insults, and a lack of power to defend against insults.

We will also use the events of the Attica prison riot to demonstrate the connection between self-esteem, shame, and violence. "With the exception of Indian massacres in the late nineteenth century, the state police assault which ended the four-day prison uprising was the bloodiest one-day encounter between Americans since the Civil War" (McKay Commission 1972, xi). Our analysis is a further attempt to explain the brutal events at Attica, where prisoners rebelled, seized hostages, gained control of a large part of the prison, and held it for several days. Finally, state troopers and guards attacked, killing both hostages and inmates. Even after the inmates' power had been destroyed, violence by the guards and troopers continued. The McKay Commission reported numerous instances of "brutality and humiliation of the inmates"; prisoners were killed, wounded, and humiliated (forced to crawl naked through mud, for example).

Our reanalysis concerns the underlying emotional dynamics behind self-esteem, as it exists in the context within and between prisoners, guards, and prison administration. The continuing violence against the inmates after they were no longer a threat points to anger and hostility as a defense against shame.

The conditions at Attica before the crisis made it easy to understand the need for reform:

> For inmates, "correction" meant daily degradation and humiliation: being locked in a cell fourteen to sixteen hours a day; working for wages that averaged thirty cents a day in jobs with little or no vocational value; having to abide by hundreds of petty rules for which they could see no justification. . . . All their activities were regulated, standardized, and monitored for them by prison authorities . . . their incoming and outgoing mail was read, their radio programs were screened, their reading material was restricted, their movements outside their cells were regulated, they were told when to turn lights out and when to wake up. (McKay Commission 1972, 3)

The degrading conditions the inmates faced mark "overregulation" by the institution (Lansky 1983), a breeding ground for shame and humiliation.

The crisis at Attica began with the appointment of a new commissioner, Russell G. Oswald, an "enlightened and progressive correctional administrator," who saw the abject conditions and the necessity for improvements. Oswald's philosophy was that "an atmosphere of community life-style, even though in a confined situation, [held] greater promise for successful rehabilitation" (McKay Commission 1972, 130–131). He granted the inmates new rights, such as mail and visiting privileges, and revised censorship procedures to allow privacy with attorneys and public officials, greater access to media, and increased public knowledge of prison conditions. He also ordered that Muslim prisoners be given porkless meals and ruled that inmates were entitled to defend themselves when charged with infractions. These new policies granted civil rights to the inmates, removed some of the humiliating conditions, and gave the prisoners a greater sense of self-respect.

Although these were enlightened and necessary changes, the new policies were not well received by the guards. The commissioner's policies led to a decline in the power and status of the guards relative to the inmates.

> Attica's all-white correctional staff from rural western New York State was comfortable with inmates who "knew their place," but unprepared and untrained to deal with the new inmate. . . . Unused to seeing *their authority challenged*, officers *felt threatened* by the new inmate. Viewing the recent relaxation of rules and discipline, the interventions of the courts, and the new program for the inmates, they felt that their authority was being undermined by Albany and that *their superiors were not backing them up*. The officers became *increasingly resentful and insecure*. The result was . . . daily confrontations between the new inmate and the old-style officer. (McKay Commission 1972, 107; emphasis added)

The courts were also responsive to the inmates' complaints; for example, punitive damages were assessed against the warden on May 14, 1970, for censorship of mail to lawyers and public officials.

The reaction of the guards was intense. Guards felt that the courts were "interfering in matters in which they had no competence. Judges, they felt, knew nothing about either prisons or prisoners. . . . The decisions were wrong, guards felt, and *they—not the judges—would have to live with the consequences*" (McKay Commission 1972, 125; emphasis added). The new rules created a sense of *helplessness* for the guards, who had no voice in decisions that directly affected them. In this way, they were as powerless as the inmates had been before the new policies came into effect. The administration was being responsive to the inmates' needs, but not to the needs of the guards, because the conditions of the inmates were more visible than the problems of the guards.

Helplessness and feelings of incompetence are intrinsically connected with shame states, which were not acknowledged by the guards or administration, but which created a response of increased hostility toward the inmates. The McKay Commission reports: "Corrections officers frequently found themselves demanding adherence to rules which inmates would not accept. As the number of confrontations increased . . . so did their intensity. An officer's orders to stop talking . . . were first questioned, later ignored, and finally ridiculed" (1972, 120).

While feelings of competence and control increased among the inmates, feelings of incompetence and shame increased among the guards. Greater attempts to control the inmates, who responded with less tolerance for disrespect, led to increased hostility and lack of respect on the part of the guards. The guards began concentrating on inmates who were considered "troublemakers," searching for behavior that would justify discipline, harassing inmates who advocated prison reform, searching cells, and locking up men for investigation.

Under new contracts, more experienced guards began taking posts that involved the least contact with inmates. The less experienced guards were closer in age to the inmates, which caused resentment. The inmates faced not only inexperienced officers but also new ones. The new guards did not have "supervisory training or experience; they were totally unprepared for the jobs. . . . The inmates could never learn what was expected of them from one day to the next," and the officers had difficulty ascertaining what caused the inmates' uncooperative behavior, leaving both sides with few incentives to "establish any *rapport* or *respect*" (McKay Commission 1972, 126, 127; emphasis added). There was no opportunity or desire to develop mutual understanding. The lack of social bonds, as indicated earlier, breeds shame; separation and shame are intricately connected. Thus the tensions and conflict between inmates and guards steadily increased.

Hostile behavior and lack of respect by both sides grew more serious. When a guard attempted to regulate a prisoner, the inmate punched him lightly in the chest. This defiance was supported by other inmates, and the guard, powerless to do anything, backed away. The inmate was placed in special custody the next day, a punishment that other inmates perceived as excessive. Violence by the guards increased, in response to the humiliating situation of the previous day. With no way to verify the facts, a rumor spread among the inmates that the prisoner in special custody had been brutally beaten.

In response to the rumor, inmates attacked guards and began to take over the prison. The guards responded with the sense that they were helpless to do anything commensurate with the seriousness of the outbreak; nor did they immediately inform the administration. The takeover quickly escalated: keys were taken from guards, inmates found and improvised weapons. The takeover involved five cell blocks, shops, the

auditorium, the school, the commissary, and forty-two officers and ci-
vilian hostages. Even the warden admitted to being helpless. These developments were spontaneous; the McKay Commission found no evidence that the uprising was planned.

The staff expected the prison to be retaken immediately. Instead, ne-
gotiations developed, causing further resentment among the staff, for
the tradition in correctional institutions is to refuse to negotiate with
inmates holding hostages. Guards arrived with their own weapons, but
they were restrained by their superiors, causing more bitterness. The
guards were angered not only by the increase in inmate power and
the mistreatment of the hostages but also by the recognition given to the
prisoners, "as if they were equals." The guards felt that they were not
being given recognition by the administration or the media. They
watched as the inmates denounced them on television. No one stood up
for the guards; they were ignored.

Although the governor ordered that corrections officers should be excluded from the assault force because of their emotional involvement,
the order never reached the state police or correctional supervisors. The
result was a bloody massacre.

In the aftermath of the assault, hundreds of inmates were stripped
and brutalized by corrections officers, troopers, and sheriffs' deputies.
The suffering of wounded inmates was prolonged by failure to make
adequate arrangements for medical attention.

Stotland's analysis, that the "guards' and troopers' self-esteem must
have suffered by the rise in status and power of the inmates" (1976, 93),
can be interpreted further. The guards were shamed by their powerlessness relative to the inmates and the administration. Feeling that they had
no one to turn to and being humiliated by both sides, the guards engaged in angry attempts at control that finally ended in brutal violence.

An analysis of the deference/emotion system (Scheff 1988) may be
used to explain the sequence of events. The administration, guards, and
inmates were involved in a complex emotional tangle, with the guards
caught between the other two factions. The guards were shamed the
most—both by the administration, who failed to consult them before
making changes, and by the inmates, who challenged their authority.
Shown a lack of respect by both sides, the guards were in a position to
enter the shame/rage spiral, which led to further disrespectful acts toward the prisoners; this in turn trapped them in their own spiral, and so
on, in a repetitive loop of insult, humiliation, revenge, back and forth
between guards and prisoners.

Although the commissioner's new policies had been more humane, giving inmates more rights, the guards had never been consulted, and they had not been trained to deal with the new level of inmate rights. Thus they reacted with old disciplinary actions. Under the old rules, the inmates' behavior could be viewed as disrespectful. The tension between guards and inmates increased in part because of the perceived lack of respect shown to the guards by the inmates and the resulting humiliation felt by the guards. The prisoners in turn perceived the guards' behavior as lack of respect; the prisoners knew they had been given new rights and felt that they did not deserve to be treated in the old style. To reciprocate this lack of respect, the inmates humiliated the guards further by questioning, ignoring, and ridiculing them.

The situation can be interpreted as a triple shame/rage spiral (Scheff 1987). The guards were shamed by the behavior of the administration and the inmates, were powerless to confront the administration, and became hostile toward the inmates, who in turn were shamed by the guards' lack of respect and reacted with an angry lack of respect toward the guards. The theory predicts no limit to the intensity of the emotions generated in this chain reaction, a prediction amply borne out in this case.

To summarize our interpretation: First, the initial level of self-esteem of the prisoners was unacceptably low; prison policy and the informal system used by the guards combined to constantly humiliate the inmates. Second, reforms were introduced in a way that humiliated the guards, because they were not allowed to participate in the changes. The riot itself appears to have been a result of changes in the level of self-esteem of the guards. Perhaps because these changes were not acknowledged, the humiliation they caused led to blind rage and violence.

Short-Range and Long-Range Policy Implications

Our analysis may have implications for social policy. The level of self-esteem of those involved with social agencies, both staff and clients, may be crucial not only in explosive crises but also in day-to-day operation. If we construe self-esteem to involve the management of shame, then a host of issues that are usually unnoticed become important.

This review suggests that both formal and informal policies should consider the material well-being of staff and clients and the level of respect that is being accorded to them. Because issues of pride and shame typically go unacknowledged, reorienting policy along these new lines is not a simple matter.

At the policy level, it may be possible to make changes that would upgrade the level of self-esteem of both staff and clients. Lansky (1983, 1984) has proposed that mental hospital units need to avoid what he calls *overregulation* of patients. He suggests that overregulation humiliates clients and interferes with their rehabilitation. His experience as an administrator shows that policy changes can be made without alienating staff, by continuing education and by including staff in the planning of change.

Lansky's unit has established what seems to be something of a record for successful treatment. For example, in more than fourteen years of dealing with openly suicidal patients, none of the approximately 350 inpatients or recent discharges originally admitted in acute suicidal crisis has actually committed suicide or even made a serious attempt. Although we cannot provide records of comparable units, it appears to us that the effectiveness of Lansky's unit may be unparalleled in this respect.

In addition to training the staff to be sensitive to shame and shaming, Lansky's unit calls in families to participate in the treatment program. Family participation in treatment of suicidal patients appears to be extremely important. By commenting on and interrupting a family shaming process and by bringing the family into treatment, the unit can successfully take what seem to be great risks: "We often allow such patients to go on weekend passes after management sessions with family, or go to jobs, even while they are suicidal" (Lansky 1983, 108). The policy of avoiding overregulation, as carried out in Lansky's unit, seems to be effective.

At the level of state policy, Lansky's unit could be used as a model to train staff at other mental hospitals. Lansky has apparently been successful at helping staff understand the patients' intense need for respectful treatment, avoiding overregulation of patients' activities, and training staff to notice and comment on the shame process. Perhaps lectures and videotapes concerning Lansky's techniques could be used to construct a training program.

It may also be possible to build on Lansky's methods so that they would be applicable to any kind of social agency. Self-esteem workshops could be made available for prisons, mental hospitals, and welfare agencies, sensitizing staff to the relationship between pride and shame, respectful treatment, and self-esteem.

For the sake of brevity, we will give only one example of the kind of training we have in mind. In order to maintain and build client self-esteem, staff must be acutely aware of the fact that signals of respect and disrespect are carried less by *what* is said than by *how* it is said. That is, respect is signaled much more by our *manner* than by the *content* of what we say. In routine contacts, we often forget that our facial expression, bearing, and intonation can be disrespectful, even though our words are proper. Clients, who are already in a disadvantaged position, are likely to be extremely sensitive to an insulting or demeaning manner, no matter how subtle.

Even with only brief training, staff members seem to learn that becoming aware of their own manner is advantageous both to them and to the clients. For example, staff who are unaware of the difference between content and manner may tend to be somewhat embarrassed to talk openly about the gritty details of a client's situation. But avoiding the details works to the disadvantage of the client. First, it interferes with resolving the client's problems. Second, the lack of acknowledgment or resolution of staff-client embarrassment helps to perpetuate the client's already low level of self-esteem, as explained by the theory reviewed above.

Becoming aware of the importance of their own manner often has a liberating effect on staff members' ability to deal with clients. Staff may quickly realize that if their manner is respectful, they are free to talk about anything with little risk of embarrassment. This change may be extremely valuable, because it promotes cooperation in solving the client's real problems and also may help in increasing the client's level of self-esteem.

The self-esteem workshops and policy changes suggested here are both short-range interventions that could be introduced into social policy very quickly. Both interventions would involve upgrading the professional standing of staff through policy changes and continuing education. Both changes could be instituted with very little cost, requiring only relatively small changes in the relevant laws and organizational policy, as well as brief training programs.

The idea that the self-esteem of both staff and clients is a key ingredient in the effectiveness of social programs also suggests the possibility of long-range changes in policy. For example, the upgrading of the status of social agency staff through policy changes and continuing education is limited by certain features of the existing framework of social programs. One such feature involves the centralization and isolation of mental hospitals, prisons, and similar social agencies, relative to the communities from which their staff and clients are drawn. The isolation of these units seems to affect not only the self-esteem of the inmates but also that of the staff. As long as staff and inmates are separated from their communities of origin, those communities can emotionally disown them, treating them as aliens rather than as members, reducing the social status of both staff and inmates. This can certainly serve as a brake on any proposed program to increase their status and self-esteem.

With respect to mental hospitals, a proposal to change the framework has already been made. The Task Force on the Seriously Mentally Ill has submitted a proposal to the state of California that calls for decentralizing the mental health system along the lines we have suggested above: small treatment units that can be located in or near the community from which their staff and clients are drawn. If our analysis of self-esteem, crime, and violence proves to be valid, then the same reasoning should also apply to the corrections system. The day of the huge centralized prison is probably over. Small units located in or near the communities they serve may be the wave of the future.

No doubt the long-range changes in the mental health and corrections system advocated here would be expensive initially. Given the relationships we have discussed between self-esteem and program outcomes, however, it is possible that in the long run the initial investment would be more than repaid by increases in the efficiency and humaneness of the new programs. Perhaps both the short-range and long-range changes might be tried out first on a small scale, with careful studies to evaluate their effectiveness. If they proved effective in the small trial units, this record could encourage their introduction on a large scale.

Bibliography

Adler, A. 1956. *The Individual Psychology of Alfred Adler.* Edited by H. Ansbacher and R. Ansbacher. New York: Basic Books.

Bandura, A., and R. Walters. 1959. *Adolescent Aggression.* New York: Ronald Press.

Berkowitz, L. 1962. *Aggression: A Social Psychological Analysis.* New York: McGraw-Hill.

Bowlby, J. 1969. *Attachment and Loss.* Vol. 1, *Attachment.* New York: Basic Books.

Buss, A. H. 1961. *The Psychology of Aggression.* New York: Wiley.

Bynner, J. M., P. M. O'Malley, and J. G. Bachman. 1981. "Self-Esteem and Delinquency Revisited." *Journal of Youth and Adolescence* 10(6): 407–444.

Cohen, A. R. 1959. "Some Implications of Self-Esteem for Social Influence." In *Personality and Persuasibility,* by I. L. Janis et al., 102–120. New Haven, Conn.: Yale University Press.

Cooley, C. H. 1902. *Human Nature and the Social Order.* New York: Scribner.

Crandall, R. 1973. "The Measurement of Self-Esteem and Related Constructs." In *Measures of Social Psychological Attitudes,* edited by J. P. Robinson and P. R. Shaver, 45–168. Ann Arbor, Mich.: Institute for Social Research.

Darwin, C. 1872. *The Expression of Emotion in Men and Animals.* New York: Philosophical Library.

Diggory, J. C. 1966. *Self-Evaluation: Concepts and Studies.* New York: Wiley.

Dollard, J., L. Doob, N. Miller, O. Mowrer, and R. Sears. 1939. *Frustration and Aggression.* New Haven, Conn.: Yale University Press.

Edelman, R. 1989. "Self-Reported Expression of Embarrassment in Five European Cultures." *Journal of Cross-Cultural Psychology,* forthcoming.

Epstein, S., and S. P. Taylor. 1967. "Instigation to Aggression as a Function of Degree of Defeat and Perceived Aggressive Intent of the Opponent." *Journal of Personality* 35:265–289.

Feshbach, S. 1971. "The Dynamics and Morality of Violence and Aggression." *American Psychologist* 26:281–292.

Geen, R. G. 1968. "Effects of Frustration, Attack, and Prior Training in Aggressiveness upon Aggressive Behavior." *Journal of Personality and Social Psychology* 9:316–321.

Glueck, S., and E. Glueck. 1950. *Unraveling Juvenile Delinquency.* New York: Commonwealth Fund.

Goffman, E. 1967. *Interaction Ritual.* New York: Anchor.

Gottschalk, L., C. Winget, and G. Gleser. 1969. *Manual of Instructions for Using the Gottschalk-Gleser Content Analysis Scales.* Berkeley and Los Angeles: University of California Press.

Horowitz, M. 1981. "Self-Righteous Rage and the Attribution of Blame." *Archives of General Psychiatry* 38:1233–1238.

Jackson, M. 1984. *Self-Esteem and Meaning: A Life-Historical Investigation.* Albany, N.Y.: SUNY Press.

Kaplan, H. B. 1975. *Self-Attitudes and Deviant Behavior.* Pacific Palisades, Calif.: Goodyear.

———. 1980. *Deviant Behavior in Defense of Self.* New York: Academic Press.

Kaplan, H. B., R. J. Johnson, and C. A. Bailey. 1986. "Self-Rejection and the Explanation of Deviance: Refinement and Elaboration of a Latent Structure." *Social Psychology Quarterly* 49(2): 110–128.

———. 1987. "Deviant Peers and Deviant Behavior: Further Elaboration of a Model." *Social Psychology Quarterly* 50(3): 277–284.

Kaplan, H. B., S. S. Martin, and R. J. Johnson. 1986. "Self-Rejection and the Explanation of Deviance: Specification of the Structure Among Latent Constructs." *American Journal of Sociology* 92:384–411.

Katz, J. 1988. *The Seductions of Crime.* New York: Basic Books.

Kingsbury, S. J. 1978. "Self-Esteem of the Victim and the Intent of Third-Party Aggression in the Reduction of Hostile Aggression." *Motivation and Emotion* 2(2): 177–189.

Kohut, H. 1977. "Thoughts on Narcissism and Narcissistic Rage." In *The Restoration of the Self,* by H. Kohut, 124–160. New York: International Universities Press.

Lansky, M. 1977. "Establishing a Family-Oriented Inpatient Unit." *Journal of Operational Psychiatry* 8:66–74.

———. 1983. "The Role of the Family in the Evaluation of Suicidality." *International Journal of Family Psychiatry* 3:107–118.

———. 1984. "Violence, Shame, and the Family." *International Journal of Family Psychiatry* 5:21–40.

———. 1987. "Shame and Domestic Violence." In *The Many Faces of Shame,* edited by D. Nathanson. New York: Guilford.

———. n.d. "Murder of a Spouse: A Family System Viewpoint." Typescript.

Lewis, H. 1971. *Shame and Guilt in Neurosis.* New York: International Universities Press.

———. 1981. *Freud and Modern Psychology: The Emotional Basis of Mental Illness.* New York: Plenum.

Lynd, H. 1958. *Shame and the Search for Identity.* Glencoe, Ill.: Free Press.

McCarthy, J. D., and D. R. Hoge. 1984. "The Dynamics of Self-Esteem and Delinquency." *American Journal of Sociology* 90:396–410.

McCord, W., J. McCord, and A. Howard. 1961. "Familial Correlates of Aggression in Nondelinquent Male Children." *Journal of Abnormal and Social Psychology* 62(1): 79–93.

MacDougall, W. 1908. *An Introduction to Social Psychology.* London: Methuen.

McKay Commission (New York State Special Commission on Attica). 1972. *Attica: A Report.* New York: Praeger.

Matsueda, R. C. 1982. "Testing Control Theory and Differential Association." *American Sociological Review* 47:489–504.

Piers, G., and M. Singer. 1953. *Shame and Guilt: A Psychoanalytic and Cultural Study.* New York: Norton.

Retzinger, S. 1987. "Resentment and Laughter: Video Studies of the Shame-Rage Spiral." In *The Role of Shame in Symptom Formation,* edited by H. Lewis, 151–182. Hillsdale, N.J.: Erlbaum.

———. 1988. "Marital Quarrels: The Role of Emotion." Ph.D. dissertation, University of California, Santa Barbara.

————. 1989. "Marital Conflict: The Role of Emotion." *International Journal of Family Psychiatry*, forthcoming.

Rosenbaum, M. E., and R. deCharms. 1962. "Self-Esteem and Overt Expressions of Aggression." In *Decisions, Values, and Groups*, vol. 2, edited by N. F. Washburne, 291–303. New York: Pergamon.

Rosenberg, M. 1988. Personal communication to T. Scheff.

Satir, V. 1972. *Peoplemaking*. Palo Alto, Calif.: Science and Behavior Books.

Savin-Williams, R. C., and D. H. Demo. 1983. "Conceiving or Misconceiving the Self: Issues in Adolescent Self-Esteem." *Journal of Early Adolescence* 3:121–140.

Scheff, T. 1984. "The Taboo on Coarse Emotions." *Review of Personality and Social Psychology* 5:146–169.

————. 1985. "The Primacy of Affect." *American Psychologist* 40:849–850.

————. 1986. "Micro-Linguistics and Social Structure: A Theory of Social Action." *Sociological Theory* 4:71–83.

————. 1987. "Interminable Quarrels: Case Study of a Shame-Rage Spiral." In *The Role of Shame in Symptom Formation*, edited by H. Lewis, 109–149. Hillsdale, N.J.: Erlbaum.

————. 1988. "Shame and Conformity: The Deference/Emotion System." *American Sociological Review* 53:395–406.

————. 1989. "Cognitive and Emotional Components in Anorexia: Reanalysis of a Classic Case." *Psychiatry*, forthcoming.

Scheff, T., and S. Retzinger. n.d. "Hiding Behavior: Toward Resolution of the Controversy over Shame." Typescript.

Stotland, E. 1976. "Self-Esteem and Violence by Guards and Troopers at Attica." *Criminal Justice and Behavior* 3:85–96.

Stotland, E., and J. Martinez. 1976. "Self-Esteem and Mass Violence at Kent State." *International Journal of Group Tensions* 6:4–54.

Toch, H. 1969. *Violent Men*. Chicago: Aldine.

Tomkins, S. 1963. *Affect/Imagery/Consciousness*. Vol. 2, *The Negative Affects*. New York: Springer.

Wells, L. E. 1978. "Theories of Deviance and the Self-Concept." *Social Psychology Quarterly* 41(3): 189–204.

Wells, L. E., and G. Marwell. 1976. *Self-Esteem: Its Conceptualization and Measurement*. Beverly Hills, Calif.: Sage.

Wells, L. E., and J. H. Rankin. 1983. "Self-Concept as a Mediating Factor in Delinquency." *Social Psychology Quarterly* 46(1): 11–22.

Worchel, P. 1958. "Personality Factors in the Readiness to Express Aggression." *Journal of Clinical Psychology* 14:355–359.

Wurmser, L. 1981. *The Mask of Shame*. Baltimore: Johns Hopkins University Press.

Wylie, R. C. 1979. *The Self-Concept*. Vol. 2, *Theory and Research on Selected Topics*. Rev. ed. Lincoln: University of Nebraska Press.

Self-Esteem and Chronic Welfare Dependency

Leonard Schneiderman, Walter M. Furman, and Joseph Weber

Introduction

California State Assembly Bill 3659, the act that created the California Task Force to Promote Self-Esteem and Personal and Social Responsibility, identifies chronic welfare dependency, along with crime and violence, alcoholism and drug abuse, teenage pregnancy, child abuse, and educational failure, as "intractable social problems" of major concern to the citizens of California. It declares that the most cost-effective and humane solution to such social problems is to "discover, address, eradicate, and thereby prevent" their causes. This legislation calls specific attention to low self-esteem as a possible root of these social problems:

> Low self-esteem may well have a wide-ranging, negative influence on individual human conduct, the costs of which both in human and societal terms are manifested in a number of ways, many of which convert into significant expenditure of state moneys. If so, these human costs and the costs to government could be reduced by raising the self-esteem level of our citizenry.

This chapter will review the scholarly literature linking self-esteem and chronic welfare dependency. At least three possibilities exist:

1. Variations in levels of self-esteem are related to variations in welfare dependency. That is, low self-esteem "causes" prolonged dependence on public assistance. Or, high self-esteem allows resistance to negative public attitudes and bureaucratic obstacles and "causes" indi-

200

viduals to use welfare benefits on a long-term basis when no other means of support is available.

2. Chronic dependence on welfare affects recipients' levels of self-esteem. Dependence on welfare "causes" feelings of helplessness and loss of control and lowers self-esteem. Or, dependence on welfare may enhance self-esteem through providing basic resources and improving living conditions (Nichols-Casebolt 1986).

3. No scholarly evidence links self-esteem to chronic welfare dependence.

All available research on the relationship between chronic welfare dependency and self-esteem necessarily rests on certain assumptions about the nature and causes of poverty and dependency. One set of assumptions holds that poverty and dependency are the consequences of external events over which affected persons can exercise little control, such as an economic system that does not provide opportunities for all to earn an adequate income. Another view assumes that poverty reflects a lack of ability or other personal deficiencies (perhaps low self-esteem) among the poor themselves and is the result of their failure to take advantage of existing opportunities (Gilder 1981; Murray 1984).

Differences also exist concerning the relative importance of public policies designed to reduce *poverty* and public policies designed to reduce *dependency.* To the extent that individuals do not have enough income to maintain an adequate standard of living, they are thought to be "poor." To the extent that individuals receive income from government transfers, they are thought to be "dependent." Some advocate public transfers (hence dependency) to reduce or eliminate the injurious effects of poverty, based on the conviction that an affluent society has a moral obligation to those in need. Others oppose using government transfers to reduce poverty, based on the conviction that such aid will undermine character and weaken self-sufficiency.

Reducing poverty and reducing dependency are compelling goals of social policy, but they are clearly not fully compatible. Different legislatures, in different times, with different leadership have seen these problems in different ways and have advocated different public policy responses (Morris and Williamson 1987).

Liberals and conservatives have tended to divide according to the explanations of poverty they find most convincing and the relative priority they assign to poverty reduction and dependency reduction, although recent signs indicate decreasing polarization and increasing consensus.

Both systemic and individual factors appear to play a role in reducing poverty, often interacting in complex ways. There is growing recognition that both liberals and conservatives share the goals of independence and self-sufficiency, although they may differ on public policies designed to promote the achievement of these goals. Liberals have generally held that adequate levels of income achieved through nonstigmatizing public income transfers and services (i.e., job creation and training, education, health and social services) may increase dependency in the short term but will lead to self-reliance in the long term. Conservatives hold that limiting transfer income may increase poverty in the short term but will be more likely, in the long term, to lead to adequate incomes through strengthened self-sufficiency; dependence on government is seen as the greater problem.

Across the political spectrum, concern that we have not been doing enough to aid the poor has been joined by a fear that we may be doing the wrong things. As a consequence, there has been a resurgence of interest in redesigning welfare programs (especially the program of Aid to Families with Dependent Children), with the aim of providing more adequate assistance to the poor without reinforcing or inducing values and habits that encourage prolonged dependency (Novak et al. 1987).

To what extent are persistent poverty and chronic welfare dependency associated with character deficiency and the failure of personal initiative, responsibility, and self-sufficiency? To what extent does relieving poverty through public income transfers have a detrimental effect on self-esteem and personal and social responsibility? To what extent can enforced self-reliance, accompanied by poverty, promote the long-term enhancement of independence, self-esteem, and personal and social responsibility? Can self-esteem prosper in an environment of material deprivation and limited opportunity? Do programs that improve material conditions and open new opportunities enhance self-esteem? What is the appropriate role of government in ensuring adequate incomes?

Questions so deeply enmeshed in personal values and ideology cannot be fully resolved through scientific inquiry, but there are some findings, drawn from available research, that can help us understand and approach the problem. In the pages that follow, we discuss "welfare" and attempt to delimit the social problem of primary concern here, that is, chronic welfare dependency. We look especially at the program of Aid to Families with Dependent Children and examine its role as the major public program designed to address the poverty of families and children in the United States and as the program most commonly thought of as "welfare." We then look at the dynamics of welfare utilization, patterns of entering and leaving the welfare system, and characteristics of the chronically dependent. We discuss the concept of self-esteem and then review evidence linking self-esteem to patterns of welfare utilization. We end with suggestions for research regarding chronic welfare dependency and discuss public policy implications emerging from the review.

Chronic Welfare Dependency as a Social Problem

Assembly Bill 3659 identifies the long-term use of legislatively created entitlements (welfare benefits) as an "intractable social problem." Unlike the other social problems listed in the bill, however, welfare dependency could not exist without legislatively mandated programs and legislatively authorized expenditures. Welfare benefits exist to fulfill the legislature's intention to relieve the poverty of those in dire need. In the case of the program of Aid to Families with Dependent Children (AFDC), welfare benefits are targeted to meet the needs of children who are deprived of parental support.

Why, then, does the California legislature regard the use of entitlements it has itself created as a problem? What is "welfare dependency," and at what point does the use of welfare become excessive? To answer these questions, we begin with a brief review of the range of social welfare benefits offered under governmental auspices in the United States.

Total public spending (federal, state, and local) for social welfare in the United States in 1984 amounted to $672 billion, or 18.2 percent of the gross national product (Social Security Administration 1986). Social insurance programs designed to protect against the loss of income as a result of old age, disability, death, or unemployment accounted for approximately 51 percent of the total. Health and medical programs (excluding Medicare and Medicaid) amounted to 6 percent, veterans' programs to 4 percent, education 23 percent, and public aid to the poor only 13 percent (Social Security Administration 1987).

The percentage of government spending devoted to social welfare has been declining steadily at federal, state, and local levels since 1979 (Social Security Administration 1987, 31). Excluding trust-fund social insurance programs, federal social welfare expenditures for public aid (including AFDC) have fallen sharply as a percentage of all federal spending, from 13.7 percent in 1979 to 10.5 percent in 1984, a 24 percent reduction in spending.

Of the approximately $90 billion in public aid targeted for the poor in 1984, $14.5 billion, or 16 percent, was expended as cash benefits through AFDC. The remaining 84 percent of the total went to the needy aged, blind, and disabled, to provide health benefits and food stamps. Put another way, of the $672 billion expended for social welfare purposes under public auspices in 1984, some $14.5 billion, or 2.2 percent of the total, went to AFDC, the one program usually identified as welfare (Social Security Administration 1986).

The enormous amount of attention given to so small a part of the nation's total social welfare effort reflects the symbolic importance of "welfare" and the deeply held public attitudes and values concerning it. It could be argued that all human beings are dependent to a greater or lesser extent on other people and on institutions. In a population of some 245 million Americans, for example, approximately 115 million are in the labor force. More than half of all Americans are therefore "dependent" on the productivity of others for the goods and services they need and want.

Such an example treats dependence as normative and basically benign. Ample evidence exists, however, that public attitudes toward dependence vary with its presumed degree of "legitimacy." If a particular group—such as children or the aged or disabled—is not expected to be self-supporting, or if a particular person's loss of independence is seen as involuntary, society views the dependence as legitimate. But if dependence occurs among people who are expected to be self-reliant, the public view is negative (Rainwater 1982).

Chronic welfare dependency is viewed as an intractable social problem to the extent that such dependence is not regarded as legitimate. Although dependence on the largest and most costly of the nation's welfare programs (Social Security) is largely seen as legitimate, this is not generally the case for the program of aid to poor children and their families. It is the question of legitimacy, and not just the dollars expended or the duration of benefits received, that defines welfare dependency as a problem and that led to our decision to confine this review of welfare dependence to the AFDC program.

Views about AFDC—whether dependence on the program is legitimate, for example, or whether such dependence lasts too long (that is, becomes chronic)—are powerfully influenced by how society feels about women as heads of households. If women who head families with children are expected to hold jobs and to be economically independent, even a short period of dependency may seem too long. If women who head families are not expected to participate in the labor force, then duration and degree of economic dependence may not seem like an intractable social problem.

Maternal employment has until recently been viewed negatively, because it may reduce the mother's participation in the child's educational activities and emotional development, as well as her monitoring and supervision of the child's activities. According to this argument, single mothers who are employed disadvantage their children doubly: such children spend less time with absent fathers *and* less time with their mothers. Our current AFDC program was enacted at a time when the prevailing judgment was that mothers should stay at home and be full-time caretakers of their children. Although this view is still strongly held, nearly everyone also agrees that heads of households should support their families. Thus, when a woman voluntarily assumes this role, she implicitly assumes the same obligations. This presents an unresolvable contradiction in values: single mothers should both hold jobs and stay at home (Garfinkel and McLanahan 1986).

Today, more than half of married mothers work outside the home at least part of the day. Given this change in the pattern of women's participation in the labor force, it is not surprising that welfare recipients are often viewed as lazy and undeserving and that welfare dependency is viewed as a problem. Despite the increasing expectation that women should hold jobs, the AFDC program continues to reflect ambivalent public attitudes by operating in a manner that discourages employment. Benefits are drastically reduced as earnings increase, and earnings replace rather than supplement welfare payments, often leaving those who are employed in a situation that is no better—and is sometimes worse (without medical care, for example)—than the situation of those who remain entirely dependent on AFDC. Sawhill (1976) found that women on welfare in the early 1970s had very low earning capacity; even if they had worked full time, more than half would still have earned less than they received in welfare grants. Schneiderman et al. (1987a) found that 90 percent of AFDC recipients in Los Angeles County in 1986 were totally dependent on AFDC benefits for their incomes.

A study by Ellwood (1986b) reports that only one woman in five who left welfare was able to do so as a result of increased income from earnings and that earnings adequate for self-support required year-round, full-time work at the level of two thousand hours annually. Using data from the Panel Study of Income Dynamics (Survey Research Center, Institute for Social Research 1984) for the late 1970s, Ellwood shows that only 8 percent of all wives (poor and nonpoor) with preschool children actually worked full time, with an additional 15 percent working between fifteen hundred and two thousand hours per year. If self-sufficiency based on earnings requires nearly full-time work, and if only one-quarter of all wives with young children work three-fourths of the time or more all year, complete self-sufficiency through earnings for single-parent households may not be a realistic goal for AFDC recipients with small children.

The strength of the legitimacy issue and its impact on the provision of benefits for women and children is evident when one compares public benefits available to widows and their children with benefits available to single mothers (divorced, separated, never married) and their children. Whereas 51 percent of all families headed by single mothers are poor, only 34 percent of families headed by widows are poor. Some of this difference is related to discrepancies between those social welfare benefits most commonly involving men and those in which women are predominantly involved—that is, differences between Social Security survivors' insurance, the program that aids widows and orphans, and AFDC, the program that aids primarily families headed by single mothers. Among whites, nearly 90 percent of all widows receive survivors' insurance, as do 70 percent of all widows among blacks. Only 23 percent of white divorced women and 34 percent of black divorced women receive AFDC, and the percentage of separated and never-married women, both white and black, who receive AFDC ranges from 40 to 59 percent. Yet it is difficult to argue that the financial needs of children living in these female-headed households are different from the needs of children in families headed by widows. In addition, the average Social Security survivors' insurance benefit is nearly twice the AFDC benefit among whites and more than double the AFDC benefit among blacks (Garfinkel and McLanahan 1986, 26).

> The division between social insurance and public assistance has bifurcated social welfare across class lines. With a strong, articulate, middle-class constituency, social insurance, especially social security, carries no stigma, and its expanded benefits have reduced drastically the amount of poverty among the elderly. Public assistance, which has become synonymous with welfare, is, of course, restricted to the very poor. Its recipients carry the historic stigma of the unworthy poor, and, as a consequence, they are treated meanly. Their benefits, which do not lift them out of poverty, remain far below those paid by social security. (Katz 1986, ix)

Williamson (1974), in a study of 375 men and women in the Boston area in 1972, tried to determine how well informed people were on a number of factual issues related to welfare. He asked respondents, "What percent of welfare recipients are able-bodied unemployed males?" Statistics compiled by the U.S. Department of Health, Education, and Welfare (HEW) for 1971 showed the official government estimate of this group to be less than 1 percent of the total number of recipients. But the mean estimate in Williamson's sample was 37 percent. He also asked, "What percent of welfare recipients lie about their financial situation?" HEW reported in 1971 that "suspected incidents of fraud or misrepresentation among welfare recipients occur in less than four-tenths of one percent (0.4 percent) of the total caseload in the nation." The mean response among the sample was 41 percent. Concerning the question of how many children under eighteen there were in the average AFDC family, official HEW figures showed 2.6 children per family. The mean response among the sample was 4.8. Williamson's data show evidence of negative misconceptions about welfare held by respondents at all levels of income and education. Surprisingly, even welfare recipients themselves shared these misconceptions.

Poverty and AFDC

Families headed by single women with children are the poorest of all major demographic groups in the United States, regardless of how poverty is measured (U.S. Bureau of the Census 1985). Their economic position relative to that of other groups, such as the aged or the disabled, has declined steadily during the past two decades.

Children being raised by their mothers alone are four times as likely to be poor as children with both parents at home. The poorest children are those with never-married mothers. (See Table 6.1.) More than 70 percent of children of never-married mothers—black, white, or Hispanic—lack enough money to reach the poverty level (U.S. Congress, Congressional Research Service and Congressional Budget Office 1985). Whether poverty is measured before or after government transfer payments and whether the income counted includes or excludes noncash benefits and money paid as taxes, poverty rates among children rose sharply from 1979 to 1983.

Roughly two-thirds of the nation's poorest families gained at least some of their income in 1985 from their own earnings. Welfare payments (principally AFDC) were the most frequent source of nonwage income for the poor; 37 percent received such income (U.S. Bureau of the Census 1985).

Table 6.1.   Who Are the Poor Children?
              by Family Structure

	Share of All Poor Children	Percentage Who Are Poor
In families headed by mothers who are		
Divorced or separated	31%	49%
Never-married	17	77
Widowed	5	39
Married, but spouse absent	1	54
All mother-headed families	54	53.6
In married-couple and other male-present families	46	11.7
All families	100	20.1

SOURCE: "Welfare and Poverty Among Children" 1987, 7.

Inadequate income levels can have important consequences for the well-being of children and families. Health, nutrition, and access to pre-natal and postnatal care are all associated with income level. Schneider-man and his colleagues (1987b) found in their study of 1,046 families receiving AFDC in 1986 that 18 percent of AFDC family cases and 29 percent of AFDC-UP (two-parent household) cases reported health-related conditions considered severe enough to interfere with em-ployment.

AFDC is the only federal program explicitly designed to provide cash assistance to impoverished families with children. Maximum benefit levels for a single-parent, two-child family with no income vary in the forty-eight contiguous states, from 16 percent of a 1986 poverty-level income (Alabama) to 85 percent (California).* (See Figure 6.1.) In fiscal year 1986, AFDC monthly enrollment averaged 11 million persons, 7.3 million children in 3.8 million families (U.S. Congress, Congressional Research Service and Congressional Budget Office 1985).

The AFDC program is targeted specifically for children who are de-prived of parental support because of the absence or disability (and in some cases unemployment) of a supporting parent. The size of the tar-geted population can be appreciated when we recognize that half of all American children born today will spend part of their childhood in a

* Only in Alaska and Hawaii do the combined AFDC and food stamp benefits exceed the poverty level. The national poverty level, however, is not corrected for the cost of living in a particular state, and the cost-of-living indexes in these two states tend to be quite high.

Figure 6.1.   Combined AFDC and Food Stamp Benefits for a Family of
                Three with No Income, January 1987

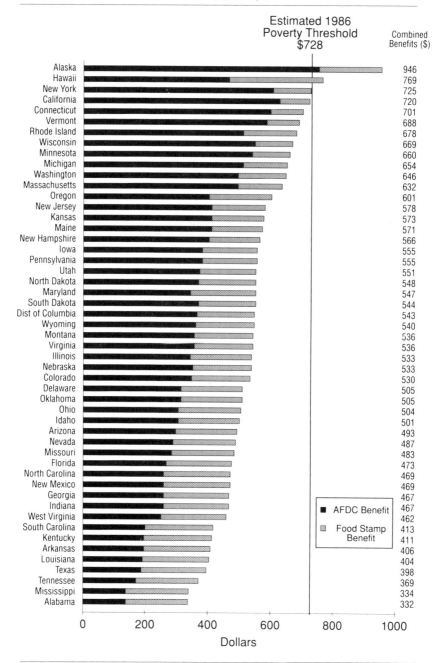

SOURCE: "Welfare and Poverty Among Children" 1987, 6.

family headed by a mother who is divorced, separated, unwed, or widowed. About half of all such families are poor and dependent on welfare (Bumpass 1984). To some extent, these dependent families are in periods of transition (between marriages or jobs, for example), averaging five years for white families and seven years for black families. From the child's point of view, these are long periods of time. Furthermore, a large and growing minority of black children are being born to never-married women and can expect to spend their entire childhood in a mother-only family (Garfinkel and McLanahan 1986, 7). Whereas 45 percent of white children will spend part of their youth in a family headed by a woman, the estimate for black children is 86 percent (Bumpass 1984).

The number of families in the AFDC program has been relatively stable since the mid-1970s, rising slightly during the recession of 1980. The number of children per family has declined, however. Consequently, the actual number of children receiving AFDC benefits has dropped steadily, but children still account for two-thirds of all recipients (U.S. Congress, House Select Committee on Children, Youth, and Families 1987, 86).

In 1984, 38.2 percent of children receiving AFDC were deprived of parental support as a result of divorce or separation, 46.4 percent as a result of being born out of wedlock, 1.9 percent because of the death of the father, 8.6 percent because of the father's unemployment, and 3.6 percent because the father was incapacitated (U.S. Congress, House Select Committee on Children, Youth, and Families 1987, 29). Schneiderman et al. (1987b) found in their June 22, 1986, sample of Los Angeles County AFDC recipients that 9.7 percent of those AFDC cases involved families of unemployed workers. Seventy percent of all the AFDC recipients were children.

How effectively were poor children and their families assisted by the AFDC program? In 1985, the national child poverty rate was reduced 4 percent by cash welfare benefits. Even though Social Security imposes no means test for eligibility, it reduced the child poverty rate by 6 percent in 1985 ("Welfare and Poverty Among Children" 1987). Because of sharply differing public attitudes, however, children and their caretaker parents who depend on Social Security benefit programs are not defined as being among the "chronically welfare dependent," regardless of the degree or duration of their reliance on Social Security payments.

The number of AFDC-assisted children as a percentage of all poor children grew until 1974, when the number of AFDC children per 100 poor children started dropping (U.S. Congress, Congressional Research

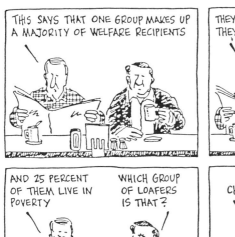
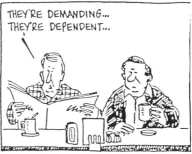
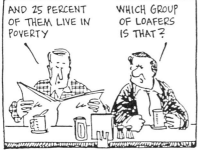
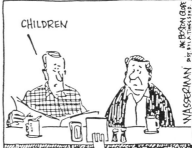

Service and Congressional Budget Office 1985, 212). The average number of children on AFDC per 100 children in poverty increased from 13.4 in 1960 to 83.6 in 1973; the number then declined continually from 77.5 per 100 in 1977 to 53.3 per 100 in 1983.

These figures suggest that concern about chronic welfare dependency must be balanced with concern about the destructive impact of the chronically unrelieved poverty of a shockingly large proportion of the nation's children. Increasing the number of poor children aided and increasing the level and adequacy of the benefits will necessarily relieve poverty and increase dependency. Limiting dependency through restrictive eligibility and inadequate benefit levels will discourage reliance on public benefits and contain cost but will also leave poverty essentially unrelieved. Questions of value and choice are involved here, which research findings can amplify but not resolve.

Who Are the Welfare Dependent?

Understanding chronic welfare dependency requires a review of patterns of welfare use over time—that is, the dynamics of entering and leaving the welfare system. The AFDC caseload is not static; daily, people enter and exit the program. Point in time, or cross-sectional, studies of welfare populations cannot adequately address factors that cause welfare dependency, cannot accurately measure past welfare use by a household or how long a current welfare episode will last. Cross-sectional studies do give an accurate picture of the characteristics of the caseload at a particular time, but that picture reflects the preponderance at any point of long-term welfare recipients and underestimates the amount of cycling on and off welfare that occurs among short-term recipients (Bane and Ellwood 1983; Wiseman 1985). For this reason, our analysis focuses on longitudinal studies of welfare and the lessons that have been learned from observing large samples over many years—decades, in some instances.

The two primary sources for longitudinal data on patterns of welfare dependency are the Panel Study of Income Dynamics (Survey Research Center, Institute for Social Research 1984), widely known as the PSID, and the National Longitudinal Survey (Center for Human Resource Research, Ohio State University 1980), known as the NLS. The first portion of the NLS was conducted in 1968 and sampled approximately five thousand women between the ages of fourteen and twenty-four. The PSID, conducted under the direction of the Survey Research Center at the University of Michigan, began in 1968 with a nationally representative sample of 2,930 households, plus another 1,872 households drawn from a previous census study (the Survey of Economic Well-Being) that concentrated on low-income households.

The analysis of information from the longitudinal surveys has involved different methods of characterizing the degree of welfare dependency. These methods include (1) simply counting years in which welfare was received at a criterion level (e.g., $250 per year) during the period of observation; (2) computing "spells" of welfare use; and (3) estimating "careers" of welfare use, including not only single spells but also probabilities of recidivism (Ellwood 1986a).

Each of these methods yields a somewhat different picture of the characteristics of individuals, assistance programs, and labor market conditions that affect entry into the welfare system, exits from welfare, and becoming chronically welfare-dependent. There is, however, no agreed-upon criterion in the empirical literature to delimit when a case is termed chronic or, as some analysts prefer, "persistently dependent" (Ellwood 1986a). In addition to the purely temporal measure of duration (length of time during which assistance is received), the extent of the family's reliance on AFDC for its household income (AFDC as a percentage of total income) is also often considered as a measure of dependency. Several analysts (Rein and Rainwater 1978; Coe 1981) note from the PSID data that income from AFDC for a family on aid generally constituted less than half of the entire household income reported in the multiyear period. (Rein and Rainwater found that two-thirds of the households receiving aid in at least four of the seven years observed received less than half of their entire income in the period from welfare.) In contrast, as mentioned earlier, recent research on AFDC recipients in Los Angeles County revealed that 90 percent of recipients had no income other than AFDC (Schneiderman et al. 1987a), a finding supported by Garfinkel and McLanahan's observation that about 85 percent of women with children do not work during any month in which they receive aid (1986, 38).

How then shall we define chronic welfare dependency? Depending on the method used to analyze total time on welfare, various authors (e.g., Coe 1981; O'Neill et al. 1984; Ellwood 1986a) have characterized persistent dependence as starting from two to ten years after the initial receipt of welfare aid. Most analysts view receiving welfare for five years or more as chronic or persistent dependency, and we will accept this rough guideline for delimiting the characteristics of the population chronically dependent on AFDC. (But we will apply it with some flexibility in reviewing work concerning the relationship between self-esteem and chronic welfare dependency.)

Going on Welfare

We have already noted that AFDC families become eligible for aid as a result of divorce or separation, out of wedlock births, or the father's unemployment, incapacity, or death. In our recent cross-sectional survey of the Los Angeles County caseload, the officially coded reasons for eligibility included 43.9 percent listed as separation, divorce, or desertion; 37.2 percent as an "absent parent" (i.e., children needing support in a household in which the parents never were married or lived together); 8.8 percent as loss of work (most of these cases were in the AFDC-UP program); and the remainder in various categories such as death or disability of a parent (Schneiderman et al. 1987b, 79–80).

These data point to the overwhelming primacy of changes in family or household composition, as opposed to changes in income levels, as the factors that precipitate welfare episodes. Bane and Ellwood ana-

Table 6.2.   Beginning Types for Spells of AFDC

	Percentage of All Beginnings
Wife became female head	45.2
Unmarried woman without child became female head with child[a]	30.4
Female head's earnings fell	12.1
Other	
Fall in other's earnings	3.0
Fall in other income	1.1
Family size grew	2.5
Moved	0.2
Unidentified	5.4

SOURCE: Bane and Ellwood 1983, 18.
[a]Unmarried women include those who are single, divorced, widowed, or separated.

lyzed the PSID sample data for women who had ever received AFDC (N = 676) to investigate reasons associated with going on welfare; their findings from the 554 observations of new welfare episodes are shown in Table 6.2. The authors conclude that "three-fourths of all spells of AFDC begin with a relationship change whereby a female-headed family with children was created. Only 12 percent of beginnings can be traced to earnings decreases" (1983, 19).

Short-Term AFDC Use

Although the subject of this analysis is chronic welfare dependency and its relationship to self-esteem, an aside about short-term welfare use provides a valuable context for the discussion. The NLS and PSID analyses focusing on welfare dynamics have promoted a new understanding that most welfare assistance is temporary and that a fairly large proportion of the general population (an estimated one-quarter) has at some point received welfare assistance (here defined to include AFDC, General Assistance, SSI, or food stamps received by the household head or spouse [Duncan and Hoffman 1987, 4]). Coe (1981, 140) shows that in the PSID sample only 25.8 percent of the individuals who ever received welfare between 1969 and 1978 received aid for more than five years during that period. And although it has been estimated that one-quarter of the general population has received welfare at some time, only an estimated 6.5 percent received it in six or more years during the ten-year period of observation. A recent summary of the body of evidence on welfare dynamics concludes: "Occasional welfare receipt is common, persistent welfare receipt is not. Movement on and off welfare rolls is widespread" (Duncan and Hoffman 1987, 3). Clearly, then, most welfare assistance does *not* involve chronic welfare dependence, and any policy or programmatic efforts to alter and reform the AFDC program must consider the large volume of short-term reliance on AFDC.

Leaving AFDC

Most analysis directly relating to welfare dependency concerns factors that differentiate short-term from long-term AFDC recipients. Ellwood (1986a) presents data from the PSID on "the primary reason for spell completion" for all observations of completed spells in the sample (Table 6.3). These data reveal that "becoming a wife is the primary reason that women leave welfare" and that "earnings gains account for only 21 percent of all exits" (1986a, 55–56). Other common reasons for terminating an AFDC episode are children reaching the age of eighteen (11.2 percent) and increases in other transfer income (14.2 percent—representing alimony, child support, Social Security [such as survivors' or disability benefits], and other transfers).

Table 6.3.   Percentage Distribution of Completed AFDC Spells, by Reason for Spell Completion

Primary Reason for Spell Completion	Percentage of All Persons Questioned[a]
Marriage, remarriage, or reconciliation	34.6
No longer had children under age eighteen[b]	11.2
Increase in own earnings	21.3
Increase in transfer income other than AFDC	14.2
Increase in earnings of other family members	4.9
Other change in family size	2.4
Moved	1.8
Unidentified or other	9.4

SOURCE: Ellwood 1986a, 57.
NOTE: These reasons were checked and tabulated in the order presented. That is, an individual who both got married and had a change in earnings of other family members was assigned "married" as the primary reason for the spell completion.
[a]Because of a rounding error, this column does not total exactly 100 percent.
[b]AFDC ended when children under age eighteen no longer resided in the household.

Table 6.4.   Probability of Remaining on Welfare Beyond a Given Number of Years: Results from Different Data Sets

Sample	Spell Duration (Years)									
	1	2	3	4	5	6	7	8	9	10
PSID[a]										
Bane and Ellwood 1983										
(N = 554)	.71	.52	.43	.38	.34	.20	.17	.15	N.A.	N.A.
Urban Institute										
(N = 787)	.53	.38	.28	.21	.17	.16	.12	.12	.11	.05
NLS[a]										
All races (N = 1,124)	.50	.39	.30	.24	.18	.16	.12	.10	.08	.07
Black[b] (N = 650)	.68	.54	.46	.37	.31	.27	.23	.19	.16	.16
White[b] (N = 474)	.42	.32	.22	.17	.13	.12	.08	.07	.05	.04
AFDC Case Records[c]										
1965 cohort	.59	.41	.32	.26	.22	.18	.16	.13	.11	.09
1970 cohort	.54	.36	.26	.21	.16	.13	.11	.09	.07	.05
1975 cohort	.50	.31	.21	.16	.12	.09	.07	—	—	—
1980 cohort	.45	.26	—	—	—	—	—	—	—	—

SOURCE: O'Neill et al. 1984.

NOTE: The PSID and NLS data include only welfare recipients who are adult women with children. The PSID data are further restricted to female heads of household, whereas the NLS data include women with children living in households where the women are not the heads. AFDC case record data cover all cases, including families headed by an unemployed father.

[a] Spell duration is derived from weighted data.
[b] Includes other races, except black.
[c] Data were not available for calculating survivorship beyond 1982. Probabilities are obtained from regression results.

O'Neill and her colleagues (1984) analyzed the PSID and the NLS data, as well as national AFDC caseload statistics between 1965 and 1982, in order to estimate durations of AFDC spells and to identify variables associated with long-term dependency. Table 6.4 shows the probability of remaining on welfare after a given number of years (post–case opening), as found in the three data sources. This table also presents results from Bane and Ellwood (1983), using a slightly different criterion for receipt of aid during the year.

The probability of remaining on welfare beyond five years was .34 in Bane and Ellwood's 1983 analysis, .18 for all races in the NLS data, and .22 for the cohort starting AFDC in 1965, but it was .16 and .12, respectively, for the 1970 and 1975 AFDC cohorts, indicating a reduction in long-term dependence over the time period. These findings are for single-spell durations, however, and ignore the effect of recidivism on the total welfare career of a recipient. Given this limitation, the authors note that they were able to piece together a distinct profile of recipients who "are likely to have long or short spells, based on their characteristics at the start of a welfare spell" (O'Neill et al. 1984, 10–11). The following independent variables were associated with this distinctive profile and thus with duration of welfare dependency:

1. *Market productivity.* Histories of work and high earnings led to quick exits from AFDC.

2. *Children.* A larger family size led to a slower exit.

3. *Education.* More years of schooling were associated with earlier exits, particularly exits resulting from marriage.

4. *Being a teenager when first child is born.* Although this variable in fact did *not* directly affect exit rates, we will later show that it seems indirectly associated with greater dependency.

5. *Race.* Longer durations were found for black women, even when other relevant factors were controlled.

6. *Attitudinal factors.* Attitudinal factors (in particular, the Rotter locus of control measure, which we will discuss below) were weakly related to spell duration.

7. *Welfare grants.* The authors noted mixed evidence tying increased grant levels to lower probabilities of exit.

Ellwood's (1986a) analysis of the PSID data appears to be the most comprehensive identification of recipient characteristics associated with careers of long-term AFDC dependence. Using the multiple-spells approach, Ellwood found that earlier analyses had underestimated the extent of persistent welfare dependence and that more than 40 percent of welfare recipients had multiple spells of welfare receipt. When multiple spells are considered,

> fifty percent of those who ever receive AFDC will receive it for no more than four years. Yet nearly 25 percent will eventually use AFDC in ten or more years. The estimated average total period of AFDC receipt is nearly seven years. . . . The majority of those who receive welfare do not receive it for very long. Nonetheless, a sizable minority appear to have very long periods of receipt. Consequently, of those who are on AFDC at any point in time, almost 60 percent are in the midst of periods of welfare use that will include ten or more years of receipt. (Ellwood 1986a, 25)

Table 6.5 presents Ellwood's marginal and aggregate findings concerning factors associated with length of time on welfare. Marginal findings show the influence of a factor by itself, with all other factors remaining equal. The aggregate analysis allows factors to naturally covary, so that, for example, changing marital status at spell beginning may also then change mean age.

Ellwood summarizes the findings on the marginal effects of recipient characteristics: "Education, marital status, number of children, work experience, and disability status are all closely correlated with first-spell durations. These same variables generally have substantial influence on recidivism and later-spell durations as well" (1986a, 31). As to the aggregate duration estimates, marital status seems to be associated with the most difference in the expected length of time during which women receive assistance. Never-married women averaged 9.3 years of AFDC receipt, whereas divorced women averaged less than 5 years. Ellwood also notes that race and work experience distinguished different subgroups of AFDC recipients and that education also seemed to affect total duration on aid. Although AFDC benefit levels are not individual characteristics, Ellwood did note that "persons in high-benefit states averaged longer spells and were likely to return to welfare" (1986a, 32) when all else was held constant.

Intergenerational Welfare Dependency

The transmission of welfare dependency between generations is a topic of both theoretical and policy interest. Views of poverty and wel-

Table 6.5.   Marginal and Aggregate Effects of Recipient Characteristics
on Duration of AFDC Receipt

Recipient Characteristics at Time of Spell Beginning	Marginal Findings: Average Duration of the First Spell (years)	Aggregate Findings: Average Number of Years of AFDC Receipt
Age		
Under 22	3.7	8.23
22–30	4.4	7.08
31–40	5.4	5.15
Over 40	4.6	5.23
Race/Ethnicity		
White	4.1	5.95
Black	4.9	8.14
Other	2.8	6.94
Years of education		
Less than 9	5.6	6.81
9–11	5.2	7.65
More than 11	3.7	6.33
Marital status		
Single	7.3	9.33
Divorced	2.9	4.94
Separated	3.9	6.80
Widowed	2.4	4.37
Number of children		
0–1	4.2	7.71
2–3	4.1	6.04
More than 3	6.2	6.83
Age of youngest child		
Under 3	4.8	8.09
3–5	4.2	6.79
6–10	3.2	4.51
Over 10	3.6	4.71
Work experience		
Worked during the two years prior to AFDC receipt	3.9	6.53
Did not work during the two years prior to AFDC receipt	5.2	8.00
Disability status		
No disability	4.1	6.85
Disability limits work	5.5	6.97
Total sample	4.3	N.A.

SOURCE: Ellwood 1986a, 104.

Table 6.6.   Intergenerational Patterns of AFDC Receipt

Dependence of Parents	Dependence of Daughters			Unweighted Number of Cases
	None	Moderate	High	
None	91%	6%	3%	811
Moderate	62	22	16	127
High	64	16	20	147

SOURCE: Duncan, Hill, and Hoffman 1988, 469.

fare dependence that hold individual failings responsible for the problems often describe the transmission of a parent's dysfunctional values and attitudes to a child through early socialization as the operative mechanism that induces "doomed to fail" attitudes.

The dynamics of this aspect of chronic welfare dependency are less well understood than are the various factors causing individuals to enter and exit AFDC. Only recently have reliable findings on the association between the welfare dependence of parents and that of their adult children become available. Table 6.6, compiled from the PSID data base over a nineteen-year period of observation, shows the relationship between the welfare dependence of parents (when the female child was thirteen to fifteen years old) and the child's subsequent welfare dependence between the ages of twenty-one and twenty-three.

The table reveals a clear relationship between parents' dependence and that of children, but it also reveals that 64 percent of daughters from highly dependent families (defined as receiving welfare in all three study years) were not at all dependent during the follow-up period. Duncan, Hill, and Hoffman (1988, 469−470) point out that although women from welfare backgrounds have a higher incidence of welfare dependence than do women whose parents did not receive welfare (20 percent of the former group were classified as highly dependent, as opposed to 3 percent of the latter group), the analysis did not control for other factors related to receiving welfare, such as the lack of material resources available to children in impoverished mother-only families. The authors conclude that "the welfare dependence of these daughters is affected by factors other than the welfare dependence of their parents, but as yet more elaborate attempts to estimate the extent to which welfare dependence is transmitted between generations, controlling for other factors, have been inconclusive" (1988, 470).

*Patterns of Welfare Use and
Social-Psychological Variables*

We possess a considerable body of evidence regarding factors—both personal and programmatic—that affect entering and staying in the welfare system. It is apparent that psychological or social-psychological variables such as self-esteem are not highlighted in these analyses. Goodwin argues that these studies are conducted by economists and that the data sources say "virtually nothing about the social-psychological experiences of respondents" (1983, 8). O'Neill and her colleagues did find that locus of control exercised some influence on exit probabilities, with those individuals who had a greater internal locus of control being more likely to exit quickly from welfare, but they note that this association is weak (1984, 14). Before reviewing the evidence implicating self-esteem in chronic welfare dependency, we must first discuss the theoretical and measurement issues pertaining to self-esteem (and related constructs) as used in this literature.

The Concept of Self-Esteem

Self-esteem is currently an ambiguous and poorly defined construct in the literature. Numerous conceptualizations, operational definitions, and measurement methodologies exist and often vary depending on the theoretical orientation of the researcher, the context of measurement, and the research goals. Crandall (1973) argues that self-esteem has been found to relate to a wide variety of other variables at one time or another and has no agreed-upon theoretical or measurement definition. Wells and Marwell state that "self-esteem is a deceptively slippery concept about which there is a good deal of confusion and disagreement" (1976, 5). In a compilation of thirty major self-esteem inventories (Robinson and Shaver 1973), little common ground and few consensus findings are noted among the tests reviewed.

Despite the ambiguity in the research literature, there are certain common elements normally understood as "self-esteem." These core elements include (1) a notion of *reflexivity* in the self, with the self necessarily divided into an observing component and an object of that observation; (2) a notion of *evaluation* as the self is viewed as an object; and (3) a notion of *affective response* to the evaluation, whereby the individual has feelings and cares about the evaluation.

Despite these common elements, the research literature is characterized more by diversity than by convergence. The lack of consistent definition is evident in the diversity of names used for self-esteem and its cognates. Coopersmith (1967) employs the term *self-attitudes;* Wylie (1968, 1974) uses *self-regard* and *self-worth*. Other terms include self-confidence, self-efficacy, ego-acceptance, self-acceptance, self-concept, self-affection, self-appreciation, self-evaluation, self-description, and so on. The sparsity of empirical tests of association makes it difficult to determine whether these various constructs converge into what is commonly called self-esteem. As we will see later, the evidence in support of empirical convergence is weak. Thus, in the absence of good reliability and validity tests, we cannot confidently assume that studies examining self-efficacy, for example, are indeed measuring a component or covariate of self-esteem (Crandall 1973). Nevertheless, many of the above constructs are often used interchangeably with self-esteem in the literature, even though tests for convergent construct validity are lacking.

Regardless of the diverse measurement methodologies and the weak evidence for measurement convergence, there is considerable *conceptual overlap* among the various theoretical perspectives on self-esteem. In general, theories stress the importance of the individual's immediate social context—particularly the family—in determining self-esteem. Rosenberg's reference group theory (Rosenberg 1965, 1967; Rosenberg and Pearlin 1978) emphasizes the immediate reference groups that individuals employ in making self-evaluative social comparisons. Coopersmith (1959, 1967) assumes that similar groups largely determine the parameters of individual notions of personal success and aspiration. The emphasis is generally on the affect received from significant others within the individual's most immediate social context, with the attitudes and values of those external to this context—the society at large—being less important for self-esteem. Minority children and adults in objectively impoverished conditions, for example, can demonstrate a relatively high level of self-esteem, even higher than that demonstrated by individuals in far better economic conditions (Rosenberg and Pearlin 1978).

Almost all approaches assume a compelling drive to maintain one's level of self-value, or self-worth, even if this requires perceptual distortion, denial, rationalization, or other defense mechanisms. Rosenberg (1965) suggests that the motive to achieve and maintain self-esteem is possibly the most powerful in the entire human repertoire.

A third area of general consensus concerns the affective, evaluative nature of self-esteem. Self-esteem is seen as a function of the individual's feelings about the self, feelings that may be independent of what could be called self-knowledge. It is possible to be aware of negative objective aspects of the self without actually feeling poorly about oneself. To the extent that self-esteem is determined by the feelings of significant others, negative self-knowledge may indeed be peripheral to self-esteem.

The widely held assumption that low self-esteem has predictable behavioral consequences that are necessarily associated with low motivation or lack of initiative or social responsibility is not supported by the empirical literature. Indeed, evidence suggests that some individuals with low and moderate levels of self-esteem may be more driven, competitive, and motivated than individuals with high self-esteem (Wells and Marwell 1976; Graf and Hearne 1970). Cohen (1959), for example, suggests that those with high self-esteem employ more defensive strategies and repressive tendencies, which prevent challenging or personally threatening information from entering into the self-concept. Consequently, Cohen argues, people with high levels of self-esteem are less open to change, because of their rigid thought patterns and excessive use of psychological defenses. Similarly, Taylor and Brown (1988) concur that individuals with low self-esteem are most likely to maintain more accurate and reality-based impressions of their abilities, potential, and self-image. Other research suggests that persons with low self-esteem have greater social competence (Achenbach and Zigler 1963) and higher interpersonal stability (Neuringer and Wanake 1966). In sum, this research concludes that common assumptions regarding the relationship between self-esteem and behavior are not unequivocally correct. Neither, however, is there unequivocal support for a positive relationship between low self-esteem and pro-social behavior. On balance, the relationship as studied to date seems indeterminate.

Related Constructs

Numerous psychological and social-psychological concepts that refer to the self have been shown to relate to self-esteem in both theoretical and, to a lesser extent, empirical domains. Again, the reported empirical associations vary depending on the particular definition of self-esteem employed.

Coopersmith (1967) suggests that one's sense of efficacy and ability is highly related to self-esteem, in terms of the influence of self-esteem on the individual's perceptions of personal success. Utilizing data from both face-to-face interviews and a series of objective personality tests, Coopersmith operationalizes personal efficacy as individual competence in dealing with social, academic, and personal matters and reports that self-esteem was consistently positively related to the various indices of personal efficacy. Other research supports this finding, though less convincingly. For example, Woodworth (1958) suggests that efficacy and self-esteem are conceptually interrelated, but provides little supporting evidence.

A sense of personal effectiveness in dealing with life's challenges and obstacles undoubtedly affects how individuals evaluate themselves. But, as Korman (1970, 1976) suggests, there may be various types of self-esteem that are localized around specific behaviors or tasks confronted by the individual. He suggests that there are at least three independent kinds of self-esteem, which are differentially derived from social interaction, task-specific performance, and more general evaluations of the self. From this perspective, it is likely that an individual who is effective in one domain will have high self-esteem specific to that area of performance, whereas other domain-specific areas of self-evaluation will be unaffected.

Another construct related to self-esteem involves Rotter's (1966) notion of internal or external locus of control, which suggests that individuals differ in ascribing causality for personally relevant events. Some believe they are personally responsible for their successes and failures and are labeled "internals." Others tend to externalize the causes of events and are labeled "externals." One might expect that "internals" would feel more competent than would those individuals who believe that life events are controlled by outside forces, a belief that could lead to feelings of helplessness and inadequacy. Hesketh (1984), reviewing a number of studies measuring the association between self-esteem and locus of control, reports a range of correlations between .24 and .30 and suggests that the two variables are only moderately related. In general, it has been found that those with high self-esteem tend to have an internal locus of control, whereas those with low self-esteem are more external (Bhagat and Chassie 1978; Kishor 1981). It would appear that a moderate but statistically significant relationship does exist between the sense of personal control and efficacy and measures of self-esteem. Wells and Marwell (1976), however, suggest that many researchers use the locus of control and sense of efficacy measures as expedient "proxy measures" of self-esteem, although the substitution is not entirely justified, given the relatively low levels of association between the two constructs. Nevertheless, numerous studies do present conclusions regarding self-esteem that are derived from items designed to measure either internal/external locus of control or personal efficacy.

The reported low levels of empirical association between self-esteem and certain related constructs does not necessarily imply that personal efficacy and locus of control are not components of self-esteem. Given the relatively loose association between the various indicators of self-esteem, it is not surprising to find that various conceptually related constructs bear a weak empirical relationship to commonly employed measures of self-esteem. It may be, once again, that these related constructs are highly associated with specific components or types of self-esteem (i.e., social self-esteem, or task-specific self-esteem), as Korman (1976) suggests, but the relationships may be obscured in empirical tests employing global self-esteem indices.

Relating Self-Esteem to Chronic Welfare Dependency

Only a small body of research exists that is directly relevant to the relationship between self-esteem and the related psychological and social-psychological constructs and chronic welfare dependency. Some of these studies are strictly cross-sectional (e.g., Carson 1967; Druga 1986; Goodban 1985; Jayaratne et al. 1980; Bishop 1974); others are based on longitudinal data (Handler and Hollingsworth 1969; O'Neill et al. 1984; Hill et al. 1985; Nichols-Casebolt 1986; Goodwin 1983). Duncan, Hill, and Hoffman point out the difficulty in making causal associations between welfare dependence and "values and attitudes" (1988, 239). They note that cross-sectional association between attitudes and welfare receipt is inadequate for gauging a link between welfare dependency and psychological characteristics. They suggest that three criteria are required to find a consistent link between receiving welfare and psychological variables:

1. Recipients should have values and attitudes that are measurably "worse" than those of nonrecipients;

2. Attitudes and values should be adversely affected by welfare receipt; and

3. Initially worse values and attitudes should increase the likelihood of future dependence.

In this formulation, the authors ignore possible positive relationships between receiving welfare and psychological variables such as self-esteem, although as a whole their review of welfare dependence clearly identifies the positive consequences of welfare benefits for recipients. Duncan and Hoffman (1987) note that most analyses of welfare dependence and its effects have only crudely estimated the characteristics of the welfare system itself that potentially affect the recipient's behavior and that most research has not adequately addressed the nonwelfare alternatives available to the recipient.

Cross-sectional evidence for a relationship between self-esteem and welfare dependence is inconclusive. Carson (1967) tested relationships between welfare receipt (yes/no) and self-esteem, using the Social Vocabulary Index (SVI) with 81 welfare and 116 nonwelfare clients applying for services at the Utah Division of Vocational Rehabilitation. According to Carson, the SVI yields scores relating to self-concept, self-acceptance, ideal self-concept, and concept of others. This early study found no differences between welfare recipients and nonrecipients on the SVI measures. To further test the relationship, length of time on welfare was subdivided into short, intermittent, and long (more than three years) and tested as an independent variable in relation to SVI scores. Again, expected variations in self-concept among subgroups were not found. The author offers a post hoc explanation that the excessive defensiveness of welfare clients may keep them from admitting to a lowered self-concept, a view that Carson finds corroborated by the fact that chronic welfare clients scored highest on scores of self-concept and self-acceptance.

Bishop (1974), in a study of 231 black women who had been on welfare at least once, did find expected differences—with current welfare recipients evidencing lower self-esteem. Druga (1986) also looked at length of time on aid (but measured at a particular point) as it related to the social-psychological makeup of a sample of 75 AFDC recipients. The long-term recipients (on AFDC for six consecutive years) were not found to differ significantly from the shorter-term recipients on eleven items chosen from Rotter's (1966) locus of control scale. Druga concludes from these data that welfare use may best be understood by examining systemic rather than personal variables.

Goodban (1985) analyzed certain psychological effects of receiving welfare assistance among a group of one hundred single, black AFDC recipients in New Haven, Connecticut. (Fifty-five had been on aid more than five years.) Self-esteem was defined with a single item asking a woman "whether welfare made her feel differently about herself" (1985, 415). Fifty-five percent of the respondents stated that welfare did indeed make them feel differently about themselves. Goodban reports a relationship between this self-attitude and (1) lower subjective social class; (2) a belief in not having control over going on welfare; and (3) a belief that opportunities are generally available in America. Goodban summarized her data as attesting to the extreme psychological (and economic) hardship of the welfare role, presumably also referring to the fact that a majority of respondents reported being stigmatized (embarrassed or ashamed) by being on welfare and receiving food stamps. Although more than half of the respondents had been on aid for six years or more, no data are reported tying length of time on aid to the social-psychological variables. Furthermore, the self-esteem measure used in the study is suspect—we are unclear as to how the item references the self-esteem concept, to say nothing of the reliability or validity of the measure. Nevertheless, based on her finding that recipients who believe in individualistic explanations for going on welfare and who report feeling a high degree of control over going on welfare are more affected in terms of their self-esteem, Goodban concludes that this constellation of attitudes is counterproductive in that it discourages legitimate activism by the recipients (i.e., seeking all legitimate entitlements and possibly joining a welfare rights organization).

Longitudinal or experimental studies are more appropriate than strictly cross-sectional studies for analyzing questions about relationships between self-esteem and chronic welfare dependency. Analyses of both PSID and NLS data, as well as two studies that collected data at two points in time only (Handler and Hollingsworth 1969; Goodwin 1983), are discussed below.

Handler and Hollingsworth (1969) investigated feelings of stigma, other attitudes, AFDC program use, and the probability of leaving welfare among a sample of 767 AFDC recipients in Wisconsin over a period of approximately two years, beginning in June 1967. Stigma was conceptualized as (1) feeling embarrassed or uncomfortable when interacting with people who do not receive AFDC; and (2) a generalized feeling held by the recipient about the community's degree of understanding or hostility toward AFDC recipients. More than half of the subjects reported feeling stigmatized in both respects. Although this is not a direct measure of self-esteem, the idea of stigma (Goffman 1963) incorporates both the devaluation of individual attributes by society and the internalization of this general opinion, reflected in a devalued self-estimation. Handler and Hollingsworth note that recipients who reported feeling stigmatized differed in several respects from the nonstigmatized group, feeling less satisfied with the AFDC program and less accepting of unannounced home visits by the caseworker. But the authors report apparently paradoxical findings, for stigmatized recipients were more aggressive in asserting their rights to a variety of program benefits, were likely to leave the welfare system sooner than those recipients who did not report feeling stigmatized, and were more likely to exit AFDC as a result of their own efforts (including finding work and getting married). The authors conclude that "feelings of stigma . . . seem to reflect an independent cast of mind. Recipients who have these feelings are upset about being on welfare. . . . Moreover, they do something about their situation" (1969, 17–18).

Goodwin (1983) studied AFDC recipients enrolled in the Work Incentive Program (WIN) in 1978, as well as a comparison group of individuals receiving unemployment insurance in New York and Chicago. Goodwin expressly attempted to uncover the attitudinal and social-psychological factors associated with both economic and attitudinal outcome measures from a one-year follow-up. Regrettably, he was able to achieve only a 57 percent reinterview rate. Among the attitudinal measures included were (1) "expecting economic independence"—intending or expecting to work and not receive aid at a later time; (2) feeling that it was proper to support one's family by working; and (3) a measure of general self-confidence incorporating items seemingly related to locus of control and to self-esteem. Two items from Goodwin's self-confidence scale provide the flavor of this measure: "When I make plans, I am almost certain that I can make them work"; "I am able to do most things as well as other people" (1983, 23).

Goodwin found achieving economic independence at time-2 to be related to several factors at time-1: the expectation of achieving independence, the length of time spent on aid, and previous job status. The self-confidence measure was *not* reported as significant in the regression model. Further, Goodwin noted a spiral of causation, in which expectations for independence at follow-up were influenced both by the earlier level of those expectations and by the independent influence of having achieved economic independence in the interim. Again, the self-confidence variable was found to be irrelevant.

Several analyses of the large-scale longitudinal data bases—the NLS and the PSID—have attempted to uncover the relationships between psychological factors and economic mobility. One study (Hill et al.

1985), while not limiting its research to welfare cases, reviewed the PSID findings on motivation and economic success. The PSID employed Atkinson's theory of motivation (Atkinson 1964, cited in Hill et al. 1985), differentiating between more basic motives (including need for achievement, need for affiliation, and need for power, as well as the negative motivation, fear of failure) and expectancies (defined as the "individual's assessment of the chances that his or her own performance will, in fact, lead to a desired outcome" [Hill et al. 1985, 4]). This motivation theory holds that action is precipitated by the stable basic motives plus an expectation that action can affect an outcome in a particular set of circumstances. To measure expectancy in the PSID, a personal efficacy index was constructed, consisting of two items asking respondents whether they "usually felt pretty sure their life would work out the way they wanted" and whether, "when they made plans ahead, they usually carried them out" (PSID items cited in Hill et al. 1985, 28). These items seem to connote some certainty about controlling outcome, making this efficacy index seem more akin to a locus of control concept than to the generalized self-evaluation suggested by self-esteem.

The findings on motivation and economic well-being show expected correlations (rather weak) between the efficacy index and the other motivational indices and current measures of economic well-being, with the exception that welfare income correlated negatively with the motivational measures. These data support an inference that receiving welfare is related to motivational and efficacy states. As the authors note, however, causality was indeterminate in this analysis. To measure the direction of causation between attitudes and economic status, the authors constructed a model testing the effects of prior motivational levels on subsequent economic well-being. With this procedure, "no more than modest and usually insignificant effects of basic motives on economic outcomes [were found] and . . . no consistent effect of expectancies on outcomes" (Hill et al. 1985, 7). Rather, changes in the efficacy index seem to be predicted by "various economic and non-economic events" (77). Thus, when the cross-sectional correlations are subject to longitudinal causal analysis, it appears (in the PSID) that the attitudes (expectancies) are more reflective than predictive of economic status.

O'Neill et al. (1984) analyzed the contribution of psychological factors to welfare dependency in both the PSID and the NLS samples. As previously noted, the PSID contained an efficacy index, and the NLS contained items from Rotter's locus of control inventory that the O'Neill study equates with the PSID efficacy index, with internal control denoting greater efficacy, that is, certainty that plans will turn out as intended. For the NLS (Rotter scale) data, a more external attitude was associated with a greater degree of welfare dependency, although the effect was not significant. Furthermore, locus of control affected welfare dependency in the case of welfare exit as a result of earnings only (with external outlook decreasing the probability of exit as a result of earnings), but it did not affect exits that occurred because of marriage. Replicating that analysis in the PSID sample produced equivalent results: the efficacy index (in the weighted regression) had the right sign in relation to welfare dependency, but the result was not statistically significant.

In these studies, the factors delineated earlier in our discussion of welfare dynamics (individual factors such as education, marital status at first birth, labor market experience, and disability, as well as program factors) are the variables that seem to control long-term dependence on aid, with the efficacy index as measured not contributing significantly to the observed outcomes over time. The O'Neill et al. study, however, despite controlling for a variety of relevant variables, was unable to account for the effect of duration itself on subsequent duration. In an attempt to discover whether an individual might "lose motivation and self-confidence as a result of being on welfare and [whether] these attitudes . . . perpetuate welfare dependency" (1984, 85), an analysis was conducted of the effects of enrollment in AFDC on attitudes over time. The effect of AFDC was, as expected, negative on efficacy, but again the effect was not statistically significant. Analyses with both the PSID and the NLS data yielded similar results on this question.

Nichols-Casebolt (1986) conducted an analysis similar to that reported by O'Neill et al. (1984) with the PSID, focusing her entire inquiry on the psychological effects of income-tested programs (those which provide assistance to low-income clients only), in order to evaluate the "stigma" argument—that recipients "incorporate the general negative views of themselves held by others, thus reducing the recipient's feelings of self-worth" (1986, 288). The psychological concept employed was "psychological well-being" (PWB), measured by four PSID items covering satisfaction with self and sense of control over intended outcomes. This conceptualization seems to blend a notion of self-esteem with the concept of locus of control. Nichols-Casebolt, however, argues that these dimensions of self-satisfaction and personal competence "incorporate essential elements in overall PWB" and relate to the major arguments about the effects of stigma as they focus "on the loss of self-esteem and the increased dependency of recipients" (1986, 289).

As did O'Neill et al., Nichols-Casebolt presents both cross-sectional

Table 6.7.   Means of PWB Variables for Each Income-Support Category
              for Blacks and Whites

| | Personal Competence[a] | | Self-Satisfaction[b] | |
Sample	Mean	N[c]	Mean	N
Blacks				
AFDC	2.35	151	.533	156
Survivors' insurance				
(Social Security)	2.92[d]	23	.537	31
Neither	2.63[d]	125	.675[d]	133
Whites				
AFDC	2.58	32	.504	34
Survivors' insurance				
(Social Security)	3.51[d]	32	.631	35
Neither	3.44[d]	114	.693[d]	114

SOURCE: Nichols-Casebolt 1986, 291.
NOTE: The means are weighted. Pooled sample for 1968–1972.
[a]Scored with 1 = low, 5 = high.
[b]Scored with 0 = low, 1 = high.
[c]Sample sizes vary across measures because of missing data.
[d]Significantly different from AFDC (p < .05).

and longitudinal findings. Table 6.7 reproduces her findings for cross-sectional data by race for a subgroup of PSID subjects (female heads of household less than fifty-four years old, with children under the age of eighteen, from data collected between the years of 1968 and 1972) for different categories of income support. As before, cross-sectional data support the implication that income-tested support is associated with a decrease in PWB in a statistically significant fashion. To test the causal relationships in the data, a panel model was used that incorporated data on all welfare cases, short-term as well as long-term,* and evaluated change in PWB as a function of (1) change in AFDC status in the prior year, and (2) possible changes in other personal characteristics during that time (income, number of children, age of youngest child, and work status). In this model, PWB was differentiated into its two measured components, self-satisfaction and personal competence, and the analysis was conducted separately for blacks and whites. Results reveal that entering AFDC had a statistically significant impact in lowering feelings of self-satisfaction and personal competence for blacks, but not for

* Nichols-Casebolt proposes that a test of the model using changes in PWB during an AFDC spell would be advisable; in fact she ran such an analysis and reported that the "results were in the expected direction—increasing years on AFDC was related negatively to PWB—but the coefficient was not significant" because of sample sizes (1986, 302n.20).

whites. Six of eight coefficients for blacks and whites were, however, in the expected direction.

Nichols-Casebolt concludes that these results, taken together with the cross-sectional data, show that for blacks the lower psychological well-being of AFDC recipients was a result of being on AFDC. She also argues that her data may underestimate the effects of AFDC on PWB, because of the method of analyzing each year of aid as a distinct entity, and that initial AFDC receipt may capture a "relief" phenomenon, presumably associated with the lessening of stress the recipient experiences when benefits are first received. Nichols-Casebolt speculates that "once the financial crisis is alleviated, however, the negative psychological consequences of AFDC begin to be felt" (297). We should point out that no data are presented in the analysis to either confirm or reject this speculation and that the data concerning effects on PWB subsequent to exiting AFDC, in which one would predict improved PWB as the negative stimulus ends, do not support that interpretation.

Has the Relationship Between Self-Esteem and Chronic Welfare Dependency Been Tested?

From the available evidence, we conclude that there has been only a partial test of a possible relationship between self-esteem and chronic welfare dependency in the empirical literature. Adequate testing would include (1) adequate measurement of self-esteem in the mainstream tradition of that literature; (2) a focus that allows us to differentiate between chronic and nonchronic welfare use, as these populations differ considerably; and (3) relatively clear causal paths that help to resolve the problem of what comes first, attitudes or dependency. We might also wish for a measure of welfare dependence that takes into account nonwelfare income and for a data set that allows us to understand how variations in AFDC programs influence observed differences in self-esteem and chronic use.

Given these criteria, we can see the limitations in the evidence available to judge self-esteem's contribution to this social problem. Perhaps the most severe drawback is in the measurement of the self-esteem variable. Jayaratne and colleagues note that although the concept of self-esteem is widely studied in social psychology, "very little information is available on adults in general, and *virtually none on welfare recipients*" (1980, 285; emphasis added). The cross-sectional studies all used different measures of self-esteem, and, as we have noted, studies measuring locus of control and efficacy are not equivalent to self-esteem studies, for associations between these constructs are weak. The longitudinal studies use explicit theories of motivation (needs and expectancies) to guide their instrumentation. Although these theories try to identify the *most likely* attitudinal or motivational contributors to economic outcomes, they do not provide direct measures of self-esteem.

Taken as a whole, the studies have included a roster of approximations for measured self-esteem, ranging from single items about whether individuals feel "different" about themselves or are satisfied with themselves to multiple-item clusters representing efficacy, psychological well-being, stigmatization, evaluative self-concept, and self-esteem. All told, the record of inquiry includes a dozen or so studies of evaluative self-attitudes and how these relate to receiving welfare. A number of the studies, especially those which by design delve into the causal paths, may contain not self-esteem measures but efficacy measures. Some authors (e.g., Nichols-Casebolt) maintain that these measures directly pertain to self-esteem. Our review of self-esteem measurement leads to the conclusion that these measures are not synonymous but appear to be conceptually related. Although it appears that not a single study adequately measured the self-esteem variable, this is probably true precisely because no consensus or rationale for adequate measurement of the ambiguous concept has emerged.

Does Level of Self-Esteem Cause Welfare Dependency?

We have reviewed the major direct evidence on this question and find that although cross-sectional studies might lean toward positing a relationship between low self-esteem and dependency, the longitudinal data generally negate the observed finding. It is true that the longitudinal data bases provide less adequate measures of self-esteem than do certain of the cross-sectional studies. Goodwin (1983), however, did include a self-concept scale in his follow-up research and did not conclude that self-attitudes were important for later status and expectations of independence.

As to the possibility that *high* self-esteem causes welfare dependency, the evidence to evaluate this relationship seems inadequate. Two theoretical avenues have been suggested. The first argues that individuals must have considerable persistence and resilience to overcome the bureaucratic barriers associated with the welfare system and that these traits should accompany high self-esteem. The second suggestion, more theoretical, is based on certain research findings that more aggressive and "driven" individuals may have lower self-esteem. But the data are inadequate to test these assertions, although the study by Handler and Hollingsworth (1969) does in fact suggest that lower self-esteem (measured as part of a "stigma" concept) is associated with earlier exit from welfare. We find no evidence relevant to the idea that high self-esteem allows an individual to cope with the public welfare bureaucracy.

Does Welfare Dependency Affect Self-Esteem?

The evidence implicating chronic welfare dependency in the lowering of self-esteem, though essentially still inconclusive, seems stronger than the evidence linking prior self-esteem to the likelihood of chronic welfare dependency. Some investigators note that welfare provides material benefits that, at least in the short run, reduce uncertainty and may resolve an economic crisis for the individual initially qualifying for aid. Thus any decrease in self-esteem as a result of long-term welfare use would appear over a longer period and may at first be masked by this short-term relief. As Nichols-Casebolt (1986) notes, however, no data set exists with which to test this hypothesis. Duncan, Hill, and Hoffman (1988) point out that research has generally avoided analyzing the positive contribution welfare makes to individual and family circumstances and that the overall social judgment of the program should include the benefits in education, nutrition, health care, household stability, assistance with child-rearing, and so forth that are received especially by children.

Several analysts summarize the evidence in this area as mixed but generally indicating some deterioration in self-esteem as a result of welfare dependency. Rainwater (1982) argues that the stigmatizing effects of receiving welfare may be evident not only in the lowering of measured self-esteem but also in depression, denial, and defining oneself as sick or disabled, areas not subject to clear-cut observation by written self-esteem tests. Nichols-Casebolt (1986) points out the surprising lack of evidence addressing this deeply held belief that welfare stigma undermines psychological well-being (including self-satisfaction). She finds in her PSID research that, for blacks, receiving AFDC does result in lowered psychological well-being. In general, Nichols-Casebolt believes that many research designs tend to be biased against finding any relationship at all between the variables (principally because of measurement and time-lag problems); thus she views the emergence of even weak findings as suggestive of a trend implicating welfare dependence in lowered psychological well-being. O'Neill and colleagues (1984), however, while noting some findings tying overall exposure to AFDC with lowered efficacy, conclude that the relationship is not strong enough to support the idea of a causal relationship between AFDC and efficacy.

Although the evidence linking chronic welfare dependency to a loss of self-esteem remains inconclusive, certain trends in the data, combined with the methodological drawbacks of the existing research, lead us to conclude that some weak effect of welfare dependence on the variables of sense of control and personal efficacy deserves further exploration. As yet, no finding ties persistent welfare dependence to a generalized loss of self-esteem.

Theoretical and Research Directions

Further research on self-esteem and welfare dependency depends on two features: improved measurement of psychological variables and adequate longitudinal data. Experience to date reveals that when either feature is lacking, few findings of value emerge. Based on the concept of self-esteem as an overall evaluative self-attitude, which is strongly affected by social context and which individuals possess a powerful drive to sustain at a functional level, there is little reason to believe that self-esteem is a strong influence on chronic welfare dependency. If parenthood (single or otherwise), possible adherence to deviant attitudes, or membership in social groups that do not stigmatize welfare dependence can sustain self-esteem—and theoretically there is no reason to suspect that they cannot—then self-esteem per se is unlikely to emerge as a strong causative factor in predicting which individuals will become chronically welfare dependent.

Learned Helplessness.   There is weak evidence to suggest that certain psychological factors do play a role in persistent welfare dependency. Research on caseload dynamics has found that duration of welfare itself influences the probability of remaining on aid. This is true even when the research controls for all of the other factors related to duration, such as family size, educational level, labor market involvement, and so forth. It is certainly reasonable to assume that chronic material deprivation below the poverty level (AFDC standards are consistently below the poverty level), coupled with the external controls associated with welfare dependency, may have psychological consequences. According to Kane (1987), victimization and the loss of control associated with chronic poverty may breed dysfunctional psychological coping mechanisms, which are best explained by the theory of reactance/learned helplessness.

The reactance/learned helplessness model (Wortman and Brehm 1975; Taylor and Reitz 1968), which has substantial empirical support in the social-psychological literature, describes how individuals differentially react to threats to their personal control. The theory suggests that individuals, when faced with uncontrollable situations, initially react with anger and aggression, symptoms of "reactance," in efforts to reassert personal control. If the loss of control persists despite individual initiatives, the individual will experience helplessness, which is eventually internalized after prolonged repetition and can become a generalized chronic state. The helpless state is characterized by motivational deficits, apathy, resignation, and an inability to recognize and respond to new opportunity (Seligman 1975).

Pettigrew (1980) and Kane (1987) argue that the reactance/helplessness cycle helps to explain certain behaviors often characteristic of welfare recipients. These authors suggest that welfare clients who are most active, motivated, and assertive are representative of "reactive types," whereas others (possibly those chronically dependent on welfare) suffer from the motivational deficits induced by a conditioned sense of helplessness, which prevents them from taking advantage of opportunities when they do occur. Kane argues that the poor in general, and many welfare recipients in particular, experience nonresponsive bureaucratic environments over which they have little control. Such prolonged lack of control eventually generalizes even to situations where control *can* be asserted but is not. Learned helplessness may thus prevent welfare recipients from recognizing new opportunities. By implication, then, this view predicts that structural changes alone may not be sufficient to move chronically welfare-dependent individuals to a state of independence.

Further research using the reactance/learned helplessness paradigm may help to explain why chronic welfare dependency extends for a duration unexplained by any other measured factors.

Conclusion

Is welfare dependency caused by the attitudes and values of welfare recipients? Are welfare dependency and the attitudes and values of welfare recipients the products of the persistent experience of economic disadvantage and powerlessness, including the experience of welfare itself? The data needed to answer these questions with confidence do not exist. We do know that the major immediate cause of chronic welfare dependency is chronic income deficiency. Those who are chronically welfare dependent constitute a diverse group, but they all share this basic overriding characteristic of too little income.

Only four lawful sources of income are available to Americans: (1) employment; (2) membership in a family with income to share; (3) capital ownership; and (4) transfers. Overcoming income deficiency means increasing income from one or more of these sources.

Nearly 50 percent of all Americans are in the labor force. The vast majority are able to exchange their labor for an income above the poverty level. About 6 percent of the labor force is involuntarily unemployed. Others are underemployed or employed at wages so low they cannot support their families at or above the poverty level. Still others are "discouraged workers," that is, they have ceased looking for work because of repeated failures in finding employment. Although employment is a significant source of income for most Americans, it is an income source now not fully available to all. There is little evidence that low self-esteem is a major barrier to participation in the labor force.

The largest group of Americans not in the labor force is composed of the nation's children. Although most children are members of families with income to share, changes in patterns of marriage, divorce, out of wedlock childbirth, and the structure of the (increasingly contingent) labor force have created growing numbers of families (particularly female-headed families) with income deficits. Clearly, not all Americans hold membership in families with income to share.

Capital ownership, in the form of dividends, rent, and interest, is a source of income for many Americans. But a family of four would need working capital in excess of $150,000 to generate an income at the poverty level from this source, and only a very small fraction of all American families have such capital holdings.

Transfers (Social Security and related public benefit programs) are an important income source for many Americans. Many elderly persons and dependent children are taken out of poverty by these programs. But others may not be entitled to assistance from any existing program or may receive benefits that are below the poverty level and thus do little to relieve economic need or promote independence.

When income is pooled from these several sources, some 13.6 percent of all Americans are still left with income insufficient to meet their own and their families' needs. In 1983, 58 percent of all impoverished families with children in the United States received benefits from the AFDC program.

Social policy related to such poor children and their families is dominated by two conflicting objectives—to reduce their poverty by providing material benefits above a defined standard of health and decency, and to reduce or prevent their dependence on government. Efforts to reconcile these conflicting objectives within a single "welfare" program have left the nation with a very high level of unrelieved child poverty and a very substantial level of long-term dependence among welfare recipients. The program of Aid to Families with Dependent Children reduced the national child poverty rate by only 4 percent in 1985. More than half of all recipients depended on this aid for more than four years. The average length of dependence on AFDC benefits was almost seven years; slightly less than 25 percent of recipients depended on cash payments for ten or more years. The AFDC program has essentially functioned as a cash payment program, doing little to assist recipients in overcoming barriers to self-sufficiency (deficient language skills, lack of job skills, child care needs, poor health) and also doing little to relieve child poverty. Furthermore, some research plausibly suggests that long-term welfare dependence may undermine an individual's perceived capacity to exercise control over events in his or her personal life.

Public policies that fall so far short of their intended goals—to relieve poverty and to reduce dependency—are clearly in need of change. An effective public policy response should include both the provision of income adequate to bring poor children and their families above the poverty level and efforts to promote self-sufficiency. Much of the current debate on welfare reform has focused on public policy initiatives designed to reduce poverty and dependency by changing the mix of income sources available to poor families from employment, family support, and income transfers.

Employment

The current interest in "workfare" has as its focus a desire to remove long-term welfare recipients from the welfare rolls and to replace their welfare benefits with earnings. It seems clear that, with assistance (child care, education, training, job placement, counseling, and so on), potential exists to increase income from employment for some welfare recipients, though that increase will, at best, be modest (Gueron 1988). Such programs often include motivational components designed to alter the attitudes (including self-attitudes) of participants. Efforts to change motivation are logical components of a work training program for welfare recipients, but no good research is available that tests their effectiveness. Achieving the dual goals of reducing dependency and poverty requires balanced attention to ensure that earnings—or some combination of earnings and public benefits—are at or above the poverty level.

Family Support

The AFDC program was conceived as a program to protect the children of dead or disabled fathers. Today, it also serves the children of absent fathers, who often contribute little to the support of their children. Child support programs are now being advocated to reduce both poverty and dependency through increased parental support. Uniform levels of child support awards, financed by an income tax on the absent father, have been identified and are being tested in pilot and demonstration programs (Garfinkel, McLanahan, and Wong 1988). When fully implemented, such programs could have a modest impact on the size of the AFDC caseload.

Income Transfers

The Tax Reform Act of 1986 made an important step forward by removing most poor families from the income tax rolls and reducing the extent to which marginal families are taxed into poverty. Additional tax reform proposals that might use our tax structure to help alleviate poverty are now under discussion. Among these proposals, the replacement of the $2,000 personal exemption (a regressive tax feature) with a per capita refundable tax credit is the most far-reaching.

Workfare programs could, of course, have their greatest immediate impact on income from salaries and wages. Education, training, improved health care, and social services offered as part of such programs could also have a long-term beneficial impact on children and parents who care for them that is not work-specific. Added income from employment and from child support programs could relieve the poverty and dependency of many families. Better-targeted support to poor families through the income tax system would add substantially to their incomes and avoid the dangers of stigmatization, bureaucratic control, the disincentive effects of high marginal tax rates on earnings, and the high administrative costs of welfare programs.

These tax-based reforms, together with programs designed to assist employable welfare recipients, could have a considerable impact on poverty and dependency. Nevertheless, many families would still suffer income deficits that leave them below the poverty level. The profound problems of education, training, health, housing, and child care that welfare recipients face suggest that solving the problem of chronic welfare dependency will require a comprehensive, urgent effort by every one of our human service institutions to address the extraordinary needs of these families. It will also require conscious efforts to open new job opportunities for those excluded from the labor force or only marginally employed.

Even with improved access to income from employment, family support, and transfers, a residual income-tested welfare program will be needed to meet the income deficits of some poor families. The new opportunities envisioned in these policy directions presuppose a target population with the motivation and ability to take advantage of opportunities. As suggested earlier, chronic welfare dependency and its associated chronic poverty may leave some recipients with neither the hope nor the confidence that different behaviors will be differently rewarded. Some will need help in overcoming learned behaviors that are no longer functional in an environment of new opportunity. Psychological services directed to enhance client motivation and ability may be useful under such circumstances. But such services are not likely to succeed as substitutes for genuinely expanded opportunities.

Future Research

This review of the research literature indicates that substantially more work needs to be done in conceptualizing and investigating the major variables identified. We have only a beginning understanding of the dynamics of poverty and welfare dependency and the psychosocial implications of those states for the individuals and families involved. More research is needed to inform policy responses to questions that are of increasing public concern and interest. Several promising research directions have been suggested.

Unfortunately, there is no quick pathway through the process of study and analysis. There is a desperate need for longitudinal data that can help us understand the movement of individuals and families across the life span and the factors that influence participation in the civic, social, and economic life of the community. Much more will have to be invested in studies and in pilot and demonstration projects to test new ideas and approaches before moving to full implementation of new policies.

In Assembly Bill 3659, the California legislature called public attention to the problems of chronic welfare dependency, crime and violence, alcoholism and drug abuse, teenage pregnancy, child abuse, and academic failure. Although we have some idea of the number of people involved in each problem area, we have little knowledge about whether these are discrete or overlapping populations. Recently, increasing attention has been paid to the possible existence of an "underclass" in American life—a class of people who are outside the nation's economic and social mainstream. There is no rigorous or accepted definition of the term *underclass,* but Reischauer (1987) has summarized the most widely agreed-upon characteristics of the group as (1) persistently low income; (2) a weak attachment to the labor force; (3) a lack of education and skills exemplified by functional illiteracy and dropping out of school; (4) a sense of alienation from mainstream society, possibly accompanied by substance abuse, criminal activity, participation in the underground economy, fathering or bearing a child out of wedlock, or long-term welfare dependency; (5) membership in a minority group that is discriminated against; and (6) residence in a neighborhood with a high concentration of disadvantaged or dysfunctional behavior.

According to Reischauer (1987), if the underclass is defined as the nonaged, nondisabled population that has persistently low income, lacks skills or an education, and has a limited attachment to the labor force, it could represent as much as 2.4 percent of the nation's population and 15.8 percent of its poor. If one subtracts from this group those who are not black or Hispanic and who do not live in a large city, the size of the underclass shrinks to 0.8 percent of the total population and 5.6 percent of the nation's poor. Although these numbers may underrepresent single young black males, the homeless, and those engaged in illegal activities, the size of the problem population may be relatively small. But the profile of deprivation and disadvantage and its implications for public policy are very great.

It is important that problem-specific analyses of the "intractable problems" identified in Assembly Bill 3659 not lead us to overlook their overlapping existence in a single population group or the search for broader concepts of causation. Obviously, we know very little and need to know much more. Legislative support of research and testing relevant to public policies addressing these problems is needed.

Bibliography

Achenbach, T., and E. Zigler, eds. 1963. *Projective Psychology: Clinical Approaches to the Total Personality.* New York: Knopf.

Anastasi, A. 1961. *Psychological Testing.* New York: Macmillan.

Atkinson, J. W. 1964. *An Introduction to Motivation.* Princeton, N.J.: Van Nostrand.

Bane, M. J., and D. T. Ellwood. 1983. *The Dynamics of Dependence: The Routes to Self-Sufficiency.* Cambridge, Mass.: Urban Systems Research and Engineering.

———. 1986. "Slipping Into and Out of Poverty: The Dynamics of Spells." *Journal of Human Resources* 21(1): 1–23.

Bhagat, R. S., and M. B. Chassie. 1978. "The Role of Self-Esteem and Locus of Control in the Differential Prediction of Performance, Program Satisfaction, and Life Satisfaction in an Educational Organization." *Journal of Vocational Behavior* 13:317–326.

Bishop, E. S. 1974. "The Self-Concept of the Welfare Mother: Some Sociological Correlates." *Wisconsin Sociologist* 2(1): 10–16.

Branch, A., J. Riccio, and J. Quint. 1984. *Building Self-Sufficiency in Pregnant and Parenting Teens.* New York: Manpower Demonstration Research Corp.

Brehm, J. W. 1966. *A Theory of Psychological Reactance.* New York: Academic Press.

Bumpass, D. L. 1984. "Children and Marital Disruption: A Replication and Update." *Demography* 21 (February): 71–82.

California. State Assembly Bill 3659. 1986. *An Act to Create the California Task Force to Promote Self-Esteem and Personal and Social Responsibility.* September.

Carson, G. L. 1967. "The Self-Concept of Welfare Recipients." *Personnel and Guidance Journal* 45(5): 424–428.

Center for Human Resource Research, Ohio State University. 1980. *Findings of the National Longitudinal Survey of Young Americans, 1979.* Youth Knowledge Development Report 2.7, Research on Youth Employment and Employability Development. U.S. Department of Labor. Washington, D.C.: Government Printing Office.

Coe, R. D. 1981. "A Preliminary Examination of the Dynamics of Welfare Use." In *Five Thousand American Families: Patterns of Economic Progress,* vol. 9: *Analyses of the First Twelve Years of the Panel Study of Income Dynamics,* edited by M. S. Hill, D. H. Hill, and J. H. Morgan, 121–168. Ann Arbor, Mich.: Institute for Social Research.

Cohen, A. R. 1959. "Some Implications of Self-Esteem for Social Influence." In *Personality and Persuasibility,* by I. L. Janis et al., 102–120. New Haven, Conn.: Yale University Press.

Coopersmith, S. 1959. "A Method of Determining Types of Self-Esteem." *Journal of Abnormal and Social Psychology* 59:78–88.

———. 1967. *The Antecedents of Self-Esteem.* San Francisco: Freeman.

Crandall, F. 1973. "The Measurement of Self-Esteem and Related Constructs." In *Measures of Social Psychological Attitudes,* edited by J. P. Robinson and P. R. Shaver, 45–159. Ann Arbor, Mich.: Institute for Social Research.

Danziger, S. 1988. "Antipoverty Policy and Welfare Reform." Paper prepared for the Rockefeller Foundation Conference on Welfare Reform, Williamsburg, Va., February 16–18.

Druga, G. S. 1986. "Locus of Control and Patterns of Welfare Use." Ph.D. dissertation, Case Western Reserve University.

Duncan, G. J., M. S. Hill, and S. D. Hoffman. 1988. "Welfare Dependence Within and Across Generations." *Science* 29 (January): 467–471.

Duncan, G. J., and S. D. Hoffman. 1987. "The Use and Effects of Welfare: A Survey of Recent Evidence." Institute for Social Research, University of Michigan, Ann Arbor. Typescript.

Ellwood, D. T. 1986a. *Targeting "Would-Be," Long-Term Recipients of AFDC.* Princeton, N.J.: Mathematica Policy Research.

———. 1986b. "Working Off Welfare: Prospects and Policies for Self-Sufficiency of Female Family Heads." John F. Kennedy School of Government, Harvard University. Typescript.

Fish, B., and S. Karabenick. 1971. "Relationships Between Self-Esteem and Loss of Control." *Psychological Reports* 29:784.

Fitch, G. 1970. "Effects of Self-Esteem, Perceived Performance, and Choice on Causal Attributions." *Journal of Personality and Social Psychology* 16(2): 311–315.

Fitts, W. 1964. *Manual for the Tennessee Self-Concept Scale.* Nashville, Tenn.: Counselor Recordings and Tests.

———. 1970. *Interpersonal Competence: The Wheel Model.* Nashville, Tenn.: Counselor Recordings and Tests.

Garfinkel, I., ed. 1982. *Income-Tested Transfer Programs: The Case For and Against.* New York: Academic Press.

Garfinkel, I., and S. McLanahan. 1986. *Single Mothers and Their Children: A New American Dilemma.* Washington, D.C.: Urban Institute Press.

Garfinkel, I., S. McLanahan, and P. Wong. 1988. "Child Support and Dependency." In *Beyond Welfare: New Approaches to the Problem of Poverty in America,* edited by H. R. Rodgers, Jr., 66–85. Armonk, N.Y.: M. E. Sharpe.

Gilder, G. 1981. *Wealth and Poverty.* New York: Basic Books.

Goffman, E. 1963. *Stigma: Notes on the Management of Spoiled Identity.* Englewood Cliffs, N.J.: Prentice-Hall.

Goodban, N. 1985. "The Psychological Impact of Being on Welfare." *Social Service Review,* September, 403–422.

Goodwin, L. 1983. *Causes and Cures of Welfare.* Lexington, Mass.: Lexington Books.

Graf, R., and L. Hearne. 1970. "Behavior in a Mixed Motive Game as a Function of Induced Self-Esteem." *Perceptual and Motor Skills* 31:511–517.

Gueron, J. M. 1988. *Reforming Welfare with Work.* Occasional Paper 2. Ford Foundation Project on Social Welfare and the American Future. New York: Ford Foundation.

Handler, J., and J. Hollingsworth. 1969. "Stigma, Privacy, and Other Attitudes of Welfare Recipients." *Stanford Law Review* 22:1–19.

Hesketh, B. 1984. "Attribution Theory and Unemployment: Kelly's Covariation Model, Self-Esteem, and Locus of Control." *Journal of Vocational Behavior* 24:94–109.

Hill, M., S. Augustyniak, G. Duncan, G. Gurin, P. Gurin, J. Liker, J. Morgan, and M. Ponza. 1985. *Motivation and Economic Mobility*. Ann Arbor, Mich.: Institute for Social Research.

Jayaratne, S., W. A. Chess, J. Norlin, and J. Bryan. 1980. "Demographic Correlates of Self-Esteem Among Black and White AFDC Recipients." *Journal of Sociology and Social Welfare* 7(2): 285–297.

Kane, T. J. 1987. "Giving Back Control: Long-Term Poverty and Motivation." *Social Service Review*, September, 405–419.

Katz, M. B. 1986. *In the Shadow of the Poorhouse: A Social History of Welfare in America*. New York: Basic Books.

Kishor, N. 1981. "The Effect of Self-Esteem and Locus of Control in Career Decision-Making of Adolescents in Fiji." *Journal of Vocational Behavior* 19:227–232.

Korman, A. K. 1966. "Self-Esteem Variable in Vocational Choice." *Journal of Applied Psychology* 50:479–486.

———. 1970. "Toward an Hypothesis of Work Behavior." *Journal of Applied Psychology* 54:31–41.

———. 1976. "Hypothesis of Work Behavior Revisited, and an Extension." *Academy of Management Review* 1:50–63.

Maslow, A. 1968. *Toward a Psychology of Being*. New York: Van Nostrand Reinhold.

Morris, M., and J. B. Williamson. 1987. "Workfare: The Poverty/Dependence Trade-Off." *Social Policy* 18(1): 13–17.

Murray, C. 1984. *Losing Ground: American Social Policy, 1950–1980*. New York: Basic Books.

———. 1987. "In Search of the Working Poor." *Public Interest* 89 (Fall): 3–19.

Neuringer, C., and L. Wanake. 1966. "Interpersonal Conflicts in Persons of High Self-Concept and Low Self-Concept." *Journal of Social Psychology* 68:313–322.

Nichols-Casebolt, A. 1986. "The Psychological Effect of Income Testing Income-Support Benefits." *Social Service Review*, June, 287–302.

Novak, M., et al. 1987. *The New Consensus on Family and Welfare: A Community of Self-Reliance*. Washington, D.C.: American Enterprise Institute for Public Policy Research.

O'Neill, J., D. Wolf, L. Bassi, and M. Hannan. 1984. *An Analysis of Time on Welfare*. Washington, D.C.: Urban Institute Press.

Pettigrew, T. F. 1980. "Social Psychology's Potential Contributions to an Understanding of Poverty." In *Poverty and Public Policy*, edited by V. T. Covello. Cambridge, Mass.: Schenkman.

Platt, J., R. Eiseman, and A. Darbes. 1970. "Self-Esteem and Internal-External Control: A Validation Study." *Psychological Reports* 26:162.

Quarantelli, E. L., and J. Cooper. 1966. "Self-Conceptions and Others: A Further Test of Median Hypotheses." *Sociological Quarterly* 7 : 281–297.

Rainwater, L. 1982. "Stigma in Income-Tested Programs." In *Income-Tested Transfer Programs: The Case For and Against,* edited by I. Garfinkel, 19–46. New York: Academic Press.

Rein, M., and L. Rainwater. 1978. "Patterns of Welfare Use." *Social Service Review,* December, 511–534.

Reischauer, R. D. 1987. "America's Underclass." *Public Welfare* 45(1): 7–31.

Ricketts, E. R., and I. V. Sawhill. 1986. "Defining and Measuring the Underclass." Paper presented to the annual meeting of the American Economic Association, New Orleans, December 28.

Robinson, J. P., and P. R. Shaver, eds. 1973. *Measures of Social Psychological Attitudes.* Ann Arbor, Mich.: Institute for Social Research.

Rosenberg, M. 1963. "Parental Interest and Children's Self-Conceptions." *Sociometry* 26(1): 35–49.

———. 1965. *Society and the Adolescent Self-Image.* Princeton, N.J.: Princeton University Press.

———. 1967. "Psychological Selectivity in Self-Esteem Formation." In *Attitude, Ego-Involvement, and Change,* edited by C. Sherif and M. Sherif, 26–50. New York: Wiley.

Rosenberg, M., and L. I. Pearlin. 1978. "Social Class and Self-Esteem Among Children and Adults." *American Journal of Sociology* 84 : 54–77.

Rosenberg, M., and R. G. Simmons. 1972. *Black and White Self-Esteem: The Urban School Child.* Washington, D.C.: American Sociological Association.

Rotter, J. B. 1966. "Generalized Expectancies for Internal vs. External Control of Reinforcement." *Psychological Monographs* 80 : 1–28.

St. John, N. 1975. *School Desegregation: Outcomes for Children.* New York: Wiley.

Sawhill, I. V. 1976. "Discrimination and Poverty Among Women Who Head Families." *Signs: A Journal of Women in Culture and Society* 2 (Spring): 201–211.

———. 1986. "Anti-Poverty Strategies for the 1980s." Discussion Paper, Changing Domestic Priorities Project. Washington, D.C.: Urban Institute Press.

Schneiderman, L., W. Furman, P. Lachenbruch, M. B. Welch, and I. Chow. 1987a. "GAIN Participant Needs Assessment: A Profile of Recipients of Aid to Families with Dependent Children in Los Angeles County." Center for Child and Family Policy Studies, School of Social Welfare, University of California, Los Angeles.

Schneiderman, L., W. Furman, P. Lachenbruch, E. Fielder, M. B. Welch, and I. Chow. 1987b. "GAIN Participant Needs Assessment: Report Two." Center for Child and Family Policy Studies, School of Social Welfare, University of California, Los Angeles.

Schorr, A. 1986. *Common Decency: Domestic Policies After Reagan.* New Haven, Conn.: Yale University Press.

Seligman, M. E. P. 1975. *Helplessness: On Depression, Development, and Death.* San Francisco: Freeman.

Sherwood, J. J. 1965. "Self-Identity and Referent Others." *Sociometry* 28(1): 66–81.

Silber, E., and J. S. Tippett. 1965. "Self-Esteem: Clinical Assessment and Measurement Validation." *Psychological Reports* 16:1017–1071.

Simmons, R. G., L. Brown, D. M. Bush, and D. A. Blyth. 1978. "Self-Esteem and Achievement of Black and White Adolescents." *Social Problems* 26:6–96.

Social Security Administration. 1986. *Social Security Bulletin*, Annual Statistical Supplement. Washington, D.C.: U.S. Department of Health and Human Services.

Social Security Administration. 1987. *Social Security Bulletin*, Annual Statistical Supplement. Washington, D.C.: U.S. Department of Health and Human Services.

Sullivan, H. S. *The Interpersonal Theory of Psychiatry*. New York: Norton.

Survey Research Center, Institute for Social Research. 1984. *User Guide to the Panel Study of Income Dynamics*. Ann Arbor, Mich.: Inter-University Consortium for Political and Social Research.

Taylor, J., and W. Reitz. 1968. "The Three Faces of Self-Esteem." Research Bulletin no. 80. Department of Psychology, University of Western Ontario.

Taylor, S. E., and J. D. Brown. 1988. "Illusion and Well-Being: A Social Psychological Perspective on Mental Health." *Psychological Bulletin* 103(2): 193–210.

U.S. Bureau of the Census. 1985. "Money Income and Poverty Status of Families and Persons in the United States: 1984." *Current Population Reports*, Series P–60, no. 149. Washington, D.C.: Government Printing Office.

———. 1987. "Consumer Income." *Current Population Reports*, Series P–60, no. 158. Washington, D.C.: Government Printing Office.

U.S. Congress. Congressional Budget Office. 1985. *Reducing Child Poverty*. Washington, D.C.: Congressional Budget Office.

———. Congressional Research Service and Congressional Budget Office. 1985. *Children in Poverty*. Report prepared for the House Committee on Ways and Means. Washington, D.C.: Government Printing Office.

———. House. Select Committee on Children, Youth, and Families. 1987. *U.S. Children and Their Families: Current Conditions and Recent Trends, 1987*. Washington, D.C.: Government Printing Office.

Warren, P., and D. Maxwell-Jolly. n.d. "How California's Welfare Dynamic Affects Work Programs Such as GAIN." Office of the Legislative Analyst, Sacramento, Calif. Typescript.

"Welfare and Poverty Among Children." 1987. *Congressional Research Service Review* 8, no. 7 (July).

Wells, L. E., and G. Marwell. 1976. *Self-Esteem: Its Conceptualization and Measurement*. Beverly Hills, Calif.: Sage.

Williamson, J. B. 1974. "Beliefs About the Welfare Poor." *Sociology and Social Research* 58:163–175.

Wiseman, M. 1985. "The Welfare System." In *California Policy Choices*, vol. 2, edited by J. Kirlin and D. R. Winkler, 133–202. Los Angeles: University of Southern California, School of Public Administration.

Woodworth, R. 1958. *Dynamics of Behavior.* New York: Holt, Rinehart & Winston.

Wortman, C. B., and J. W. Brehm. 1975. "Responses to Uncontrollable Outcomes: An Integration of Reactance Theory and the Learned Helplessness Model." In *Advances in Experimental Social Psychology,* vol. 8, edited by L. Berkowitz, 277–336. New York: Academic Press.

Wylie, R. C. 1968. "The Present Status of Self-Theory." In *Handbook of Personality Theory and Research,* edited by E. F. Borgatta and W. W. Lambert, 728–787. Chicago: Rand McNally.

———. 1974. *The Self-Concept.* Vol. 1, *A Review of Methodological Considerations and Measuring Instruments.* Rev. ed. Lincoln: University of Nebraska Press.

Ziller, R., J. Hagey, M. Smith, and B. Long. 1969. "Self-Esteem: A Self-Social Construct." *Journal of Consulting and Clinical Psychology* 33:84–95.

Alcohol and Drug Use and Self-Esteem: A Psychological Perspective

Rodney Skager and Elizabeth Kerst

Introduction

In the fall of 1987, a network television commercial gave us a putative insider's view of creative thinking in the auto industry. The setting was a meeting of attractive young executives struggling to define what people wanted from their automobiles. The group was casually arranged around a conference table. Various signs suggested that it was near the end of the working day: the men's ties were loose, while the women sported unruly wisps of hair.

Each participant haltingly tried to capture the essence of what people were looking for. One attempt after another fell short. Finally, one of the young men hit pay dirt. "This may sound like a cliché," he said, "but you are what you drive." Here was our message. We are what we drive.

Apt as it may be for our times, the commercial is merely an example of how we define ourselves by things in our environment, especially possessions visible to other people. According to this view, who we think we are and how we feel about who we are are based on what we believe others think of us. But there is also an opposite conception, one that internalizes identity and its associated sense of self-worth. Within this perspective, the person who derives his or her sense of self primarily from the reactions of others is unlikely to achieve a firm sense of identity. If it is really a central structural element of personality, personal

The authors are deeply grateful to David Shannahoff-Khalsa for his many perceptive suggestions and comments on drafts of this chapter.

identity must be stable and self-maintaining in the mature person. Otherwise, how are we to account for the autonomous human being? Autonomous people can endure being ignored or even devalued by others, because they are supported by a strong inner sense of self that sustains independent thought and action.

Self-esteem is the *experience* of one's personal self-worth. It is a mental indicator, as body temperature and blood pressure are physical indicators. But the analogy has limits. Self-esteem tends to be experienced as either present or absent, rather than in precise gradations. Some people, especially those who are abnormally dependent on others for praise and recognition, may experience significant shifts in self-worth, depending on how much support they receive from other people. Although such individuals may be described as lacking self-esteem, it would be more accurate to characterize them as having a weak sense of self, which is revealed through shifts in self-esteem. People of this type often need constant admiration and validation from others. They cannot get enough of what some observers like to call "narcissistic supplies," literally, fuel for self-love.

When their self-esteem is very low, some people are depressed and apathetic, sometimes even suicidal. Others repeatedly form nonsupportive relationships in which they are devalued and demeaned. Suicidal behavior and the need for self-destructive relationships suggest serious problems with self-concept. But so do narcissistic disorders in which people appear to have very high levels of self-esteem, while behaving with arrogance and disregard for others. Unhealthy self-esteem may also be associated with grandiose and delusional thinking among people suffering from psychoses. This kind of self-esteem can be described as the pathological result of a failed attempt to develop a stable, cohesive self or identity.

Pathological conditions result from defects in personality development occurring early in life. People who suffer from such conditions attempt to maintain self-esteem through processes that are different from, or are serious distortions of, those used by people who developed in a relatively normal way. Healthy people do seek out and maintain social contacts that support or enhance their sense of self-worth. But they do not require constant praise and recognition from others, and they are uncomfortable about unearned praise.

In people who have achieved extraordinary levels of personal development, high self-esteem and humility coexist. Such people have a strong, enduring sense of personal identity, accepting in themselves the

personal inadequacies and failures that exist in all of us. Most important, their strong, but realistic, sense of self does not have to be sustained at the expense of others. They do not need to control or humiliate
other people. Rather, their strong identity allows them to treat others
with fairness and consideration.

Psychological theories usually assume that personality structures
maintaining self-esteem originate early in life. These theories also allow
for further development in social and other situations encountered
throughout life. For example, in Mahler, Pine, and Bergman's (1975) or
Kohut's (1977) theories, structures that maintain self-esteem are gradually internalized through a process of appropriate parenting.

There is no doubt that self-esteem is central in the consciousness of
troubled human beings. Psychotherapists report that those who seek
help typically suffer from low self-esteem. Jerome Frank has characterized the mental state of those who seek psychotherapy as one of personal demoralization: "A plausible hypothesis is that patients seek psychotherapy not for symptoms alone, but for symptoms coupled with
demoralization: subjective incompetence, loss of self-esteem, alienation,
hopelessness (feeling that no one can help), or helplessness (feeling that
other people could help, but will not)" (1982, 16).

This description applies equally well to the alcoholic. The book *Alcoholics Anonymous,* for example, describes the mental state of the alcoholic seeking help as a state of "pitiful and incomprehensible demoralization" (1976, 30). The first step of the Alcoholics Anonymous (AA)
program of action asks recovering persons to accept the proposition,
"We were powerless over alcohol; our lives had become unmanageable."

The themes of "powerlessness" and "unmanageability" recur in the
literature of AA and other support groups modeled on its program.
Members of AA believe that the alcoholic or other addict finally turns to
others for assistance when denial and rationalization give way to a profound sense of helplessness in the face of a life that has spun out of control. AA describes this crisis as "hitting bottom." More than anything
else, hitting bottom is a state of negative self-worth, a vacuum where
self-denigration replaces self-esteem.

Theories of Self-Concept and Identity

If self-esteem is an indicator or sign of the quality of an internalized
structure we call "the self," then it needs to be related to behavior
through a theory about personality. This anticipates the basic assump-

tion of this chapter: *the relationship between substance use and self-esteem is not a simple causal relationship but, rather, one that is mediated through an organized aspect of the personality we choose to call "self-concept" or "identity."*

Self-Concept and Self-Esteem

Markus and Wurf (1987) have recently contributed a comprehensive review of research on *self-concept*. They make an observation that, from the perspective of a book on self-esteem, is somewhat disquieting: "The majority of self-concept research could best be described as an attempt to relate very complex global behavior, such as delinquency, marital satisfaction, or school achievement, to a single aspect of the self-concept, typically self-esteem" (1987, 300).

In other words, the self-concept is now understood not only to incorporate self-esteem, but also to have considerably broader meaning. Markus and Wurf show that research on self-concept over the past decade has progressed beyond studying self-esteem to an emphasis on self-concept as a "dynamic interpretive structure," which mediates both *intrapersonal processes* such as information processing, affect, and motivation and *interpersonal processes* such as choice of social partner and situation, interaction strategy, and reaction to evaluations from others.

Marsh and Shavelson (1985) have demonstrated that self-concept is multidimensional. That is, it is composed of various self-representations that differ from one another in importance and, according to Markus and Wurf (1987), even in whether or not they have been achieved. Unachieved selves, termed *possible selves*, may be desirable or undesirable. They function as incentives for behavior in the sense of being end states to achieve or avoid. Higgins (1983) extends this conception by suggesting three classes of self-representations: the *actual* self; the *ideal* self, or self that the individual would like to achieve; and the *ought* self, or self that an individual or others think one should achieve. Discrepancies between actual and ideal self-conceptions are associated with depression, those between actual and ought associated with anxiety. Alternatively, self-conceptions may be divided into good and bad. The latter are readily identified with depression (Sullivan 1953; Beck 1967), which is a clinically defined state characterized by abnormally low self-esteem.

According to Markus and Wurf, identity is "an image of the self that one tries to convey to others" (1987, 325). It is thus both a self-conception and an "entity out in the world." Depending on their goals and the audience, people try to construct different identities. This is an important way in which self-representations influence human behavior. Self-representations are not always directly manifest in overt actions, however; they are often seen indirectly in "mood changes, in variations in what aspects of the self-concept are accessible and dominant, in shifts in self-esteem, in social comparison choices, in the nature of self-presentation, in choice of social setting, and in the construction and definition of one's situation" (Markus and Wurf 1987, 300). These observations are consistent with our view that self-esteem is an experiential state that varies as a function of an underlying self-representation within a situational context. The goals of the individual within a situation, as well as the individual's life history, mediate the relationship.

None of this denies the significance of self-esteem, as long as it is understood as a state that reflects the quality or adequacy of a self-representation. The self-representation takes on an organizing function in the personality. It accounts for how an individual interprets a situation in personal terms, and it focuses, organizes, and directs behavior in that situation.

The recovering alcoholic develops an explicit self-representation that is also an identity (a public self-concept). When speaking at an AA meeting, he or she learns to say, "I am an alcoholic." During recovery, this initially negative self-representation is transformed, becoming to its holder a positive self-representation incorporating the ideas of sobriety and recovery. The new identity incorporates a set of organizing principles for living. Sober alcoholics are people who do not take the first drink, who stay out of "slippery places," who value abstinence (unlike the society they live in), who reinforce their own sobriety by helping other alcoholics, and who have achieved a sense of place and belonging in a supportive community. These achievements transform self-derogation into self-esteem through the creation of a substantial, positive self-representation.

This example suggests that efforts to replenish self-esteem without regard to developing a healthy self-representation or identity are misdirected. People who continually seek praise and adulation to bolster their self-worth are only temporarily satisfied. They desperately need instead to engage in a process of personal growth that allows them to internalize their sense of self, so that they can feel self-worth without continuous bolstering from others or from alcohol and drugs.

In order to understand the relationship between self-esteem and substance use, a theory about how self-esteem is generated and maintained in the personality is needed. To simply ascertain that people drink or use drugs excessively because they have low self-esteem tells us nothing about prevention and remediation unless we also understand the origins of self-esteem.

The Self in Object Relations Theory

Object relations theories have developed within psychodynamic psychology as alternatives to the more mechanistic formulations of psychoanalytic theory, especially the Freudian concept of drives. In contrast to the latter, with its emphasis on internal sexual and aggressive forces and the mechanisms that control them, object relations theory is concerned with how parents and other caretakers shape the psychological development of the infant and child.

"Objects" are usually, but not always, other people. For example, the most celebrated "object" may be Linus's blanket in the "Peanuts" comic strip. In object relations theory, the blanket and the class of childhood objects it represents are referred to as "transitional objects," which smooth the transition from dependence on the soothing function of an adult, ordinarily the mother, to a state of separation and individuation in which the child becomes increasingly self-sufficient emotionally. The child uses the soothing provided by the transitional object to replace that originally provided by the parent. The behavior of children in relation to their transitional objects has been described by one theorist as very much like the behavior of addicted adults in relation to the "object" of their addiction (Tolpin 1971).

Although many theorists and researchers have played significant roles in the development of object relations theory, the contributions of Heinz Kohut and Margaret Mahler are most relevant to abusive or addictive use of alcohol and other drugs. Kohut (1977) conceives of the development of the self in terms of relationships with early "self-objects," especially the mother. Self-objects are other people over whom an infant (or adult) feels a sense of *control*. According to Kohut, this sense of control has a special quality, resembling the control experienced over one's own self. There is a merged quality in the relationship; the infant does not perceive a self-object as a separate person.

The idea that an infant "controls" an adult may seem farfetched, but it is based on sound clinical observation and reasoning. Adequately cared-for infants *do* control the adults around them, at least with respect to having their personal needs met. The infant's sense of controlling the parent is accurate within its own perspective. As maturation proceeds and the developing child's needs and capabilities become more complex, the sense of control over the self-object is gradually lost, at least in normal development. The process of separating and individuating is the major developmental task of early childhood.

Kohut's theoretical work evolved around the theme of the development of the self in relation to early self-objects. For example, maternal and other adult self-objects model organizing and soothing functions, which are gradually internalized by the child ("the hurt will go away in a minute").

When parents and others give recognition and praise to a very young child, they are engaging in a process called "mirroring." Their mirroring helps the child define an early self or identity. Under conditions of adequate parenting, this early self is grandiose, even omnipotent. Wise parents do not criticize toddlers or arrange experiences of failure in an attempt to teach extremely young children to develop a realistic view of their own capabilities. Mahler, Pine, and Bergman, who conducted long-term observational studies of mothers and children, characterize this period of development as the "practicing subphase" of a much longer process of *separation* from the primary parental self-object and *individuation* through achievements, "marking the child's assumption of his own individual characteristics" (1975, 4). The essential scenario of this practicing subphase casts the toddler as the recipient of recognition and praise for every act of individual achievement—hence the grandiosity of the earliest self-structure, according to the object relations theorists.

If the self is a grandiose construction, then self-esteem must be high, as long as other people are supportive. But this kind of self-esteem does not have a stable base. It is easily upset by frustration and failure, which soon occur in the life of every normally developing child. In Mahler's developmental scheme, the practicing subphase is associated with the period of crawling and early walking (from ten or twelve months to sixteen or eighteen months) and is followed by a "rapprochement phase," in which the child begins to perceive the reality of being small and inept. If, for various reasons discussed by object relations theorists, the child is prevented from negotiating this next phase of development, he or she will fail to develop a more mature self-organization or will at least retain elements of grandiosity and omnipotence that deter or distort later development.

This failure is the origin of the *narcissistic personality*, which Kohut and Wolf (1978) and others have associated with addictive behavior. Narcissistic individuals often show an inflated sense of self-worth, but one that is unstable and not self-sustaining, that is, it is highly dependent on a sustaining environment for its replenishment. Narcissistic people are exceptionally sensitive to failure, criticism, and being ignored or slighted. They also tend to relate to others primarily in terms of how well those others contribute to the satisfaction of personal needs. A narcissistic personality involves a sense of "entitlement," under which other people may be used and then discarded when they no longer prove useful. It is an abnormal or unrealistic self-representation (and associated self-esteem) that mediates such callous, insensitive behavior and disregard of the rights of others.

People who successfully negotiate later developmental phases develop a self that is stable and, in Kohut's terms, "firm and coherent." They can tolerate criticism, failure, and devaluation by others, because they possess a self-structure that remains constant even in situations of devaluation or failure. In this process of development, they were assisted by parents who not only gave support when needed but who also knew when to stand aside and let children learn to deal with life's problems. In Bandura's (1984) terms, they maintained conditions under which a child could develop a sense of self-efficacy, one of the conditions important to the development of a healthy self. Existential psychologists refer to a similar idea in the concept of "hardiness" (Kobasa 1979), which they see as a precondition to achieving autonomy as an adult.

Kohut (1977) concluded that a firm and coherent self fails to develop when a child does not achieve either an initial mirroring relationship with a parental self-object (usually the mother) or a later identification with an idealized parental figure (either the mother or the father). Chelton and Bonney (1987) suggest that an addiction reactivates emotions associated with the developmental stage at which a critical failure in object relationship occurred. The addictive use of alcohol or drugs may be viewed as an abortive attempt to recreate a primitive mental state, from which interrupted growth can begin anew. Addiction, of course, is a flawed solution.

Ego States and the Fragmented Self

Kohut's (1977) descriptions of the fragmented or noncohesive self are paralleled in the work of object relations theorists using a more traditional terminology. Kernberg (1966) helped lay a theoretical foundation for the observation that changes in personality often occur in people who are under the influence of alcohol or other drugs. For example, even when they are only moderately drunk, quiet and shy people may become outgoing and daring in social interactions, the meek may become assertive, the asexual sexual, and so on. Occasionally, complete changes of identity occur in alcoholic "blackouts," dissociative states that are walled off from ordinary consciousness by forgetting (amnesia).

These phenomena can be interpreted as changes in self or identity. As such, they represent alternative "ego states," or, in Kernberg's terms, "compartmentalized psychic manifestations" (1966, 236). Such states originate in response to inconsistencies in parental behavior that remain unresolved during later development. Primitive self-organizations arise in response to such inconsistencies, each corresponding to representations of the parental object, the associated "part-self," and emotional states associated with each. For example, a child with an alcoholic parent usually experiences dramatic changes in that parent associated with whether he or she is drunk or sober. Alternative selves develop accordingly, with the two part-selves defensively separated, so that feelings associated with one parental self-object do not spill over into the other. The "good parent" object is thus internally protected from the fear, rage, or grief associated with the "bad parent" object. These coexisting part-selves are in turn buried under a superordinate personality structure that continues to develop. Because the part-selves remain separated, the succeeding personality structure has the potential for fragmentation, such as that occurring in multiple-personality disorders or other dissociative phenomena.

The clinical literature on addiction contains many case studies of ego states associated with part-selves. Wurmser (1985) presents an in-depth analysis of a single case that illustrates the views just presented. A drug addict whose alcoholic mother was perceived "both as a friend in childhood and as a vicious, nasty, alcoholic tormentor who had no ability to see him as an individual" (1985, 89) developed part-identities corresponding to his "two" mothers. Drug-taking was associated with a "defiant, arrogant, angry, even murderously furious man and addict," and the sober state with a "good boy, who is bending over backwards, giving in, compliant, 'well-adjusted'" (91). Especially important is the fact that *extreme fluctuations in self-esteem characterized shifts from drug-taking to sobriety.* Fear of rejection and consequent shame precipitated drug use. Contrition and remorse "in the form of massive shame and guilt" brought about temporary sobriety, during which "reparation, expiation, and grandiose fantasies undoing the perceived flaws" (93) were the order of the day.

This brief vignette illustrates the central conception of this chapter: self-esteem is indeed involved in addictive substance use, but in relation to self or identity structures. Case studies do not prove theories. Yet there seems to be a preponderance of argument and evidence to suggest that positing a simple relationship between self-esteem and addictive drinking or drug use, such as the hypothesis that addicts and alcoholics are people with low self-esteem, is insufficient. Three generalizations seem in order:

1.   Although it is influenced by one's current situation, self-esteem usually reflects the cohesiveness and strength of self or identity structures developed during the formative years of childhood and adolescence. Dramatic changes in self-esteem observed with substance use therefore reflect actual transformations in self or identity associated with intoxication.

2.   It is further apparent that low self-esteem is not susceptible to a "quick fix," as is often assumed in prevention programs for young people. Rather, lasting enhancement of self-esteem requires the development of a positive and rigorous self-concept or identity. In the case of alcoholics and other addicts, this process requires significant changes in personality organization and associated systems of values.

3.   Working directly to change levels of self-esteem in the treatment of alcoholics and addicts is not likely to be productive. Rather, the changes in self-organization necessary for attaining the "firm and coherent self" described by Kohut demand a commitment of time and effort similar to that required in the original developmental process.

Research on Self-Esteem and Substance Use

A great deal of research has been conducted concerning self-esteem and similar concepts in relation to drug and alcohol use. For the past two decades, low self-esteem has been the most popular psychological explanation of drug and alcohol abuse and addiction (Furnham and Lowick 1984). This is apparent not only in the sheer volume of work on the topic but also in the fact that various forms of self-esteem development are so frequently incorporated into alcohol and drug prevention programs for youth.

It would be neither feasible nor particularly useful to cite all of the large body of empirical research on self-esteem and alcohol and drug use produced since the 1940s. Instead, conclusions will be drawn from representative examples of this work.

Our summary of empirical research begins with a brief description of how self-esteem is actually assessed in research studies. Empirical studies of three types will then be reviewed: (1) *nonexperimental research,* which compares alcoholics or addicts to so-called normals in measures of self-esteem or closely related characteristics; (2) *explanatory research,* which asks whether alcohol and drug use enhances or maintains self-esteem under various kinds of hostile environmental conditions; and (3) *research on consciousness,* which assesses changes in how people feel about themselves and their environment when they are "high."

Measuring Self-Esteem

The ways in which self-esteem has been measured parallel the different ways in which the concept is defined. A common approach is to ask respondents, through multiple-choice questions, whether or not they are good at various kinds of activities. This approach assumes that people who feel competent in a sufficient number of areas will as a result experience high levels of self-esteem. That is, high self-esteem is a direct function of self-competence. Both research and theory suggest, however, that perceptions of self-competence and self-esteem are not necessarily the same thing. Bandura (1984) has researched self-competence (although he prefers the term *self-efficacy*) and insists that self-competence and self-esteem are different concepts.

A second approach to measuring self-esteem, also using multiple-choice questions, is to ask respondents whether or not they *like* themselves in various ways. Sometimes, these questions are merely self-competence questions rephrased as "what I like about myself," but others, such as estimates of personal attractiveness, are not so closely tied to competence. This approach sees the self-concept as made up of many specific facets that, in adolescents, are organized hierarchically (Marsh and Shavelson 1985). In short, self-esteem as assessed by multiple-choice tests usually combines self-ratings of competency (efficacy) and self-acceptance or liking, in the belief that self-esteem is the sum of many specific self-assessments.

A third, alternative approach to measurement is to give the respondent a method of describing the self in a holistic way. Such an approach attempts to determine *who* someone is, rather than *how good* he or she is, by eliciting one or more coherent self-representations. For example, the semantic differential technique (Osgood, Suci, and Tannenbaum 1957) has respondents rate themselves on a series of bipolar adjective scales such as "strong/weak." Adjective checklists (Gough 1952) have respondents check from a list those adjectives that they feel accurately describe themselves. Finally, Q-techniques require respondents to sort a set of descriptive statements about personal characteristics according to a continuum of relevance to themselves (MacAndrew 1979; Stephenson 1953).

This third group of methods tends to mix identity, or *who* one is, with self-esteem, or how much one likes oneself. But these approaches can be used to get more directly at self-esteem by being administered twice, once concerning the actual self ("myself as I am") and once concerning the ideal self ("myself as I would like to be"). From a strictly operational perspective, the discrepancy score between actual self-concept and ideal self-concept more closely represents self-esteem as we experience it. That is, people feel self-esteem when there is little or no discrepancy between the experienced self and the ideal self. (Admittedly, discrepancy scores are associated with technical problems in measurement, however.)

Nonexperimental Studies

One way to determine whether there is a relationship between self-esteem and drug use is to assess groups of alcoholic or other addicted persons. Studying addicted subjects rather than moderate or "controlled" drinkers and drug users is logical, because self-esteem would presumably be lowest among addicts. This approach indirectly recognizes that the use of drugs—whether they are alcohol, psychoactive medical drugs, or illicit drugs—is widely promoted and accepted in our society and that it is implausible to suggest that the majority of the population suffers from a psychological deficit. For example, Schaeffer, Schuckit, and Morrissey (1976) found no relationship between self-esteem and marijuana use among college students, a finding that is hardly surprising, as experience with marijuana is very common among college students.

Case Studies. These studies are intensive examinations of individuals or groups and ordinarily do not incorporate comparisons with other individuals or groups. Most case studies have focused on alcoholics. Findings show that self-esteem among addicted persons is extremely low, often reaching a feeling of personal worthlessness (Ghadirian 1979; Hendin 1974; Stengel 1978). Gross and Adler (1970) found that both alcoholic inpatients and members of Alcoholics Anonymous scored lower on objective tests of self-esteem than did the groups for which norms had been developed. Kinsey (1966) reported that lack of self-worth was the predominant self-characterization of alcoholic women undergoing hospital treatment. A substantial proportion disagreed with the statement, "I'm the kind of person I want to be," and believed that the people they cared most about would have agreed with their negative personal assessment.

Low levels of self-esteem have also been observed among heroin addicts (Kurtines, Hogan, and Weiss 1975; O'Mahony and Smith 1984). Similar findings have been reported for adult and adolescent polydrug addicts in treatment (Lindblad 1977; Padina and Schuele 1983). Padina and Schuele also found that heavy substance users among female junior high and high school students had relatively low self-esteem, although their levels of self-esteem were higher than those of adolescents in treatment for drug problems.

Case studies generate rather than confirm hypotheses. It can always be argued that people who have experienced the humiliation, shame, and guilt usually associated with addiction, who have been labeled as alcoholics or addicts, or who find themselves in a chemical dependency treatment program suffer from low self-esteem because of their addiction rather than because of any preexisting condition.

Criterion Group Studies.   The criterion group design attempts to improve on the case study by comparing the group of interest with another group that is as similar as possible—ideally, differing only in the characteristic under study. For example, a group of alcoholics or addicts might be contrasted with a comparison group of individuals who are of the same age, educational level, and so on, but who are "normal" as far as substance use is concerned. If the matching procedure is good—and this can be a shaky assumption—this method works fairly well when the results are negative, as would be the case if alcoholics' levels of self-esteem did not differ from those of matched normals. Unfortunately, it is not much better than the case study when differences in the hypothesized direction are found. In this case, the possibility of a flawed matching process assumes great importance, for the groups could differ in some way that is unknown to the researcher but that accounts for the observed difference in self-esteem. Worse, one can still argue that the lower self-esteem of the addicted group is the result rather than the cause of the addiction.

Criterion group studies reveal that groups of problem drinkers or alcoholics score lower than normal comparison groups do on measures of self-esteem (Buhler and Lefever 1947; Button 1956a, 1956b; Maddox and Williams 1968; Schaeffer, Schuckit, and Morrissey 1976; Mayo 1979; Brown 1980). The findings are especially strong in studies comparing alcoholic and nonalcoholic women. Beckman et al. (1980) found white alcoholic women to have lower levels of self-esteem than comparable women social drinkers *and* male alcoholics. McLachlan et al. (1979) reported similar findings for women undergoing hospital treatment for alcoholism. Hoar (1983) found that the discrepancy between actual self-concept and ideal self-concept was greater for both female alcoholic inpatients and outpatients than for a nonalcoholic comparison group.

Heilbrun and Schwartz (1980) found that the scores of male alcoholics on a measure of self-esteem derived from the Gough adjective checklist (a global measure of identity) were lower than those of nonalcoholic controls. In this case, the same relationship did not hold for women, probably because of problems in the experimental design. Williams (1965) reported greater discrepancies between descriptions of actual and ideal selves on the Gough adjective checklist among college fraternity members who were problem drinkers than among members whose drinking did not pose any problems.

Beckman (1980) reported that a group of white female alcoholics believed that low self-esteem was the major cause of their drinking. College women who drank heavily held the same belief in a study by Beckman and Bardsley (1981). On this same theme, Anderson (1981) had alcoholic women describe their adolescence. These women characterized their adolescent selves as "full of self-doubt" (presumably implying low self-esteem) to a significantly greater degree than did their nonalcoholic sisters. The alcoholic subjects also reported feeling competent during adolescence, however, supporting Bandura's (1984) distinction between self-competence and self-esteem.

Blatt et al. (1984) compared opiate and polydrug addicts at the treatment referral stage with control and psychiatric patient groups. They found that the levels of self-esteem of the opiate addicts were lower than those of either polydrug users or nonaddicts, even though opiate addicts saw themselves as more competent than polydrug addicts did. Moreover, self-esteem was significantly related to use of opiates by the polydrug users, with heavier opiate users reporting lower self-esteem. Graeven and Folmer (1977) likewise found level of heroin use to be negatively related to level of self-esteem. Compared to less involved users, heavy users retrospectively reported lower self-esteem during their high school years. Finally, Blatt et al. (1984) distinguished between two types of depression, the first characterized by feelings of help-lessness and loneliness and the second by a sense of personal worth-lessness. The latter type was manifested by the opiate addicts.

Carroll (1980) found few differences in self-esteem between male al-coholics and addicts (but excluding opiate addicts). Similar results for women alcoholics and addicts were reported by Carroll et al. (1982). These findings are not surprising, if addiction itself is the primary causal factor in low self-esteem. In other words, the personal damage associ-ated with addiction to any substance is more or less the same for all substances except opiates. The deeply ingrained stigma conferred on heroin users by society, plus the dangerous and often criminal lifestyle associated with heroin, may set this group apart.

In a study assessing self-esteem in relation to identity, Gossop (1976) compared self-ratings by inpatient and outpatient drug addicts with self-ratings of nonusers through the semantic differential technique (Os-good, Suci, and Tannenbaum 1957). On the *evaluative* dimension, which used bipolar adjective scales such as "good/bad" and "important/unimportant," the discrepancy between descriptions of actual and ideal selves was greater for female addicts than for male addicts. Addicts re-gardless of gender were lower on the *potency* dimension ("strong/weak," and so on) than were controls. Silver (1977), who obtained similar re-sults, suggested that the potency dimension represents a theme of per-sonal power. In this sense, addicts felt more powerless than controls did. (The experimental design cannot rule out the possibility that this feeling may result from experiences associated with the addiction itself. But this finding also anticipates a theme that will be salient when we discuss the effects of drugs on consciousness.) Feeling powerless may be a predispos-ing condition for low self-esteem. Coopersmith (1967) tied self-esteem directly to perceived personal power, meaning control over the events that affect one's life. Personal power is thus a perception about the self that reflects the quality of the self-concept or identity.

Back and Sullivan (1978) also used a measure of identity to assess the discrepancy between "how one appears to others" and "how one would like to be" in a sample of middle-aged and elderly members of an insurance plan. They found that the larger the discrepancy, the more frequent was the use of medical drugs, many of which were psychoactive drugs. This relationship was stronger for women than for men.

Correlational/Analytical Studies.   A third nonexperimental approach uses multiple-regression methods to assess the predictive power of self-esteem in relation to other potential predictors of substance use. This approach identifies a subset of predictors, each of which makes an independent contribution. The relative importance of each predictor is also determined.

Studies by Steffenhagen and Steffenhagen (1985) on alcoholics, Reid, Martinson, and Weaver (1987) on students in fifth through eighth grades, and Kaplan and Pokorny (1977) on high school students revealed that levels of self-esteem were consistently related inversely to substance use. That is, frequent or heavy substance users and problem users had lower self-esteem. Self-esteem was itself related to other predictor variables, however, and usually was not one of the variables selected in the multiple-regression solution. For example, Steffenhagen and Steffenhagen (1985) found that depression, rather than level of self-esteem, was the most powerful predictor of alcoholism. But low self-esteem is a major distinguishing characteristic of depression as a clinical condition, and a measure of depression may thus subsume low self-esteem, as demonstrated by Blatt et al. (1984). Kaplan and Pokorny (1977) likewise found that self-esteem was correlated with many other variables, each of which also related to substance abuse.

In general, then, the findings of correlational studies are often clouded by technical issues having to do with complex interrelationships between the measures studied.

Summary of Nonexperimental Research.   Self-esteem has frequently been the focus of nonexperimental research on alcohol and drug use. There is overwhelming support for an association between low levels of self-esteem and the use of alcohol and drugs. The relationship is strong for men, especially those entering treatment programs, and strongest for women alcoholics and for opiate users regardless of sex.

Nonexperimental research designs are open to the criticism that low self-esteem in groups diagnosed as alcoholics or other drug addicts may be a result of experiences associated with the addiction rather than a preexisting or "causal" condition. The former explanation is consistent with findings that women alcoholics and opiate addicts have the lowest self-esteem among the groups studied. Female alcoholics are likely to perceive more censure and feel more shame than will male alcoholics. Likewise, opiate addicts, usually heroin users, are the most feared and despised group of drug addicts. Nevertheless, for women alcoholics and for heroin users of both sexes there is retrospective evidence of low self-esteem during adolescence, which argues that low self-esteem may be a problem that predates addiction.

Research based on measures that assess self-esteem as the discrepancy between actual self-concept and ideal self-concept suggests that addicts also experience feelings of powerlessness. These feelings, associated with self-concept or identity, may underlie the low self-esteem characteristic of addicted people.

Explanatory Studies

A second type of research attempts to explain how drug or alcohol use "works" in relation to self-esteem. In other words, to say that people drink or use drugs because they have low self-esteem does not explain how getting drunk or high deals with the problem. Simplistic explanations—for example, suggesting that people simply "forget" their problems—are often inconsistent with the facts. An elderly recovering alcoholic told one of the authors how his anger toward other people related to getting drunk: "I drank in order to remember not to forget," he explained.

Self-Efficacy. According to Bandura (1982), the desire to be competent is a fundamental human motive. In the course of his research, self-perceptions of competence, or "self-efficacy," have been shown to influence thinking, behavior, and emotional arousal. Influential within academic psychology, Bandura's work has been the basis from which *social learning theory* has evolved. This theory, in turn, has of late provided a theoretical basis for prevention education, as well as for behavioral approaches to the treatment of addiction. The principle of *modeling,* which proposes that observing successful performance on the part of others generates an expectation of self-efficacy in the observer, has been very influential: "If they can do it, I can do it." For example, adolescents, despite threats from adults about negative consequences, probably use peer and adult models of "successful" alcohol and drug use to conclude that they will have the same capacity for control.

Bandura (1984) argues that self-efficacy and self-esteem are different. Self-efficacy refers to the evaluation of one's own competencies, whereas self-esteem refers to one's sense of self-worth. One may be a competent driver, but driving a car is something that virtually anyone can do. Or, one could be a hopelessly bad golfer, yet lack any personal investment in playing golf well. Self-efficacy would simply dictate that one should avoid playing golf.

Bandura's distinction is plausible. Still, what kinds of experiences might contribute to the development of self-esteem? It is doubtful that anyone who is not competent in activities that he or she values could feel high self-esteem. If playing golf really were important to an individual, it might be connected to self-esteem in addition to self-efficacy. Thus we are confronted with an empirical question: does self-efficacy also relate to alcohol and drug use?

Bandura (1982) readily accepts the application of self-efficacy theory to the prevention of relapse in cases of smoking, alcoholism, and other drug addictions. For example, Marlatt (1985) reported that people who felt less confident about their ability to resist resuming an addiction were in fact more likely to slip (relapse) after a period of abstinence. This finding is hardly surprising, but it may not imply what it seems to imply. Psychodynamic, as opposed to behavioral, theory could interpret such lack of confidence as resistance or rationalization, which excuses in advance the resumption of a behavior about which the individual is highly ambivalent.

Social learning theory has also been applied willy-nilly to a variety of school prevention programs in which children are led to experience success in various activities, on the theory that they will feel self-efficacious and thus not want to use drugs (Tobler 1986). A comprehensive review of such programs found no positive results as far as drug use was concerned (Schaps et al. 1983). Part of the basis for these negative results may be that the activities used in the programs may not have related to anything of personal importance to the children. Moreover, such programs are misdirected when they focus on children in general, instead of on the smaller population of children who are at high risk for addiction and other problems.

What about research that attempts to link self-efficacy to problem drinking or drug use? Vaillant (1983) found that a history of personal competence did not protect men from alcoholism. A measure of personal competence collected when his subjects were children was the best predictor of all facets of adult adjustment *except* later alcoholism. Even people who were highly competent as children could become alcoholics as adults. Recall that although opiate addicts in the study by Blatt et al. (1984) had lower self-esteem than other addicts, they also described themselves as more competent than did other addict groups.

There is strong evidence that alcohol enhances feelings of personal competence. Tarbox (1979) found that male alcoholics, compared to normals, overestimated their own competence. Konovsky and Wilsnack (1982) reported that social drinkers who believed they had been drinking—both those who had actually consumed alcohol and those who had been drinking a nonalcoholic placebo—gave higher estimates of their own performance on a creativity test. Finally, anxiety about the evaluation of one's performance seems to promote more drinking. Higgins and Marlatt (1975) found that young males who were heavy social drinkers drank significantly more when they believed their performance was being evaluated by young women judges.

Perhaps these two groups of studies are complementary rather than contradictory. Vaillant's (1983) work is important because his measures were self-reports of accomplishments rather than self-ratings of competency and because the data were collected in childhood, before the onset of alcoholism. His findings support what should be obvious: highly competent people may become alcoholics or addicts. Bissell and Haberman's (1984) studies of alcoholism among professionals also document a paradox that should be readily apparent in a society in which so many talented people enter alcohol and drug treatment programs.

But *being* competent is not the same thing as *feeling* competent. The second group of studies suggests that not only alcohol but even the belief by experienced drinkers that they have consumed alcohol enhances self-estimates of competence. (By reputation, it is likely that other drugs, cocaine in particular, do the same thing.) In other words, perceived competence or self-efficacy, as contrasted to objective competence, may relate to problem drinking or drug use. Despite Bandura's plausible distinction between self-efficacy and self-esteem, it still seems likely that self-efficacy is one of the conditions that affect self-esteem, especially in relation to alcohol and drug use.

Self-Handicapping. Berglas and Jones (1978) were also interested in the relationship between alcohol use and self-efficacy, but they added the notion that people could *feel* competent only if they were able to attribute success to their own efforts. That is, accidental success is not a basis for self-efficacy. Success as a result of one's own efforts and competence elicits respect and love from others, which also helps to enhance self-esteem. But accidental success, or other good fortune for which one cannot take credit, is honored neither by one's self nor by others.

Based on these observations, Berglas and Jones proposed that people may use alcohol or other drugs to protect their self-image through "self-handicapping." If one is drunk, success may be perceived by others as even more remarkable, whereas failure may be excused. In effect, drinking enhances the positive attributions of others when the performance is successful but excuses failure when it is not.

In a series of experiments, Jones and Berglas (1978) allowed some of their subjects to achieve high scores on a task in a way that seemed accidental—that is, the subjects who did well were likely to attribute success to chance rather than to their own efforts. Male (but not female) subjects under this condition were more likely, on a second task, to take what they had been told was a performance-inhibiting drug. These researchers concluded that "alcohol and certain forms of drug usage may be facilitated by prior experiences of success unaccompanied by subjective feelings of mastery and control" (1978, 416). In other words, drug use could be a way of handicapping oneself in order to get more credit for success and to avoid blame for failure.

Adding the concept of attribution to self-efficacy produces a theory with more explanatory power than the concept of self-efficacy alone has. Self-handicapping in the interest of maintaining self-esteem may also be the basis for alcohol or other drug use in certain situations and by some people. It does not seem plausible, however, that this hypothesis could account for most alcohol and drug use, even by those who show signs of addiction.

Suppression of Self-Awareness.   Hull proposed that alcohol consumption reduces self-awareness of performance and, in so doing, renders negative self-evaluations following failure less likely. "By decreasing the individual's level of self-awareness . . . alcohol is proposed to reduce the individual's sensitivity to potentially unfavorable information about self and hence provide a potential source of psychological relief" (1981, 594). This hypothesis is compatible with self-efficacy, in the sense that self-evaluation is tied to success or failure in performance.

Hull and Young (1983) studied alcohol consumption in relation to self-consciousness (degree of awareness and concern about one's own performance) and self-esteem in an experimental task in which subjects experienced success or failure. There were two main findings. First, the "self-awareness suppression" hypothesis was confirmed only for highly self-conscious subjects who had been told they performed poorly. This group drank more during a wine-tasting than did either less self-conscious subjects or highly self-conscious subjects who were told they had been successful. Second, there was also an across-the-board difference related to self-esteem. Subjects with low levels of self-esteem drank more wine, regardless of either prior success or failure or high or low self-consciousness. Subjects who were highly self-conscious and had low levels of self-esteem also felt more hostility under the failure condition than subjects in any other group felt. In other words, this group not only drank more but also felt more anger.

The self-awareness hypothesis was thus only partially confirmed (for highly self-conscious subjects). In contrast, self-esteem appeared to affect drinking behavior, irrespective of other conditions. The study also revealed that self-consciousness affected drinking under conditions of failure.

Despite these interesting findings, the success-failure paradigm has serious limitations. In real life, drinking and drug use are not usually linked to a specific performance situation in which the drinker or user is being evaluated by others. Rather, they are associated with a variety of other kinds of situations and in many instances seem to occur spontaneously. The study by Hull and Young does indicate, however, that people who are both self-conscious and low in self-esteem are particularly vulnerable to failure and that individuals with low self-esteem may drink more heavily regardless of other conditions.

Self-Derogation. Kaplan (1975b) has developed and tested a theory that explicitly attributes deviant behavior in adolescents to low self-esteem. The theory assumes that adolescents who feel devalued and rejected by their peer group will develop negative attitudes about themselves. It further suggests that such socially rejected adolescents will associate the patterns of behavior endorsed by the peer group with their own negative self-evaluation: "When I try to do things their way, I always seem to fail." This association will promote deviance from group norms as a means of finding alternative ways to enhance self-esteem. Such adolescents are likely to join an "out-group" with different behavioral norms.

Kaplan and others have found considerable support for this hypothesis. Using a longitudinal research design, they found that children initially classified as "self-derogating" later adopted various types of deviant behavior, including drug and alcohol use and drug dealing (Kaplan 1975a, 1976, 1977). In another study, Kaplan (1978a) found that social experiences damaging to self-esteem, in combination with associated antisocial attitudes, promoted deviant behavior.

Kaplan (1978b) also found that social class was related to the kinds of deviant behavior adopted. Self-derogating middle-class youngsters subsequently adopted behaviors considered antisocial in middle-class society. Highly self-derogating working-class students, whose group norms actually sanctioned many of those same behaviors, were likely to behave differently. Because deviance is relative to the norms of a given social group, the particular behaviors adopted in response to damaged self-esteem will vary accordingly.

Finally, Kaplan (1978a) also reported that adopting deviant behaviors *worked,* though it worked mainly for males. That is, among males, deviant behaviors associated with masculine roles appeared to reduce self-derogation. Among females, for whom the same behaviors were not gender-appropriate, only narcotics use by middle-class females was significantly associated with subsequent decrease in self-derogation. Among lower-class females, there was no association between deviant behavior and enhanced self-esteem.

In a study focusing specifically on the use of alcohol, Kaplan and Pokorny (1977) again found that self-enhancing effects occurred primarily for males, presumably because of role compatibility, and much more strongly where there was corresponding evidence of a personal history of rejection by peers, family, or school. These results were partly confirmed by Newcomb, Bentler, and Collins (1982) in an eight-year longitudinal study using analyses designed to establish causal relationships. These investigators found that feelings of self-derogation and alcohol use initially were positively related in the adolescents studied, yet negatively related later on, just as Kaplan and his colleagues had predicted and in part demonstrated. Despite the fact that early alcohol use decreased self-derogation later, however, adolescent self-derogation did not influence later alcohol use, possibly because the initial assessment was made at too late an age to establish this effect.

Although it is supported by evidence from longitudinal research, Kaplan's theory is at best only a partial explanation of deviant behavior in general and substance use in particular. For one thing, people who reject the norms of their social groups because they have experienced personal devaluation may opt for socially positive deviance. For example, the adolescent who is isolated or ignored in the teen social scene may decide to be a serious student. What would account for choosing "positive," as opposed to "negative," deviance? More important, the hypothesis is significantly less applicable to the problem of substance use at a time when drug and alcohol use are no longer deviant, as is the case among teenagers and young adults today.

Despite these reservations, Kaplan's self-derogation hypothesis is relevant to at least some patterns of substance use. Frequent alcohol or drug use, multiple substance use, and the use of especially dangerous substances remain deviant, even in a population in which experimentation or occasional use of other drugs is the norm. Yet such deviant patterns of behavior *are* approved within subgroups that practice these behaviors. Coombs (1981) has demonstrated that heroin users follow a classic model of career achievement within the context of their own highly deviant subcultures. This kind of addiction requires the same total commitment that careers in the "straight" world require. The successful junkie who manages to obtain a regular supply of good quality heroin without engaging in "straight" behaviors such as working, who rigorously follows group norms that prohibit revealing insider information to outsiders, and who manages to elude the police achieves high status among other users and concomitant support for self-esteem.

Summary of Explanatory Research.   The research reviewed does suggest a number of conditions under which alcohol or other drugs may be used to protect or enhance self-esteem. The concept of self-efficacy is important to this discussion, not only because it has been so widely applied in drug and alcohol prevention and relapse prevention, but also because its relationship to self-esteem is a matter of debate.

There is no doubt that some alcoholics and addicts are highly competent people in certain aspects of their lives and that they might feel self-efficacious as a result. But being competent is not necessarily the same as feeling competent. And being competent in one area of living, such as work, is no guarantee of competence in another area, such as sexuality. There is some evidence that alcohol enhances feelings of personal competence and that men may drink more when they are worried about the quality of their performance. In other words, it is possible that low self-efficacy may be a basis for at least some problem drinking and drug use and that self-efficacy and self-esteem overlap significantly in relation to alcohol and drug use. This impression is supported by research on self-handicapping and suppression of self-awareness. In both cases, subjects have been shown to use alcohol to protect self-esteem from the effects of failure (low self-efficacy) in performance situations. Purely logical distinctions, like the one that can be made between self-esteem and self-efficacy, are not necessarily empirically valid distinctions.

There is also evidence that adolescents may respond to negative feedback from their social group by developing a condition of very low self-esteem, labeled "self-derogation," and that they may further associate the social norms of that group with their negative feelings about self. Joining a deviant group in which illicit drug and alcohol use is approved behavior may be a solution to this problem. Although this hypothesis about social factors underlying low self-esteem and consequent alcohol and drug use may have had considerable validity in the past, however, it seems less applicable during a period in which alcohol and drug use is relatively common in the dominant peer culture.

Research on Altered States of Consciousness

The effect of drugs, including alcohol, on self-esteem can be assessed directly by asking drinkers and users to report on their sense of self-worth both when they are sober and when they are high. Alternatively, their behavior when drinking or using drugs may be observed for signs of changes in self-esteem.

To the lay person, this kind of research might seem the most direct way to illuminate the relationship between self-esteem and substance use. People ordinarily use psychoactive drugs because drugs change the way they *feel*, not because they are planning to engage in some sort of task. The resulting change in consciousness may be an end in itself, or it may in addition affect the user's self-perceptions. There may be no effect on actual behavior that can be readily interpreted.

Academic psychology tends to discount or ignore research on consciousness, because it is associated with the sterile, mentalistic psychology of the late nineteenth century. Most research psychologists believe that directly observable behavioral evidence is the only evidence that counts. But this assumption is severely challenged if one assumes, as we do, that people use psychoactive drugs, including alcohol and many medical drugs, primarily to change states of consciousness.

Expectations About the Effects of Alcohol.   Brown et al. (1980) developed a survey on expectations about the effects of alcohol after initial interviews with drinkers of both sexes. The survey was administered to a large sample of nonalcoholic respondents. Analysis of the results revealed six groups of positive expectations, three of them (enhancement of sexual performance and experience, increased power and aggression, and increased social assertiveness) conceptually related to self-esteem. Heavier drinkers especially expected "sexual enhancement and aggressive arousal." A later study by Rohsenow (1983) of expectations by college students used a more refined method but drew similar conclusions. Heavier drinkers expected more positive consequences from drinking, as well as specific outcomes, such as social and physical pleasure, sexual enjoyment, aggressiveness, and expressiveness, that would be compatible with the enhancement of self-esteem. Unfortunately, neither of these studies assessed self-esteem directly.

Effects of Marijuana.   Comprehensive studies of the drug-related experiences of marijuana users have been reported by Tart (1971) and Fisher and Steckler (1974). Neither of these studies focused specifically on self-esteem; instead, they looked at a broad spectrum of possible effects. Both studies related frequency of use to the effects experienced. Tart also related level of intoxication to drug effects.

This work, in addition to a later report by Pihl, Shea, and Costa (1979), reveals that many of the effects commonly attributed to marijuana by both experienced and inexperienced users are unrelated to self-esteem or identity. These include alterations in sensory perception, space and time perception, bodily sensations, cognitive thought processes, memory, and emotional state. Many of these effects are regularly experienced and highly valued by users. The assertion that changes in self-esteem are the primary reasons normal people use marijuana does not follow.

Nevertheless, marijuana users commonly reported positive alterations in self-esteem and identity. Tart (1971) found that a frequent effect included feeling "powerful, capable, and intelligent when stoned" and that this effect was more likely in heavier users. This observation is consistent with Silver's (1977) previously cited finding that addicts commonly felt powerless. For people who are prone to addiction, drugs may be an antidote to powerlessness and associated low self-esteem. Other marijuana-induced experiences included feeling that one's conversation is more profound and interesting, that one has deep insights into others, and that one's ideas are more original. These and other feelings are consistent with feeling powerful, but they are also consistent with what users might refer to as an "expanded" awareness, associated with a less confined or ego-centered sense of self.

In the Fisher and Steckler (1974) study, positive effects related to self-esteem and self-efficacy were invariably reported with greater frequency going up the scale from past users, occasional users, and regular users to daily users. The majority of daily users associated increased self-approval with marijuana intoxication; only about a third of regular users and one in five occasional users made this association. Similar relationships were found for other effects related to both self-esteem and self-efficacy. For example, among daily users, seven of ten felt that getting high increased their self-knowledge, and more than six of ten felt more creative and more able to communicate with others.

The fact that effects related to self-esteem are reported with increasing frequency by heavier users is most significant. Yet it will not necessarily be apparent behaviorally that an individual feels heightened self-approval, self-esteem, or creativity. Unless one is willing to accept the proposition that human beings can be powerfully motivated to attain a particular state of consciousness *for its own sake,* these findings may be judged as falling outside the domain of science or simply as unimportant.

Especially interesting are Tart's findings on identity changes induced by marijuana: "At higher levels of intoxication . . . the sense of separateness, of being an individual, is often replaced by feelings of oneness with the world, of actions and experiences becoming archetypal, and, occasionally, of merging with people or objects" (1971, 212). Such altered states of consciousness were greatly valued by many of Tart's respondents. Although these experiences may sound bizarre, similar states are sought and apparently attained in various forms of meditation.

The perception that the self is merging with something larger may be a *solution* to the problem of self-esteem. In such states, the user is no longer preoccupied with self-worth or even with the idea of self, in the sense of a finite or individual identity. Although these experiences may seem illusory to an objective observer, achieving profoundly altered states of consciousness is intensely gratifying to many marijuana and hallucinogenic drug users. Such states of consciousness may be perceived as relief from the struggle to maintain a conventional sense of identity and self-esteem. These altered states may be alternative varieties of experience that transcend our culturally approved versions of self-worth, and they may be particularly appealing to users who have problems with the culturally approved concepts.

At the same time, it should be admitted that deliberately altered states of consciousness may appeal to those who wish to experience more about themselves in a purely explorative sense. Accordingly, the need to experience an expanded sense of reality may be a normal desire in human beings.

Effects of Alcohol on Power and Assertiveness.   McClelland et al. (1972) analyzed stories made up by young male subjects about pictures of people in various situations. Behavioral data on the subjects were related to themes in the stories. Participants under both drinking and sober conditions were also observed in simulated social situations. Initial findings led to a focus on needs for personal power (*n* Power) and social power (*s* Power). Participants with high *n* Power scores told stories that emphasized strong, forceful actions (including assaults, giving help or advice, and controlling other people) or that expressed strong concern about reputation or prestige. This work led to an important conclusion: "Men drink primarily to feel stronger. . . . Who drinks excessively? The man who has an accentuated need for personalized power and who for a variety of reasons has chosen drinking as an outlet for it rather than some other alternative" (1972, 334).

McClelland and his associates analyzed their respondents' stories for power imagery rather than for self-esteem. Are there grounds for assuming that this work has anything to do with self-esteem? The *n* Power score, which consistently related to drinking, was interpreted as a measure of *motivation* to attain personal power. For example, the "fantasy pattern" associated with low *n* Power was described as follows: "Explicit concern with own reputation; also mention of superior/subordinate relationships. . . . Negative anticipations, emotions about outcomes; low prestige and view of self" (1972, 118).

Men concerned with such personalized power drank more heavily. They also often engaged in activities that created a "relatively immediate, certain, and riskless *subjective feeling of power.*" Drinking was "a second-best alternative for the man who is both highly concerned about power and highly threatened or made fearful by it" (1972, 116). The *n* Power motive seems related to self-esteem; achieving *n* Power allows men to feel worthy.

In addition to the work by Tart (1971) and Silver (1977) already cited, other research supports the findings by McClelland et al. (1972) on feelings of power. Williams (1968) reported that alcohol consumption increased the differences between young men who were problem drinkers and those who were social drinkers. Problem drinkers became relatively more aggressive, self-centered, heedless of others, and exhibitionistic with higher doses of alcohol. These kinds of behaviors presumably would be released under a heightened sense of personal power and consequent self-esteem. Parker, Gilbert, and Speltz (1981) compared male alcoholics and social drinkers concerning expectations about their own assertiveness. Social drinkers expected no change when intoxicated, whereas alcoholics expected to be more assertive. (Assertiveness implies *n* Power, in the sense of influencing or controlling others.)

There seems to be little doubt that male problem drinkers, and probably users of at least some other drugs, frequently feel less powerful or even powerless and that drinking or using drugs counteracts these feelings. The inference that self-esteem also varies accordingly seems inescapable.

Effects of Alcohol on Self-Esteem and Identity.   A number of studies of the effects of intoxication have used adjective checklists, Q-sorts, or global assessments of discrepancy between descriptions of actual and ideal self. These studies provide direct evidence on changes in self-esteem associated with drinking.

Lang, Verret, and Watt (1984) assessed self-esteem for male and female social drinkers in both "dry" and "wet" party situations. For men, self-esteem was somewhat higher under the drinking condition than under conditions of abstinence, although the difference was not statistically significant. Women who drank were significantly lower on one measure of self-esteem. The difference between the sexes was interpreted as reflecting the relative compatibility of male and female sex roles with drinking in a social context. The important point is that for social drinkers personal and situational variables (set and setting), rather than alcohol alone, may also determine the effect of alcohol on self-esteem (Zinberg 1984).

MacAndrew and Garfinkel (1962), Vanderpool (1969), Berg (1971), and MacAndrew (1979) reported that discrepancies between actual self-concept and ideal self-concept were greater for alcoholics than for normals in the sober state and that these discrepancies increased in most respects with drinking (although Berg's 1971 results were a partial exception). In other words, when assessed as a discrepancy between actual and ideal selves, self-esteem may decline for alcoholics when they are drunk, a finding that requires some explanation.

When drunk, alcoholics also saw themselves as less submissive and eager to please and correspondingly more assertive and hostile. MacAndrew (1979) concluded that drunkenness allowed the alcoholic to dispense with any concern about accountability that might be associated with the sober self, replacing it with one's "other self," an ego state capable of expressing resentment without feeling anxious. This interpretation implies that drinking allows alcoholics to bypass their conventional identity. They are bad, but they do not care. The tyranny of negative self-esteem is circumvented by a change in identity. But the two identities are farther apart than they would be in the sober state, resulting in an apparent decline in self-esteem, if it is being assessed as discrepancy between actual and ideal selves.

Effects of Cocaine and Barbiturates on Self-Esteem and Identity.
Spotts and Shontz (1984a, 1984b) used Q-sort and interview methods to identify changes in consciousness associated with heavy cocaine and barbiturate use. Instead of studying large numbers of subjects, they conducted in-depth studies of a relatively few committed male users and comparable male abstainers. Their central concept was that of *ego state*, defined as the "properties of the field of consciousness within which the ego is located at a given time" (1984a, 120). (As noted earlier, the activation of an ego state incorporates an associated sense of self or identity, in addition to perceptions, emotions, and motives associated with that self-concept or identity.)

Spotts and Shontz reported that moderate users of cocaine described themselves in positive terms in the pre-drug state. In contrast, heavy users in the pre-drug state experienced "massive losses in self-regard," along with increased depression and despair and violent impulses. This state corresponded to participants' characterizations of their "worst" selves. For most of these men, cocaine blocked the emergence of the worst self and delivered "a state of exhilaration, elevation of mood, and a heightened sense of well-being and mastery" (1984a, 136). Even moderate use inflated the ego and produced "exceptional feelings of exhilaration and power."

These authors also reported that moderate cocaine users were insecure and troubled by self-doubts and feelings of inadequacy. Cocaine made them feel more self-assured and seemed to enhance social relationships. In contrast, heavy users were intense, achievement-oriented men intent on self-sufficiency, loners who equated dependence on others with weakness. Their sense of being a powerful person who did not need others was reinforced by cocaine.

Spotts and Shontz (1984b) found a different picture with users of barbiturate drugs. These substances, along with alcohol, are classified as depressants. In the pre-drug state, there was a welling up of hostility and rage accompanied by depression, anxiety, and loneliness. In the drug state, users initially felt substantially increased power and self-confidence. As this state progressed, these desired feelings were replaced by negative feelings such as hostility, arrogance, and impulsiveness. Barbiturate users became their own worst selves.

The assertiveness, hostility, and rage associated with addictive barbiturate use is reminiscent of findings in the alcohol studies cited earlier. Alcohol, cocaine, and barbiturates, though pharmacologically different, have frequently been found to dramatically enhance the male users' feelings of personal power and consequent willingness to be assertive and aggressive.

Summary of Research on Altered States of Consciousness. Studies of alcohol and other drug use reveal that self-esteem is affected by substance use, but in relation to self-concept or identity. Needs for personal power and authority appear to be associated with heavier use, almost irrespective of the drug used. Because most studies have been conducted with men, this generalization may in part reflect cultural and biological, as well as intrapsychic, influences.

It further appears that among problem drinkers and drug users the changes in self-esteem associated with intoxication may reflect a deeper transformation in self or identity. That is, the organizing principles by which the actions of others are interpreted and responded to are changed. Feelings of increased competency, aggression, and power contingent on the use of drugs thus may be derived from transformations in the perceived self. An ego state connected with intoxication replaces the ego state identified with sobriety.

For men, identity transformation may release a "bad" or "worst" self, about whom the drinker or user normally (and subsequently) feels embarrassed or ashamed. This "worst" self is less concerned about accountability and inclined to be more assertive and even hostile. Increased assertiveness suggests a concomitant increase in self-esteem. When self-esteem is assessed as a discrepancy between one's view of actual and ideal selves, however, it may appear to be lower when sober respondents reflect back on their intoxicated behavior, for the ego state associated with being drunk or high is likely to be less socially acceptable than the sober ego state.

With marijuana and some other drugs, the personality transformation may take the form of an altered state of transcendental consciousness in which the self merges with others or with the environment and in which personal identity and fixed perspectives on reality become less important. This state may in part recapitulate the early, merged state of the infant-mother relationship (Mahler, Pine, and Bergman 1975).

Finally, major or primary identity changes associated with alcohol and drug intoxication are likely to be more characteristic of problem drinkers and users, although such changes may also occur to at least some degree in social drinkers.

Self-Esteem and Recovery

The fundamental question addressed in this chapter is whether people with a weak or fragmented sense of self or identity may sustain their self-esteem through the use of alcohol or drugs and, consequently, be especially prone to "problem" or addictive use. Undoubtedly, psychological defenses such as denial—as well as other admittedly important factors, including social supports—also play a role in alcohol or drug use, although these topics cannot be covered here.

Recovering people often refer to a period in which their addiction "worked." They suggest that as long as their habit was working, there was no reason to stop drinking or using drugs. Addictions stop being functional in a number of ways, but usually there is a history of accumulating problems. Eventually, a crisis occurs, which may be precipitated by shattered relationships, serious employment or financial problems, trouble with the law, or poor health. This crisis is the moment when drinking or using drugs can no longer suppress realistic anxiety about the problems themselves or support identity structures that maintain self-esteem. There is often a precipitous fall into demoralization (Frank 1982) and despair, the "hitting bottom" described earlier. Not surprisingly, this is also the time when alcoholics and other addicts are most likely to ask for help. For example, Matefy, Kalish, and Cantor (1971) found that alcoholics seeking help had lower self-esteem than alcoholics who rejected assistance.

All of this suggests that the recovery process should facilitate developing a personal identity that can maintain self-esteem outside the supportive environments associated with virtually all professional, as well as lay, recovery programs. Our goal is not to compare or even evaluate such programs, but rather to scrutinize pertinent research for additional evidence on the relationship between self-esteem and substance use. A recent in-depth study on recovery from heroin addiction without intervention or treatment will also be examined for the same purpose.

Treatment and Recovery Programs

Recovery programs include inpatient and outpatient medical and hospital programs; individual, family, and group psychotherapy; peer-support group programs such as Alcoholics Anonymous; and therapeutic communities, which are long-term, residential drug treatment programs incorporating a variety of peer intervention strategies within a highly structured living environment. Unfortunately, sufficient research is available only on group therapy. Methadone programs, which merely replace one drug habit with another, are not relevant. Heroin itself was once used to get people to stop using opium, but no one today would define such a practice as "treatment."

Hospital Programs.   Cernovsky (1983) and Hoffman and Abbott (1970) have reported positive changes in self-esteem for inpatients in chemical dependency hospital programs. Kliner, Spicer, and Barnett (1980) reported that alcoholic physicians had higher self-esteem after hospital treatment. Other studies show less consistent results. Gross and Adler (1970) and Gross (1971) found that some aspects of self-concept related to self-esteem improved after hospital treatment, whereas other aspects did not improve or even declined. Much of this discrepancy may have resulted from differences in the measures used.

Wilson, White, and Lange (1978) compared hospital programs and community residential programs for improvement in self-esteem among skid-row alcoholics of both sexes. Significant positive gains occurred in the community programs, compared to hospital programs, although differences decreased over time. Selby (1981), studying both a hospital and a vocational rehabilitation center, found positive changes in some (but not all) aspects of self-concept that are related to self-esteem.

In a study by Heather, Rollnick, and Winton (1982), both abstainers and those who maintained "controlled" or social drinking scored higher on self-esteem measures than those who relapsed after treatment. These results were not confirmed by Wald (1980), however, who admittedly used a somewhat different research design.

With respect to changes in self-representation or identity, Armstrong and Hoyt (1963) reported that the actual or current self-perception of alcoholic males did not change during hospitalization, although the ideal self did change in the direction of a more realistic and less guilt-plagued representation. This finding is consistent with the principle that changes in identity take time. The best that could be expected from a short-term hospital treatment program, which rarely lasts more than thirty days, is the beginning of a change in who one would like to be.

In summary, there is some evidence that self-esteem increases as a result of hospital programs, although for some groups, other approaches to treatment may result in greater gains. There is also some evidence that former patients who do not return to alcoholic drinking have higher self-esteem than those who relapse.

One study (Armstrong and Hoyt 1963) identified what may have been the beginning of a positive change in self or identity with treatment. These changes occurred only in representations of the ideal self, rather than the real self, as might be expected, given the brief nature of hospital treatment programs.

Although hospital programs are now the most common method of formal treatment for substance addictions, their usefulness, from the perspective of research that concerns us here, is seriously limited, because of their short duration. We failed to find long-term, follow-up studies of patients in hospital programs.

Therapeutic Communities. Residents who remain in therapeutic communities are usually involved in the treatment program for relatively long periods, and it is therefore possible to do genuine longitudinal research with this population. Whereas most of the research on hospital programs has focused on alcoholics, most therapeutic community residents have been addicted to other drugs, including opiate drugs. Therapeutic community residents are more likely to be from a deviant or "hard-core" user population than are alcoholics in hospital programs.

Positive changes in both self-esteem and self-concept, or identity, have been found in research on residents of therapeutic communities. Preston and Viney (1984) and Page, Mitchell, and Morris (1985) reported gains in self-esteem associated with time spent in the programs. The latter study also found smaller discrepancies in descriptions of actual selves and ideal selves, again associated with time in the program. De Leon and Jainchill (1981) found that aspects of self-concept related to self-esteem improved significantly, with women showing greater gains over time than men. These results were stable during a follow-up after two years. Similar gains were reported by Wheeler, Biase, and Sullivan (1986), although gender differences were reversed.

Because the data are longitudinal in nature and reflect a long-term treatment and recovery process, research on therapeutic community residents carries much more weight than does research on hospital patients. Here, the findings unequivocally support positive changes in self-esteem, whether measured by self-ratings or by discrepancies between actual and ideal self-concepts. Moreover, the long period of treatment associated with therapeutic communities allows for the development of identity structures capable of maintaining self-esteem without excessive need for external support.

Alcoholics Anonymous.   The membership of Alcoholics Anonymous (AA) provides another research population ideal for assessing changes in self-esteem and associated conceptions of self. The membership is large (estimated at well over one million in the United States alone). There are also many members who report long-term sobriety, making it possible to detect effects that might be apparent only after considerable time. Finally, AA insists on abstinence from alcohol and other drugs, thus eliminating problems of verification with research subjects who say they are now "controlled" drinkers or users. (The same question might be raised with respect to abstinence, but the climate of Alcoholics Anonymous is such that members who relapse soon stop participating unless they wish to get back "on the program.")

Unfortunately, we found very little research on AA members. Carroll and Fuller (1969) reported that imprisoned alcoholics who had been members of AA for some time had higher self-esteem than hospital inpatients who were being treated for alcoholism. There was no difference between AA members "on the program" and non-AA alcoholic prisoners. Conner (1962) reported that AA members showed self-concepts on Gough's (1952) adjective checklist that were more positive than those of jailed alcoholics not in AA but less positive than those of nonalcoholics. The obvious problems in research design here render the results very questionable, however.

AA members have not been studied in a way, or to a degree, that sheds light on the relationship between substance use and self-esteem, despite the fact that improving self-esteem is a frequent subject in AA and other twelve-step program meetings. Moreover, members of these programs deliberately adopt the concept of "recovering alcoholic" (or recovering addict) as an identity, which they proceed to develop over a considerable period of time. Although initially this identity may be a "public self," that is, the "image of the self one tries to convey to others" (Markus and Wurf 1987), over time it is likely to become a strong, internalized self-representation as well.

Group Therapy.   In general, there is evidence that self-esteem increases although the findings are restricted to alcoholics. Gains in self-esteem have been reported by Ends and Page (1959) for client-centered therapy patients compared with a control group, and by Annis (1979) and Annis and Chan (1983) for alcoholic prison inmates. Gad-Luther and Dickman (1979) also reported gains in self-esteem for male alcoholics participating in group therapy with their spouses. Finally, Tomsovic (1976) found gains in aspects of self-concept related to self-esteem for one method of group therapy (closed encounter) but not for another (open-group eclectic).

Summary of Research on Treatment and Recovery Programs.   There is some evidence from studies of recovering alcoholics and addicts that gains in self-esteem follow various forms of treatment. There is also some reason to believe that recovering persons with higher self-esteem are less likely than others to relapse. The strongest evidence comes from studies of residents in therapeutic communities, in cases where information was collected over a relatively long period. These studies report gains in self-esteem proportional to the time residents have spent in the programs. They also report a comparable decrease in the discrepancy between residents' descriptions of their actual selves and their ideal selves, suggesting parallel development of self-concept or identity.

The lack of significant research on members of Alcoholics Anonymous and other twelve-step programs is the most glaring example of the research community's general failure to grasp the potential that this population may hold for casting light on relationships between the development of a healthy identity and associated self-esteem and recovery from addiction.

The Construction of Identity

The last, and in many respects the most illuminating, research on recovery that we will discuss comes from a study of heroin addicts who recovered without treatment. Biernacki (1986) conducted in-depth interviews of 101 heroin addicts who had been addicted for at least one year (the average was between five and six years). To be included in the study, the former addicts also had to have experienced five of the ten most common withdrawal symptoms and been free from addiction for at least two years. Finally, participants were not to have been in any formal treatment program for more than three days. This group of respondents had recovered on their own, though often with the assistance of friends or family. Their ideas about addiction and recovery represent their own interpretations of these experiences, rather than those of treatment professionals or the members of any of the twelve-step programs.

Biernacki's research focuses on the "self-concept," or "the process of making an object of one's self and the process of role taking. Ultimately, the self is acquired through interaction with significant others" (1986, 20). The implication of this view is that, by making the self an object, human beings have the capability of gaining control over their identity. That is, should we choose to do so, we have the capacity to assume roles and act them out in relation to other people. This process results in the definition of self or identity. Self is not immutable, however; rather, "in the course of the life cycle the self evolves and changes as people alter their associations and interpret and reinterpret the actions others take in relation to them" (1986, 21).

Biernacki's approach, grounded in the sociological tradition of symbolic interactionism, is nonetheless compatible with the view of the functions of self-concept presented by Markus and Wurf (1987) or the object relations theories of Kohut (1977) or Mahler, Pine, and Bergman (1975). But it is not a theory of early development. Instead, it is a perspective on the continuous development of self during adulthood. Biernacki assumes that by "objectifying" themselves, people make choices that influence the further development of their concept of self or identity. This approach obviously runs counter to the environmental determinism of much of contemporary academic psychology, as well as to the medical disease concept of addiction.

Biernacki argues that the social role of an addict incorporates an identity that may coexist with other personal identities. Like Coombs (1981), Biernacki equates the addict's "hustle," or method of maintaining and managing a habit, to a legitimate occupation in the conventional world. If the addict's "hustle" is successful, he or she attains high social status in the world of addiction. This status in turn brings a "profound influence to bear on personal estimations of self-esteem."

Biernacki's analysis in part supports and recapitulates the thesis of this chapter. Adults, consciously or unconsciously, choose and develop conceptions of self that are tested as they are responded to by other people. When these self-conceptions are successful, in the sense of being congruent with ideal selves, character is shaped and frequently reinforced through social interactions that support self-esteem. We would also add that successful identities eventually become both encompassing, in the sense of accounting for more and more of a person's behavior, and to a considerable extent self-perpetuating. A successful and long-maintained identity, we believe, is to a significant degree impervious to the ups and downs of daily life. The aged general still walks as if he were on parade.

In most cases, Biernacki's addicts developed a resolution to stop using heroin as a result of problems that grew out of the addiction. In about one-third of the cases, there was an emotional "bottoming out" experience. Nearly all of the other subjects developed their ideas about quitting through a rational process of considering actions and consequences. This process, too, followed an accumulation of negative experiences and often a particularly significant personal event.

If there is a single conclusion that follows from the case analyses presented, it is that "to change their lives . . . addicts must fashion new identities, perspectives, and social world involvements wherein the addict identity is excluded or dramatically depreciated" (Biernacki 1986, 141). Biernacki identifies three basic patterns by which alternative identities were developed: developing *emergent identities,* which were either entirely new or based on "rudimentary," preexisting identities; *identity reverting,* or returning to previous, unspoiled identities; and *extending identities,* or emphasizing and extending an identity that coexisted with the addict identity but was not contaminated by it.

These processes were universal among the addicts studied. They are illustrated by one of the examples of emergent, or new, identity. A young woman addict just released from jail had nowhere to go. Her husband was still in jail for the same drug-related offense. Her family, except for a grandmother who lived in a distant small town, had become estranged during the addiction. All of her surviving friends were practicing addicts or were in jail. With her only choices being to live with her grandmother, whom she had not seen since she became an addict, or to return to the addict culture, she took the former option.

For a considerable time, she remained in her grandmother's house, not going out because she was afraid that she would "score dope." Later, she began to leave the house, but only in the company of her grandmother. She was in an "identity hiatus," completely lacking an adult identity that could replace the identity of a drug addict. Without an adult self-conception, she remained passive, much as she would have done had she visited her grandmother's home as a child.

Eventually, her husband was released from jail and joined her. Without anything else to do, the two former big-city drug addicts went to work as laborers on a farm. After a period, they began to see themselves as living in a directionless limbo. Then a brother-in-law suggested that they go to college. Lacking any other alternative, they went along with the suggestion.

Surprisingly, being college students provided a ready-made social role. Moreover, they met other recovering students and were invited to join a campus support group. They began to identify themselves as re-covering persons rather than simply as former junkies. The extent of the development of a new identity and higher self-esteem by the time of the interview is suggested by one of the young woman's statements: "Now we're going to school. Now we feel good. Now we're really going to do something. . . . We're trying, we're kind of advertising that we're making an effort to do things that are accepted, maybe even by our parents" (Biernacki 1986, 148).

Eventually, new identities developed in the addicts studied by Bier-nacki. This was evident when they began to refer to their addictions in the past tense. Addicts often remarked that they felt strange talking about their addictions, because it "no longer was them."

Cummings (1979) devoted his presidential address to the American Psychological Association to a description of the rules and techniques he and his colleagues developed for working with addicts in San Fran-cisco's Haight-Ashbury district. Cummings stressed the vital impor-tance of encouraging the addict to recall some cherished but long-abandoned hope or aspiration for his or her life. The addict who could do this, in Cummings's experience, had found something positive to strive for through the long recovery period, something that, in our view, serves to revive a lost innocence and forms the basis for a positive, emergent identity.

A number of years ago, one of the authors heard a middle-aged re-covering alcoholic reflect on the meaning of his sobriety. "At last," he said, "I am becoming the person I was meant to be." The implications of this statement stand at the beginning of the inquiry that led, ultimately, to this chapter.

Postscript

It remains to be determined which techniques or program ingredients are most beneficial in helping alcoholics or addicts construct healthy identities and learn associated ways of behaving that together promote and maintain healthy self-esteem. It is clear that genuinely successful interventions are likely to be lengthy and to concentrate on developing personality structures that maintain self-esteem rather than on self-esteem directly. Pumping up a flat tire is an inappropriate analogy for recovery from an addiction. Rather, an internalized capability to generate self-esteem has to be developed. Recovery is no magic trick. It requires hard work in the service of significant personal development.

Bibliography

Alcoholics Anonymous. 1976. *Alcoholics Anonymous.* 3d ed. New York: Alcoholics Anonymous World Services.

Anderson, S. C. 1981. "Alcoholic Women: Personality Traits During Adolescence." *American Journal of Drug and Alcohol Abuse* 8 : 239–247.

Annis, H. M. 1979. "Group Treatment of Incarcerated Offenders with Alcohol and Drug Problems: A Controlled Evaluation." *Canadian Journal of Criminology* 21 : 3–15.

Annis, H. M., and D. Chan. 1983. "The Differential Treatment Model: Empirical Evidence from a Personality Typology of Adult Offenders." *Criminal Justice and Behavior* 10 : 159–173.

Armstrong, R. G., and D. B. Hoyt. 1963. "Personality Structure of Male Alcoholics as Reflected in the IES Test." *Quarterly Journal of Studies on Alcohol* 24 : 239–248.

Back, K. W., and D. A. Sullivan. 1978. "Self-Image, Medicine, and Drug Use." *Addictive Diseases* 3 : 373–382.

Bandura, A. 1982. "Self-Efficacy Mechanism in Human Agency." *American Psychologist* 37 : 122–147.

———. 1984. "Recycling Misconceptions of Perceived Self-Efficacy." *Cognitive Therapy and Research* 8 : 231–255.

Beck, A. T. 1967. *Depression: Causes and Treatment.* Philadelphia: University of Pennsylvania Press.

Beckman, L. J. 1975. "Women Alcoholics: A Review of Social and Psychological Studies." *Journal of Studies on Alcohol* 36 : 797–824.

———. 1978. "Self-Esteem of Women Alcoholics." *Journal of Studies on Alcohol* 39 : 491–498.

———. 1980. "Perceived Antecedents and Effects of Alcohol Consumption in Women." *Journal of Studies on Alcohol* 41 : 518–530.

Beckman, L. J., and P. Bardsley. 1981. "The Perceived Determinants and Consequences of Alcohol Consumption Among Young Women Heavy Drinkers." *International Journal of the Addictions* 16 : 75–88.

Beckman, L. J., T. Day, P. Bardsley, and A. Z. Seeman. 1980. "The Personality Characteristics and Family Backgrounds of Women Alcoholics." *International Journal of the Addictions* 15 : 147–154.

Berg, N. L. 1971. "Effects of Alcohol Intoxication on Self-Concept." *Quarterly Journal of Studies on Alcohol* 32 : 442–443.

Berglas, S., and E. E. Jones. 1978. "Drug Choice as a Self-Handicapping Strategy in Response to Noncontingent Success." *Journal of Personality and Social Psychology* 36 : 405–417.

Biernacki, P. 1986. *Pathways from Heroin Addiction: Recovery Without Treatment.* Philadelphia: Temple University Press.

Bissell, L., and P. Haberman. 1984. *Alcoholism in the Professions.* New York: Oxford University Press.

Blatt, S. J., B. Rounsaville, S. L. Eyre, and C. Wilber. 1984. "The Psychodynamics of Opiate Addiction." *Journal of Nervous and Mental Disease* 172:342–352.

Brown, R. A. 1980. "Personality Measure in Gamma and Delta Alcoholics." *Journal of Clinical Psychology* 36:345–346.

Brown, S. A., M. S. Goldman, A. Inn, and L. R. Anderson. 1980. "Expectations of Reinforcement from Alcohol: Their Domain and Relation to Drinking Patterns." *Journal of Consulting and Clinical Psychology* 48:419–426.

Buhler, C., and D. W. Lefever. 1947. "A Rorschach Study on the Psychological Characteristics of Alcoholics." *Quarterly Journal of Studies on Alcohol* 8:197–260.

Button, A. D. 1956a. "The Psychodynamics of Alcoholism: A Survey of Eighty-Seven Cases." *Quarterly Journal of Studies on Alcohol* 17:443–460.

———. 1956b. "A Rorschach Study of Sixty-Seven Alcoholics." *Quarterly Journal of Studies on Alcohol* 17:35–52.

Carroll, J. F. X. 1980. "Similarities and Differences of Personality and Psychopathology Between Alcoholics and Addicts." *American Journal of Drug and Alcohol Abuse* 7:219–236.

Carroll, J. F. X., T. E. Malloy, D. L. Roscioli, G. M. Pindjak, and J. S. Clifford. 1982. "Similarities and Differences in Self-Concepts of Women Alcoholics and Drug Addicts." *Journal of Studies on Alcohol* 43:725–738.

Carroll, J. L., and G. B. Fuller. 1969. "The Self and Ideal-Self Concept of the Alcoholic as Influenced by Length of Sobriety and/or Participation in Alcoholics Anonymous." *Journal of Clinical Psychology* 25:363–364.

Cernovsky, Z. 1983. "Dimensions of Self-Actualization and Post-Treatment Alcohol Use in Fully and Partially Recovered Alcoholics." *Journal of Clinical Psychology* 39:628–632.

Chelton, L. G., and W. G. Bonney. 1987. "Addiction, Affects, and Self-Object Theory." *Psychotherapy* 24:40–46.

Conner, R. G. 1962. "The Self-Concepts of Alcoholics." In *Society, Culture, and Drinking Patterns*, edited by D. J. Pittman and C. R. Snyder, 455–467. New York: Wiley.

Coombs, R. H. 1981. "Drug Abuse as Career." *Journal of Drug Issues* 11:369–387.

Coopersmith, S. 1967. *The Antecedents of Self-Esteem*. San Francisco: Freeman.

Cummings, N. A. 1979. "Turning Bread into Stones: Our Modern Antimiracle." *American Psychologist* 34:1119–1129.

De Leon, G., and N. Jainchill. 1981. "Male and Female Drug Abusers: Social and Psychological Status Two Years After Treatment in a Therapeutic Community." *American Journal of Drug and Alcohol Abuse* 8:465–497.

Ends, E. J., and C. W. Page. 1959. "Group Psychotherapy and Concomitant Psychological Change." *Psychological Monographs* 73(10).

Fisher, G., and A. Steckler. 1974. "Psychological Effects, Personality and Behavioral Changes Attributed to Marijuana Use." *International Journal of the Addictions* 9:101–126.

Frank, J. 1982. "Therapeutic Components Shared by All Psychotherapies." In *Psychotherapy Research and Behavior Change*, Master Lecture Series, vol. 1, edited by J. H. Harvey and M. M. Parks, 9–37. Washington, D.C.: American Psychological Association.

Furnham, A., and V. Lowick. 1984. "Lay Theories of the Causes of Alcoholism." *British Journal of Medical Psychology* 57:319–332.

Gad-Luther, I., and D. Dickman. 1979. "Psychosexual Therapy with Recovering Alcoholics: A Pilot Study." *Journal of Sex Education Therapy* 1:11–16.

Ghadirian, A. M. 1979. "Adolescent Alcoholism: Motives and Alternatives." *Comprehensive Psychiatry* 20:469–474.

Gossop, M. 1976. "Drug Dependence and Self-Esteem." *International Journal of the Addictions* 11:741–753.

Gough, H. G. 1952. *The Adjective Checklist*. Palo Alto, Calif.: Consulting Psychologists Press.

Graeven, D. B., and W. Folmer. 1977. "Experimental Heroin Users: An Epidemiologic and Psychosocial Approach." *American Journal of Drug and Alcohol Abuse* 4:365–375.

Gross, W. F. 1971. "Self-Concepts of Alcoholics Before and After Treatment." *Journal of Clinical Psychology* 27:539–541.

Gross, W. F., and L. O. Adler. 1970. "Aspects of Alcoholics' Self-Concepts as Measured by the Tennessee Self-Concept Scale." *Psychological Reports* 27:431–434.

Hawkins, J. D., D. M. Lishner, R. F. Catalano, and M. O. Howard. 1986. "Childhood Predictors of Adolescent Substance Abuse: Toward an Empirically Grounded Theory." *Journal of Children and Contemporary Society* 8:11–48.

Heather, N., S. Rollnick, and M. Winton. 1982. "Psychological Change Among Inpatient Alcoholics and Its Relationship to Treatment Outcome." *British Journal on Alcohol and Alcoholism* 17:90–97.

Heilbrun, A. B., and H. L. Schwartz. 1980. "Self-Esteem and Self-Reinforcement in Men Alcoholics." *Journal of Studies on Alcohol* 41:1134–1142.

Hendin, H. 1974. "Beyond Alienation: The End of the Psychedelic Road." *American Journal of Drug and Alcohol Abuse* 1:11–23.

Higgins, E. T. 1983. "A Theory of Discrepant Self-Concepts." New York University. Typescript.

Higgins, R. L., and G. A. Marlatt. 1975. "Fear of Interpersonal Evaluation as a Determinant of Alcohol Consumption in Male Social Drinkers." *Journal of Abnormal Psychology* 84:644–651.

Hoar, C. H. 1983. "Women Alcoholics: Are They Different from Other Women?" *International Journal of the Addictions* 18:251–270.

Hoffman, H., and D. Abbott. 1970. "Emotional Self-Descriptions of Alcoholic Patients After Treatment." *Psychological Reports* 26:892.

Hull, J. G. 1981. "A Self-Awareness Model of the Causes and Effects of Alcohol Consumption." *Journal of Abnormal Psychology* 90:586–600.

Hull, J. G., and R. D. Young. 1983. "Self-Consciousness, Self-Esteem, and Success-Failure as Determinants of Alcohol Consumption in Male Social Drinkers." *Journal of Personality and Social Psychology* 44:1097–1109.

Jones, E. E., and S. Berglas. 1978. "Control of Attributions About the Self

Through Self-Handicapping Strategies: The Appeal of Alcohol and the Role of Underachievement." *Personality and Social Psychology Bulletin* 4:200–206.

Kaplan, H. B. 1975a. "Increase in Self-Rejection as an Antecedent of Deviant Responses." *Journal of Youth and Adolescence* 4:281–292.

———. 1975b. "Sequelae of Self-Derogation." *Youth and Society* 7:171–197.

———. 1976. "Self-Attitudes and Deviant Response." *Social Forces* 54: 788–801.

———. 1977. "Antecedents of Deviant Responses: Predicting from a General Theory of Deviant Behavior." *Journal of Youth and Adolescence* 6:89–101.

———. 1978a. "Deviant Behavior and Self-Enhancement in Adolescence." *Journal of Youth and Adolescence* 7:253–277.

———. 1978b. "Social Class, Self-Derogation, and Deviant Response." *Social Psychiatry* 13:19–28.

Kaplan, H. B., and A. D. Pokorny. 1977. "Alcohol Use and Self-Enhancement Among Adolescents: A Conditional Relationship." In *Currents in Alcoholism*, vol. 4, edited by F. A. Seixas, 51–75. New York: Harcourt Brace Jovanovich.

Kernberg, O. 1966. "Structural Derivatives of Object Relationships." *International Journal of Psycho-Analysis* 47:236–253.

Kinsey, B. A. 1966. *The Female Alcoholic: A Social Psychological Study.* Springfield, Ill.: Thomas.

Kliner, D. J., J. Spicer, and P. Barnett. 1980. "Treatment Outcome of Alcoholic Patients." *Journal of Studies on Alcohol* 41:1217–1220.

Kobasa, S. C. 1979. "Stressful Life Events, Personality, and Health: An Inquiry into Hardiness." *Journal of Personality and Social Psychology* 37:1–11.

Kohut, H. 1977. *The Restoration of the Self.* New York: International Universities Press.

Kohut, H., and E. S. Wolf. 1978. "The Disorders of the Self and Their Treatment: An Outline." *International Journal of Psycho-Analysis* 59:413–425.

Konovsky, M., and S. C. Wilsnack. 1982. "Social Drinking and Self-Esteem in Married Couples." *Journal of Studies on Alcohol* 43:319–333.

Kurtines, W., R. Hogan, and D. Weiss. 1975. "Personality Dynamics of Heroin Use." *Journal of Abnormal Psychology* 84:87–89.

Lang, A. R., L. D. Verret, and C. Watt. 1984. "Drinking and Creativity: Objective and Subjective Effects." *Addictive Behaviors* 9:395–399.

Lindblad, R. A. 1977. "Self-Concept of Middle Socioeconomic Status Addicts: A Controlled Study." *International Journal of the Addictions* 12:137–151.

MacAndrew, C. 1979. "A Retrospective Study of Drunkenness: Associated Changes in the Self-Depictions of a Large Sample of Male Outpatient Alcoholics." *Addictive Behaviors* 4:373–381.

MacAndrew, C., and H. Garfinkel. 1962. "A Consideration of Changes Attributed to Intoxication as Common-Sense Reasons for Getting Drunk." *Quarterly Journal of Studies on Alcohol* 23:252–266.

McClelland, D. C., W. N. Davis, R. Kalin, and E. Wanner, eds. 1972. *The Drinking Man.* New York: Free Press.

McLachlan, J. F. C., R. L. Walderman, D. F. Birchmore, and L. R. Marsden.

1979. "Self-Evaluation, Role Satisfaction, and Anxiety in the Woman Alcoholic." *International Journal of the Addictions* 14:809–832.

Maddox, G. L., and J. R. Williams. 1968. "Drinking Behavior of Negro Collegians." *Quarterly Journal of Studies on Alcohol* 29:117–129.

Mahler, M. S., F. Pine, and A. Bergman. 1975. *The Psychological Birth of the Human Infant.* New York: Basic Books.

Markus, H., and E. Wurf. 1987. "The Dynamic Self-Concept: A Social Psychological Perspective." *Annual Review of Psychology* 38:299–337.

Marlatt, G. A. 1985. "Relapse Prevention: Theoretical Rationale and Overview of the Model." In *Relapse Prevention,* edited by G. A. Marlatt and J. R. Gordon, 3–70. New York: Guilford.

Marsh, H. W., and R. Shavelson. 1985. "Self-Concept: Its Multifaceted, Hierarchical Structure." *Educational Psychologist* 20:107–123.

Matefy, R. E., R. A. Kalish, and J. M. Cantor. 1971. "Self-Acceptance in Alcoholics Who Accept and Reject Help." *Quarterly Journal of Studies on Alcohol* 32:1088–1091.

Mayo, E. E. 1979. *The Relationship Between Self-Concept Variables and Sexual Preferences Among Male Alcoholics and Male Nonalcoholics.* Ann Arbor, Mich.: University Microfilms.

Newcomb, M. D., P. M. Bentler, and C. Collins. 1986. "Alcohol Use and Dissatisfaction with Self and Life: A Longitudinal Analysis of Young Adults." *Journal of Drug Issues* 16:479–494.

O'Mahony, P., and E. Smith. 1984. "Some Personality Characteristics of Imprisoned Heroin Addicts." *Drug and Alcohol Dependence* 13:255–265.

Osgood, C. E., G. J. Suci, and P. H. Tannenbaum. 1957. *The Measurement of Meaning.* Urbana: University of Illinois Press.

Padina, R. J., and J. A. Schuele. 1983. "Psychosocial Correlates of Alcohol and Drug Use of Adolescent Students and Adolescents in Treatment." *Journal of Studies on Alcohol* 44:950–973.

Page, R. C., S. Mitchell, and V. Morris. 1985. "Changes in Self-Perceptions of Illicit Drug Abusers Related to Time in Treatment in Two Residential Treatment Programs." *International Journal of the Addictions* 20:1741–1750.

Parker, J. C., G. Gilbert, and M. L. Speltz. 1981. "Expectations Regarding the Effects of Alcohol on Assertiveness: A Comparison of Alcoholics and Social Drinkers." *Addictive Behaviors* 6:29–33.

Pihl, R. O., D. Shea, and L. Costa. 1979. "Dimensions of the Subjective Marijuana Experience." *International Journal of the Addictions* 14:63–71.

Preston, C. A., and L. L. Viney. 1984. "Self- and Ideal-Self Perception of Drug Addicts in Therapeutic Communities." *International Journal of the Addictions* 19:805–819.

Reid, L. D., O. B. Martinson, and L. C. Weaver. 1987. "Factors Associated with the Drug Use of Fifth Through Eighth Grade Students." *Journal of Drug Education* 17:149–161.

Rohsenow, D. J. 1983. "Drinking Habits and Expectancies About Alcohol Effects for Self Versus Others." *Journal of Consulting and Clinical Psychology* 51:752–756.

Schaeffer, G. M., M. A. Schuckit, and E. R. Morrissey. 1976. "Correlation Be-

tween Two Measures of Self-Esteem and Drug Use in a College Sample."
Psychological Reports 39:915–919.

Schaps, E., J. Moskowitz, J. Malvin, and G. Schaeffer. 1983. *Napa Project Summary.* Lafayette, Calif.: Pacific Institute for Research and Evaluation.

Selby, R. B. 1981. "Effects on Self-Concept in Two Different Alcoholism Treatment Programs." *American Journal of Drug and Alcohol Abuse* 8:95–105.

Silver, A. M. 1977. "Some Personality Characteristics of Groups of Young Drug Misusers and Delinquents." *British Journal of Addiction* 72:143–150.

Skager, R. W., D. G. Fisher, and E. Maddahian. 1986. *A Statewide Survey of Drug and Alcohol Use Among California Students in Grades Seven, Nine, and Eleven.* Sacramento, Calif.: Office of the Attorney General, Crime Prevention Center.

Spotts, J. V., and F. C. Shontz. 1984a. "Drug-Induced Ego States. I: Cocaine—Phenomenology and Implications." *International Journal of the Addictions* 19:119–151.

———. 1984b. "The Phenomenological Structure of Drug-Induced Ego States. II: Barbiturates and Sedative-Hypnotics—Phenomenology and Implications." *International Journal of the Addictions* 19:295–326.

Steffenhagen, L. A., and R. A. Steffenhagen. 1985. "Self-Esteem and Primary Demographic Characteristics of Alcoholics in a Rural State." *Journal of Alcohol and Drug Education* 30:51–59.

Stengel, B. 1978. "Some Observations on Repressive Values in Drug Treatment." *Journal of Drug Issues* 8:63–73.

Stephenson, W. 1953. *The Study of Behavior: Q-Technique and Its Methodology.* Chicago: University of Chicago Press.

Sullivan, H. S. 1953. *The Interpersonal Theory of Psychiatry.* New York: Norton.

Tarbox, A. R. 1979. "Self-Regulation and Sense of Competence in Men Alcoholics." *Journal of Studies on Alcohol* 40:860–867.

Tart, C. T. 1971. *On Being Stoned.* Palo Alto, Calif.: Science and Behavior Books.

Tobler, N. S. 1986. "Meta-Analysis of 143 Adolescent Drug Prevention Programs: Quantitative Outcome Results of Program Participants Compared to a Control or Comparison Group." *Journal of Drug Issues* 16:537–567.

Tolpin, M. 1971. "On the Beginnings of a Cohesive Self: An Application of the Concept of Transmuting Internalization to the Study of the Transitional Object and Signal Anxiety." *Psychoanalytic Study of the Child* 26:316–352.

Tomsovic, M. 1976. "Group Therapy and Changes in the Self-Concept of Alcoholics." *Journal of Studies on Alcohol* 37:53–57.

Vaillant, G. E. 1983. *The Natural History of Alcoholism.* Cambridge, Mass.: Harvard University Press.

Vanderpool, J. A. 1969. "Alcoholism and the Self-Concept." *Quarterly Journal of Studies on Alcohol* 30:59–77.

Wald, H. P. 1980. "An Examination of the Relationship Between Drinking Status and the Self-Evaluation of the Alcoholic." *Drug and Alcohol Dependence* 6:285–293.

Wheeler, B. L., D. V. Biase, and A. P. Sullivan. 1986. "Changes in Self-Concept

During Therapeutic Community Treatment: A Comparison of Male and Female Drug Abusers." *Journal of Drug and Alcohol Education* 16:191–196.

Williams, A. F. 1965. "Self-Concepts of College Problem Drinkers, 1: A Comparison with Alcoholics." *Quarterly Journal of Studies on Alcohol* 26: 586–594.

———. 1968. "Psychological Needs and Social Drinking Among College Students." *Quarterly Journal of Studies on Alcohol* 29:355–363.

Wilson, A., J. White, and D. E. Lange. 1978. "Outcome Evaluation of a Hospital-Based Alcoholism Treatment Programme." *British Journal of Addiction* 73:39–45.

Wurmser, L. 1985. "Denial and Split Identity: Timely Issues in the Psychoanalytic Psychotherapy of Compulsive Drug Users." *Journal of Substance Abuse Treatment* 2:89–96.

Zinberg, N. E. 1985. *Drug, Set, and Setting: The Basis for Controlled Intoxicant Use.* New Haven, Conn.: Yale University Press.

Alcohol and Drug Use and Self-Esteem: A Sociocultural Perspective

Harry H. L. Kitano

Introduction

There is a logical relationship between one's level of self-esteem and membership in groups, cultures, and families, but there is a paucity of empirical evidence linking the two. The problem of lack of evidence is exacerbated by how difficult it is to define the variable of self-esteem.

Despite the difficulty of formulating a precise definition, however, the basic concept appears to surface in a variety of ways. For example, Michael Banton, a recent visitor from England, indicated that in his estimation self-esteem is linked to morale and that army generals are, naturally, among the first to be concerned about how to raise morale. According to Banton, the shaping of morale takes place outside the individual—it is up to the commanding officer to devise programs to deal with the problem. Contests, group achievements, group citations, and the like may give troops a feeling of accomplishment, identity, and group pride. Morale as used in this example is closely linked with group esteem. Individual self-esteem, in this view, flows from identification with a group—the more successful the group, the higher the self-esteem of its members.

One's status as a member of a minority group can also be linked to deviant behavior and the reputation and image of that group. Snyder (1955) writes that it would be negligent to simply dismiss the minority

I would like to recognize the contributions of my research assistant, Colleen Turner; her ideas, research, and editing were extremely useful in the preparation of this chapter.

status of Jews as being unimportant in studying Jewish styles of alcohol consumption; similarly, the fear of looking foolish may be an important factor in controlling drunken behavior among Asians. A combination of anticipating retaliation from the dominant group and maintaining the self-respect and reputation of one's own group may play a significant role in controlling substance abuse in certain populations.

Vander Zanden makes an important point about the value of examining self-esteem from a social, as opposed to an individual, perspective:

> According to this social psychological tradition, individuals' self-appraisals tend to be "reflected appraisals." If children are accepted, approved, and respected for what they are, they will most likely acquire attitudes of self-esteem and self-acceptance. But if the significant people in their lives belittle, blame, and reject them, they are likely to evolve unfavorable self-attitudes. On the whole, social psychological research has supported the overall postulate that we hold the keys to one another's self-conceptions and identities. (1985, 329–330)

Alcoholics Anonymous (AA), the well-known group for the treatment of alcoholism, indirectly addresses the question of self-esteem in many ways, although other terms may be used to describe it. A major goal of treatment in AA is to help individuals evaluate themselves more realistically. Through this group process, many alcoholics find a middle path between grandiosity and self-effacement, both of which are believed to reinforce patterns of excessive drinking (Alcoholics Anonymous World Services 1953).

Research on alcohol and drug use, historically focused on the individual and on animal experimentation, has begun to recognize the broader relationships involving social groups, ethnicity, and society. For example, Straus (1982), in writing about changing perceptions of the use of alcohol, suggests the need for modifying social policy and social responses to recognize the importance of sociocultural norms and group pressures.

Nevertheless, most empirical research still focuses on individual psychological aspects of self-esteem and drug or alcohol use and tends to neglect sociocultural issues. The purpose of this chapter is to assess the role of self-esteem in drug and alcohol use, in relation to the sociocultural variables of family, ethnic groups, and culture. In the process, we will discuss a brief history of alcohol and drug use, and the costs to society; selected models and theories concerning alcohol and drug use by families, ethnic groups, and cultures; and studies focusing on self-esteem and drug or alcohol use by racial and ethnic groups.

In preparing our review, we conducted a computer library search (*Psychological Abstracts, Social Science Index*, Educational Resources Information Center, UC Melvyl Medline), which revealed more than sixty-five hundred studies using the specific term *self-esteem*. In addition, more than thirty thousand journal articles and dissertations used a variety of terms related to self-esteem, including *self-concept, self-evaluation, self-perception, self-respect, self-confidence, self-awareness, self-efficacy, self-image, self-congruence,* and *self-consciousness*. Other related terms were *ideal self* and *personal control*. Using a similar search method, we also discovered another twenty thousand articles that have been published in the area of drugs and alcohol.

When we cross-indexed the two groups, the search narrowed to approximately three hundred fifty studies. Of these, only about fifty even loosely related to a sociocultural perspective, and fewer than twenty were eventually judged to be relevant. To supplement this relative dearth of information, another search was conducted to find studies relating drug and alcohol use to various social and cultural groups.

For the purpose of this chapter, we have combined the discussion of drugs and alcohol, although society often distinguishes between the two. Alcohol can be considered a more socially acceptable form of a drug.

Background

Historically, the nature and level of alcohol use in the United States have varied considerably. Data from 1850 to 1976 indicate that alcohol consumption per capita increased just after the beginning of the twentieth century and remained at a fairly high level until Prohibition began in 1920. During the period between the repeal of Prohibition in 1933 and the beginning of World War II in 1941, per capita consumption returned to pre-1900 levels. From 1960 to 1971, there was a sharp 30 percent rise, and there has been very little change since that date. Before 1900, distilled spirits were the most popular form of drink, but after the turn of the century, beer accounted for about 50 percent of the alcohol consumed. (The shift to beer was attributed to the huge number of immigrants from traditionally beer-drinking countries [Cahalan 1982, 98].)

In 1984, the estimated per capita consumption of alcohol was 2.65 gallons, the lowest since 1977 and the third consecutive annual decrease. The period from 1981 to 1984 marked the first three-year decline. Surveys by Cahalan (1982) indicate that the American public currently holds somewhat ambivalent views of drinking: a vast majority would like to see tougher treatment of drunken drivers, but few would advocate measures to limit drinking through increasing taxes or closing bars earlier.

Cahalan (1970) also describes heavy drinkers as most likely to be approximately forty years old; to be of lower social status; to be of Irish, British, or Latino extraction; and to have lived in a large city. In this description, Jews and Episcopalians had the lowest percentage of abstainers, but they had lower percentages of heavy or problem drinkers than other groups did.

The use of drugs has also gone through a variety of historical changes, from legal prescription to demonization to the rise of narcotic addiction. Narcotics use was widespread in nineteenth-century America, where it was not illegal; but it had decreased considerably by the early 1900s. The types of drugs used and the affected population had shifted, too, with opium and morphine giving way to heroin, and drug use declining among the middle class while it increased among the lower classes. The Harrison Act of 1914 and the picture of the dangers of addiction that was effectively portrayed by the Federal Bureau of Narcotics led to the eventual elimination of legally prescribed heroin. There were an estimated hundred thousand heroin addicts at the time the Harrison Act was passed, but Americans were convinced that addicts numbered in the millions.

By the 1960s and 1970s, an estimated five hundred thousand heroin addicts maintained their habits illegally. Government-supported methadone maintenance programs developed, in which addicts were given substitute narcotics to treat their dependence on drugs. Concern about heroin peaked in this era, with the Nixon administration mounting an extensive campaign against heroin suppliers and heroin use. Epstein (1977) writes that this drive was motivated by political, rather than research or humanitarian, considerations; Nixon needed a compelling campaign issue. Throughout this period, heroin use and addiction increased dramatically, both in the United States and worldwide.

Cocaine replaced heroin as the primary target during the early 1980s. President Reagan announced his war on drugs in 1982, but by 1984 the supply of "coke" had expanded, prices had fallen, and the number of dealers and users had so increased that pronouncements about "losing the war" were commonplace.

Peele describes a pattern in our public policy toward drug use: alarm and rising concern; strict laws and increased police activity, visible raids and arrests; followed by drops in drug supplies; and then a reemergence of the problem, often at a greater intensity. "Apparently there is something inherently rewarding to politician and public alike about tough drug policies. Adherents of the get-tough approach are not challenged if abuse levels set new records. They instead point to these data as signalling how appropriate and necessary their efforts were in the first place" (1985, 137).

Peele argues that the basic error is focusing on supply, rather than on demand. He asks the interesting question, "What if somehow we could shut off the supply of drugs from the outside world?" He answers that committed drug users would simply switch to available alternatives such as barbiturates and other sedatives or alcohol and synthetic substitutes.

Certainly drug use is influenced by availability, but many people choose not to use drugs, in spite of accessibility. When people do not want to acquire a drug, efforts to control the supply become less significant. It is in terms of demand that self-esteem may be important. If, for instance, individuals with high self-esteem choose not to use drugs to deal with life's events and instead employ more successful and socially desirable coping mechanisms, there would be less need for a "war on drugs." The "war" could then focus on finding meaningful individual and cultural alternatives to abusing chemical substances.

Current Facts About Alcohol and Drug Abuse

A report to Congress by the Alcohol, Drug Abuse, and Mental Health Administration (ADAMHA) (1987) summarizes current findings on alcohol and drugs.

• An estimated 18 million adults aged eighteen and older experience problems as a result of alcohol use. Of these, 10.6 million suffer from alcoholism.

• In 1983, alcohol abuse and alcoholism cost the United States $116.8 billion. Costs resulting from premature deaths were $18 billion, reduced productivity cost $65.6 billion, and treatment cost $13.5 billion.

• Two-thirds of the adult population drink; but of that group, the 10 percent who drink most heavily drink half of the total amount of alcohol consumed.

• In 1985, nearly 5 percent of high school seniors drank every day, down from 7 percent in 1979.

• Women drink significantly less than men do.

• Rates of abstention among both male and female blacks and Hispanics are higher than abstention rates among whites.

• Alcohol is a factor in nearly half of all accidental deaths, suicides, and homicides and in 42 percent of all deaths from motor vehicle accidents.

• The twenty-six states that raised their minimum drinking age between 1975 and 1984 showed an average 13 percent reduction in nighttime fatal automobile crashes among eighteen- and nineteen-year-old drivers.

• Deaths from cirrhosis of the liver, most often related to alcohol abuse, are down, but cirrhosis continues to be the ninth leading cause of death. The death rates are highest among men and nonwhites.

• More than five hundred thousand Americans were reported to be under treatment for alcohol abuse and alcoholism in September 1984. Approximately two-thirds of the treated alcoholics were reported to be improved.

• Health care costs for accidents and illnesses related to alcohol abuse were estimated at $15 billion in 1983.

• Seventy million people, or 37 percent of the U.S. population aged twelve and above, have used marijuana, cocaine, or another illicit drug at some time in their lives. According to data gathered from the 1985 National Household Survey of Drug Abuse (cited in ADAMHA 1987), twenty-three million, or 12 percent of the population, were current users. The use of marijuana and other drugs had declined since a comparable survey in 1982, whereas cocaine use had increased.

• Data from a 1986 High School Senior Survey (cited in ADAMHA 1987) show a downward trend in drug use by seniors (61 percent in 1985, 58 percent in 1986). Cocaine use was an exception: the proportion of high school seniors who had tried cocaine remained at the 1985 level of 17 percent. The first survey data on the use of "crack" indicated that 4.1 percent had used this dangerous form of smokable cocaine.

• Drug use has become widespread in the workplace. The 1985 Household Survey shows that, of employed twenty-to-forty-year-olds, 29 percent had used illicit drugs in the past year, 19 percent in the past month. Sixteen percent reported marijuana use, and 5 percent reported using cocaine.

• Current users of cocaine increased from 4 million in 1982 to 5.8 million in 1985. Three hundred ninety thousand users were twelve to seventeen years old, 2.5 million were aged eighteen to twenty-five, and 2.9 million users were twenty-six years old or older.

• The dangers of cocaine have increased because of the purity of street cocaine and the potency of "crack." Between 1982 and 1986, the number of drug-related emergency-room incidents involving cocaine more than quadrupled, from 4,243 cases to 18,202 cases. Also during this period, medical examiner reports of cocaine-related deaths rose from 217 cases to 1,080 cases.

• From 1982 to 1985, the current use of marijuana decreased, from 11 percent of the population over twelve years of age reporting that they used marijuana, to 10 percent. There was a slight decline in the use of marijuana among those between the ages of twelve and seventeen.

• There has been a change in attitude toward the use of marijuana among high school seniors. Seventy-one percent of them believe that using marijuana involves great risk, more than double the number who responded in this fashion in 1978.

• Many current users of illicit drugs are polydrug users. For example, 27 percent of current marijuana users were also current cocaine users.

• Other findings showed that 1 percent of high school seniors reported using heroin, that current use of PCP among high school seniors decreased from 2 percent in 1985 to 1 percent in 1986, and that drug abuse involving nonmedical prescriptions was relatively rare among this group.

Social Costs

Estimates of the social costs of drug and alcohol use, expressed in dollar terms, run into the billions, as indicated above. But Straus, who focuses on the use of alcohol, argues that, aside from dollar costs, alcohol use leads to "the problems of infant and child care that occur when parents drink too much; marital problems; . . . violence against children, spouses, or others; and the emotional trauma of living with problem drinkers" (1982, 146). The use of alcohol is also implicated in the problem of underachievement, in a greater risk of accidents and injury, and in a disproportionate number of hospital stays. Straus concludes: "The costs of alcohol [and drugs] involve the family, business and industry, churches, health care, welfare, criminal justice, recreation, transportation, communication, government, and politics" (1982, 146).

Theoretical Perspectives

There are three major types of theories concerning alcohol and drug use. Biologically based theories point to the importance of the user as a biological organism. Psychologically based theories emphasize variables such as the individual's personality, motivation, and self-esteem. Sociocultural explanations focus on groups and the environment, including ethnic and minority status and group norms and values. These three major theoretical orientations, with their many variations, are important because they often determine the kinds of programs and policies that are established to deal with alcohol and drug issues.

Other chapters in this volume will focus on psychologically based theories, and the biological models do not appear to be directly relevant to the question of self-esteem. Nevertheless, a few words about the disease model of alcohol use and alcoholism are in order.

Current thinking in the United States, especially among those who specialize in the treatment of alcoholics, follows the disease model. The disease of alcoholism is viewed as a recognizable unitary syndrome with certain symptoms and a predictable progression. The primary symptom is the loss of control—the inability to stop drinking. Although the etiology of alcoholism is not completely known, it is assumed to have a physical cause, as well as to involve psychological and spiritual elements. Alcoholism is seen as irreversible. One can never completely recover from the disease: "once an alcoholic, always an alcoholic." The only hope for an alcoholic, then, is total and permanent abstinence (Miller 1986).

Based on this model, the best treatment is through the fellowship of other alcoholics, in programs such as Alcoholics Anonymous. The concept of self-esteem may be related to the AA idea of turning one's drinking problem over to a "Higher Power," in that the alcoholic views himself or herself as powerless to stop drinking. It is with utter humility, as opposed to cocky self-confidence, that the alcoholic asks for help to quit. True self-esteem thus comes through admitting one's vulnerabilities.

Miller is critical of the disease model, however: "This leaves 'nonalcoholics' with the illusion that they can drink with impunity, and focuses public policy on 'diagnosis' and 'treatment' of a unique disease rather than on controlling alcohol consumption. Less bridled by a unitary disease conception, many European nations employ social policy to control alcohol use and misuse within the population at large" (1986, 125).

Miller believes that the reasons behind the support of the disease concept are complex and are a combination of several elements. First, for many years the requirement of a single primary diagnosis in older versions of the *Diagnostic and Statistical Manual* of the American Psychiatric Association was very influential. Second, political expediency in seeking third-party reimbursement for treatment and funding for research may have played a role. Other, more general elements may also have been involved, such as an identification with the programs of AA, which exemplifies successful treatment based on the disease concept. Miller also suggests that a general Western tendency toward binary thinking (yes/no, either/or) has influenced this perspective (1986, 112). The disease model may also incorporate vestiges of attitudes toward drinking carried over from the Prohibition era.

A sociocultural perspective, in contrast, emphasizes the social context of drug and alcohol use, recognizing, for example, the numerous studies that report significant differences by ethnic group or by sex in alcohol consumption and drug use. From this perspective, self-esteem is related to the power and status of a group. Sociocultural research often draws from ethnographic studies and includes such variables as subcultural norms, values, expectations, male-female roles, and the role of the family, while not denying the importance of the physiological and psychological effects of drug-taking or alcoholic behavior.

A sociocultural view emphasizes the individual only in terms of specific cultural groups. As Heath indicates, culture refers to a system of patterns of beliefs and behavior that are familiar to and are to a significant degree shared by a given population. Therefore, the sociocultural model holds that

> attitudes, values, norms, and other beliefs about alcohol and its effects shape not only the ways people drink but also the ways in which they behave while drunk, the kinds of problems, if any, that they may have with drinking, and the rate at which such problems are likely to occur. Such a view of culture emphasizes the fact that various populations not only have different beverages but also attach different meanings to them, to various acts of drinking, to various potential drinking companions, and so forth, as well as attaching different values to various outcomes of drinking. (1986, 234)

White (1982) summarizes some of the major theories concerning alcoholism from a sociological perspective. As she indicates, these approaches are more interested in group and cultural differences than in individual differences. Her models include sociodemographic, sociocultural, socialization, and social deviance theories.

Sociodemographic Theories

Variables such as age, sex, religion, and ethnicity are known to be related to alcohol consumption. Other psychosocial variables related to alcohol problems include an environment that is supportive of heavy drinking, a tendency toward impulsivity, a sense of alienation and maladjustment, unfavorable expectations about one's future, an inability to achieve goals, and lack of membership in a family or primary group.

Cahalan (1970) indicates that sociodemographic variables are related to the quantity and frequency of drinking. Levels of alcohol consumption may be determined by childhood exposure to drinking behavior; the quantity considered safe and appropriate by one's family or peer group; the symbolic meaning of alcohol in a particular culture or subculture, and the customs surrounding its use; the activities associated with drinking; the amount of pressure encouraging or discouraging drinking; and the social rewards and punishments related to drinking.

From this perspective, the issue of self-esteem can be related only indirectly to alcohol or drug problems (for example, through the concepts of alienation, maladjustment, or inability to achieve goals). Cahalan, Cisin, and Crossley (1969), in their national survey, identify a group of drinkers they label as "heavy escape." The description of individuals in this category involves elements that are usually associated with a lack of self-esteem. Their social status and income were lower than those of other drinkers, and more of them were nonwhite. They tended to be less well integrated into social activities and were low in interpersonal participation. Somewhat more of them had parents or spouses who drank. They admitted to having more than their share of problems and reported that their childhoods had been unhappy. They expressed greater dissatisfaction about attaining their life goals, about their occupation, and about the state of their health. Most of the "heavy escape" drinkers also had high scores on the Neurotic Tendencies and Alienation scales. It was expected that individuals in this category would continue to increase their drinking and to be problem drinkers in the future.

Sociocultural Theories

Sociocultural models are related to cross-cultural differences in the rates of drinking and the problems that accompany alcohol consumption. Because cultural norms define alcoholism, alcoholism in one country may not constitute alcoholism in another. For example, Jellinek (1962) observes that periodic drunkenness at fiestas, lasting for several days, was considered normal behavior for Andean Indians, whereas similar behavior in the United States might have been labeled alcoholic. In France, a drinker can become an alcoholic without ever showing signs of intoxication, whereas in England, Scandinavia, and North

America, the terms *alcoholic* and *alcoholism* tend to be associated with steady, excessive drinking as a consequence of an underlying psychological problem. Irish drinking patterns have been attributed to bachelor lifestyles and the solidarity of male drinking groups, whereas the relative absence of drinking problems among Italians and Jews in America has been explained by their traditional use of wines, the integration of alcohol into family life, and the dietary function it serves.

The role of discrimination and alienation has been used to highlight the drinking problems of American Indians and blacks, although Hispanic drinking has more often been discussed in terms of male dominance (Babor and Mendelson 1986). From these perspectives, the role of self-esteem is probably most closely linked with such concepts as alienation, discrimination, and dominance.

Cultural factors affect how alcohol problems are defined, what criteria are used to diagnose alcoholism, and how persons with alcohol problems gain access to treatment. Culture may influence the etiology of different types of alcoholism, involving beverage preferences and dietary habits. Cultural identification may also influence a patient's response to treatment.

Horton (1943), in studying primitive societies, reports a relationship between the degree of anxiety in a culture and drinking. Anxiety was related to the level of subsistence provided by the economy, to the presence or absence of hazards to one's subsistence, and to an individual's degree of acculturation into the society. The function of alcohol was to relieve tension and anxiety.

Bales (1946) studied the interaction of three sets of variables that influence alcoholism. The first set involves the degree to which a culture creates inner tensions and problems of adjustment for its members. The second describes the normative orientation of the culture's members—what are their attitudes, norms, ideas, and sentiments concerning alcohol consumption? The third measures the degree to which the culture provides alternatives to cope with acute psychic distress.

Linsky, Straus, and Colby (1985) tested the relationship between heavy drinking and stress or tension levels within social structures. Their evidence is highly compatible with the hypothesis that drinking is used to relieve stress; they found that stress alone accounted for some of the variation, without reference to normative controls.

Segal (1986), in comparing the Soviet heavy-drinking culture with the American heavy-drinking subculture, found several common social and psychological causes of excessive drinking. In both cases, there had been a lessening of social control and patriarchal taboos and a weakening of the protective role of the family and small neighborhood. Individuals had learned to drink in a nonritualistic and utilitarian fashion. These drinkers often held expectations that were greater than the available opportunities, and they were often disillusioned with ideologies, old moral values, and bureaucracies. Alcohol abuse was also related to alienation, boredom, narcissism, and the loss of a sense of belonging.

In summary, sociocultural theories emphasize cultural attitudes, purposes, motivations, and norms affecting alcohol use and alcoholism. There is little direct linkage with self-esteem.

Socialization Theories

Socialization theories focus on the values, beliefs, perceptions, and norms concerning substance abuse that are passed on to members of society. The family assumes a critical role in this process. McCord and McCord (1960) identify a number of family characteristics related to alcoholism, including mothers who alternated between active affection and rejection of a child, parents who responded to a crisis with escapist behavior, overt parental rejection, lack of supervision of children, and parents who were often in conflict with each other.

Steinglass (1980) argues that because the family is a social system, alcoholism should be considered a total family problem, rather than an individual pathology. Members of the family adapt to the alcoholic; once the alcoholic is introduced into the system, family interactions attempt to accommodate this potentially disruptive member.

Woititz, who surveyed the literature of alcoholism and the family, argues that there is no such thing as the "alcoholic home environment," although certain characteristics are more commonly associated with alcoholic homes. These characteristics include excessive dependency, emotional immaturity, low tolerance for frustration, an inability to express emotions, low self-esteem, feelings of isolation, perfectionism, guilt, ambivalence toward authority, compulsiveness, grandiosity, and confusion about one's role (1978, 18).

An alcoholic home environment is destructive to a child's emotional well-being, and it does not consistently provide the conditions essential to the development of healthy self-esteem. Alcoholic families are more likely to create emotionally unstable children; their inconsistency can "affect the sense of security and the self-esteem" of the child (White 1982, 217).

Rees and Wilborn (1983) compared twenty-six inpatient adolescent drug abusers and their parents with twenty-six nonclinical controls and their parents. Drug-abusing adolescents indicated significantly more negative attitudes toward self in social, academic, family, and personal areas than did the controls. Self-esteem as a discriminator in drug abuse was influenced primarily by the lack of agreement between parent and child about what parental behavior should be. Parental attitudes related to confidence and responsibility in child-rearing differentiated the drug-abusing adolescents from the control adolescents.

Guglielmo, Polak, and Sullivan (1985) paint a picture of a child who presents a posture of doubt about his or her worth, who offers self as valueless and is received accordingly. The child's lesson has been learned in the laboratory of the family. The parent does not receive the child enthusiastically, instead preferring selfish desires to involvement with the child. The child's efforts to elicit a positive response from the parent are met with failure. The child extrapolates a lack of self-value from parental rejection and enters the social arena already labeled "unfit."

In contrast, Coopersmith provides a picture of families that develop high self-esteem in their children:

> The mothers of children with high self-esteem are more loving and have closer relationships with their children. . . . The child apparently perceives and appreciates the attention and approval expressed by his mother and tends to view her as favoring and supportive. He also appears to interpret her interest and concern as an indication of his significance; basking in these signs of his personal importance, he comes to regard himself favorably. This is success in its most personal expression—the concern, attention, and time of significant others. (1967, 178–179)

The inadequacies of parental models are reflected in their children. Baraga (1978) compared forty children of alcoholics, nine to twelve years old, to a matched control group, using the Piers-Harris Children's Self-Concept Scale. The children of alcoholic parents scored significantly lower on the self-concept scale than the control group did. Years of separation from the alcoholic parent had a favorable impact on self-concept scores.

O'Gorman (1976), using the same scale, compared twenty-nine adolescents with alcoholic parents and twenty-three from homes with recovering alcoholics to a control group of twenty-seven from non-alcoholic homes. The subjects whose parents had severe drinking problems scored significantly lower on measures of self-concept than the adolescents from nonalcoholic homes did. The former group also reported receiving less love and attention from their alcoholic fathers than did the children from more "normal" homes.

Woititz (1977) investigated the self-esteem of 150 children in grades six through twelve, using the Coopersmith Self-Esteem Inventory. One hundred were children of alcoholics. The self-esteem scores of these children were lower than those of the children of nonalcoholic parents. The author notes that there were significant differences on the "lie scale," however; when the scores were adjusted for the lie scale, the significant differences disappeared.

Davis (1983) compared adolescent children of alcoholics to a sample of adolescents from nonalcoholic homes. In his sample of 258 subjects, he found significant differences, using both the Rosenberg Self-Esteem Scale and the Coopersmith Self-Esteem Inventory. In both cases, the children from alcoholic families scored lower on level of self-esteem.

Social Deviance Theories

Social deviance theories emphasize the solidarity and cohesiveness of communities, the integration of drinking into the community as either normative or deviant, social control, knowledge of rules and roles, and the disjunction between societal goals and the institutional means of achieving these goals (Merton 1957). Alcoholics and drug addicts may be seen as "retreatists"; they cannot attain societal goals through either legitimate or illegitimate means. The term *anomie* suggests alienation— substance abusers retreat from society because they cannot succeed. The reasons why one person chooses drinking and another drugs as a means of retreat may depend on the individual's attitude toward alcohol or drugs and initial experiences with these substances.

Stephens describes the development of a "delinquent" subculture of heroin addiction, using terms such as *role, status, role identity, norms, values,* and *physical traits.* He argues that a subculture of street addicts exists and that within it a master, or central, role has been organized around the expected use of heroin. This role of street addict provides meaningful social and personal rewards to those who play it. There are also a number of secondary roles available in the subculture, such as dealer and tout, which are organized around the master role of the street addict. All of these roles function to maintain the subculture (1985, 436). In this model, self-esteem may be seen as operating in a fashion similar to its operation in "normal" society—that is, self-esteem is tied to appropriate role functioning, even though the particular roles are seen as deviant from the perspective of the dominant society.

Marlatt and Gordon (1980) view increased alcohol consumption as a response to negative emotional states, such as the loss of self-esteem. In their model, a high-risk situation is defined as any event that threatens a substance abuser's perception of personal control. If the individual is unable to successfully cope with the high-risk situation, he or she will attempt to gain personal control through the increased consumption of alcohol. Minority status itself may be related to high risk.

Bandura (1969, 1977) hypothesizes a model based on status, power, and level of competence. The possibility that those with high power and status can "pull" others toward drinking has not been lost on advertisers, who constantly show popular figures consuming their brands of alcohol. As Collins, Parks, and Marlatt (1985) indicate, the nature of social interaction and the status of the role model represent potent social influences on alcohol consumption.

Alcohol and Drug Use
Among Specific Groups

Ethnic Groups

The National Institute on Alcohol Abuse and Alcoholism's *Third Special Report to the U.S. Congress* (1979) contained a chapter entitled "Special Population Groups," which included material on the drinking problems of Native Americans, the Spanish-speaking population, and black Americans. As Gomberg (1982b) indicates, the addition of the "special populations" section represents real progress in recognizing the complexities of alcohol problems, for previous reports had focused only on the white male alcoholic.

Any overall statistic regarding alcohol and drug use in the United States masks the considerable variation that exists among ethnic groups. Blacks, Latinos, Asian Americans, and American Indians, or Native Americans, together constitute more than 20 percent of the population, and the use of alcohol and drugs is believed to be different for each group.

Self-esteem, based on ethnicity and identification, also varies by ethnic group. Various models of race relations, such as the internal colonial perspective (Blauner 1972) and the domination model (Kitano 1985), analyze the problems and adaptations of minority groups. Minority groups lack power, face restricted opportunities, and are victims of prejudice, discrimination, and segregation. A major problem is inequality—in education, in the economic sphere, in politics, and in the social and recreational arenas. Many have had to settle for less than equal positions and be content with second-class citizenship. There is little question that norms and practices of the dominant society have an effect on the self-esteem of ethnic minorities.

Albee uses the term *damage through exploitation* to assess the importance of minority-group status. Exploitation—be it sexual, economic, or through the media—has an effect on minority-group adaptation.

> The exploited groups are not responsive to exhortations or to other quick-fix solutions. Certain kinds of exploitation result in low self-esteem and become a kind of self-fulfilling prophecy. Members of ethnic minorities and women, who learn from earliest childhood that their race or sex is regarded as inferior by the white patriarchal culture, grow up with lower self-esteem that may be exceedingly difficult to change. Feelings of powerlessness are a major form of stress. (1984, xvii)

Damage to the self-esteem of members of minority groups can be limited by cohesive families and communities, the retention of cultural styles, the availability of alternative opportunity structures, and the ability to compete in the dominant community. Theoretically, high morale within an ethnic group and healthy self-esteem among its members are related, just as low group morale can be linked with disorganization, alienation, and low self-esteem. But there is a lack of empirical data to support this assumption. And the linkage of ethnic groups to levels of self-esteem and alcohol and drug use is even more difficult to validate through empirical findings.

Culture and Ethnicity

Cultural factors play a significant role in developing and maintaining alcohol and drug abuse. Hill, Steinhauer, and Zubin (1986) note that the development of alcoholism, unlike schizophrenia, requires an eliciting agent, which is exposure to an "outside substance" such as alcohol. Therefore, it is necessary to consider sociocultural conditions in addition to psychosocial vulnerability when studying alcoholism.

An early study by Child, Bacon, and Barry (1965) compares drinking practices in a number of preliterate societies. A factor analysis of the practices led to the identification of four "styles" of drinking: integrated drinking, which included drinking at ceremonies, rituals, and in other approved settings; inebriety, primarily weighted on quantity of drinking on a specific occasion, duration of the drinking episode, approval of drinking, and boisterousness; hostility, weighted in terms of the occurrence of hostile behavior; and quantity, including general consumption of alcohol and extent of drinking.

Bacon, Barry, and Child (1965), in analyzing the four styles or factors, indicate that those societies rated high on inebriety tend to pressure their members toward achievement and to show little indulgence or dependence in infancy and adulthood. Societies rated high on quantity also tend to show little indulgence or dependence, but show strong pressures toward training children to accept responsibility. Thus, both frequent drunkenness and high consumption occur in cultures where dependency is disapproved or punished, both in childhood and adult life, and where a high degree of responsible, independent, and achieving behavior is required. Although no specific mention was made of self-esteem, the descriptions of these cultures contain elements that can be linked with the concept.

Blacks

Black Americans are the largest minority group in the United States, constituting approximately 12 percent of the population. The first empirical study concerning alcohol consumption among blacks was the 1960s drinking survey by Cahalan, Cisin, and Crossley (1969). Drinking patterns among blacks were not significantly different from those among whites, except that almost three times as many black women (11 percent) as white women (4 percent) were categorized as heavy drinkers. Comparable findings were reported in a 1979 household survey (Clark and Midanik 1982).

Harper (1976), in summarizing characteristics of drinking patterns among blacks, suggests that blacks tend to be group, rather than solitary, drinkers and that many blacks tend to drink in public or outdoor places. Problem drinking among blacks is strongly associated with health and social problems, particularly in crowded black ghettos. There was no mention of the relationship between alcohol consumption by blacks and level of self-esteem.

Lex (1987) reviewed studies on alcohol use by blacks and reports that black alcoholics were found in every class level. Drinking problems were highly associated with health and social problems in low-income areas. In these studies, blacks were reportedly more likely than whites to either abstain or drink heavily, rather than drinking in moderation; to begin drinking and become alcoholic at earlier ages; to purchase larger containers of expensive beverages; to drink on weekends; or, if manual laborers, to drink on the job. Again, the issue of self-esteem was not mentioned.

A doctoral study by Martin (1984) explores the relationship between self-concept and the drinking patterns of black youths. Seventy-three males and forty-eight females were tested, using a purposive sampling technique. The findings indicate no significant relationship between self-concept and patterns of drinking. Age, sex, and socioeconomic status were also nonsignificant.

In a doctoral dissertation, Lewis (1985) analyzes the self-concept scores of low-income black alcoholics in a variety of treatment settings. The sample was made up of thirty-five black subjects enrolled in one of two New York day programs for alcoholism rehabilitation. The Tennessee Self-Concept Scale was used, along with the Michigan Alcoholism Screening Test and the Definitions of Alcohol Scale. A bivariate analysis revealed no significant differences between the experimental and comparison groups concerning self-concept in consonant versus dissonant environments.

There is a serious lack of empirical studies concerning drug use among the various portions of the black population. In a critical summary of studies of drug use among various minorities, Trimble, Padilla, and Bell (1987) point to some of the limitations of past research, which most often compares samples of blacks and whites rather than concentrating on black subgroups. We also lack information on noninstitutionalized groups and analysis of broader variables, as well as data concerning black females and drug use. Discussion of self-esteem is rarely included in the existing research.

Rosenberg (1985) reports that the data on the noxious effects of racism on the self-concept of blacks are contradictory. On the one hand, studies show that black children who are asked to choose between black and white dolls show strong preferences for the white dolls, indicating a possible negative self-image. On the other hand, survey research data show that self-esteem among blacks is at least as healthy as that among whites.

Latinos

Individuals of Spanish ancestry make up the second largest minority in the United States. Approximately 60 percent are of Mexican origin, 15 percent are Puerto Rican, and 6 percent are Cuban. Most of the rest are from Central or South America (Lex 1987).

The national survey on drinking practices by Cahalan, Cisin, and Crossley (1969) indicated that 30 percent of all Latinos drank heavily, compared to 17 percent of whites. Problems associated with heavy drinking were reported by 43 percent of Hispanics and 11 percent of whites (Cahalan and Room 1974).

The drinking styles, values, and behavior of Latinos in one area of the country cannot be compared to those of Latinos in other geographic areas. For example, in Texas, beliefs, values, and norms indicated a greater toleration for intoxication and drinking behavior than was found among a California sample (Cahalan 1970). Drinking styles vary not only by region, but also by sex, age, marital status, occupation, and the recency of migration to the United States.

Trimble, Padilla, and Bell (1987) look at drug abuse among three groups of Hispanics: Mexican Americans, Puerto Ricans, and Cuban Americans. Existing information on the use of drugs by each of these groups is spotty. Knowledge is generally limited to epidemiologic studies among adolescents, and there is little or no information on the drug use and abuse patterns of adults, the elderly, refugees, the homeless, women, or families as a unit. What little data we have indicate that alcohol is a more widespread problem than drugs among Hispanics.

Perez et al. (1980) studied the extent of the use of alcohol, marijuana, inhalants, and PCP in a group of 339 Mexican American youths from East Los Angeles housing projects. (A stratified random sample of four hundred respondents was initially selected, but events external to the study [e.g., local raids by immigration authorities, increased police patrols] caused parents to become suspicious and to deny permission for interviews. Generalizations based on these data should therefore take into account the lack of randomness.) The use of marijuana, PCP, and inhalants was "clearly shown to be affected not only by sociodemographic and cultural variables but also by self-concept factors" (1980, 633). Self-concept variables played an important role in defining the populations of users and nonusers, as well as in differentiating the high, moderate, and low users. One particular measure of self-concept ("I have as many friends as most people; I can be trusted as much as anyone; I often let other people have their way; I am not doing as well in school as I would like to") seemed to be especially important. Individuals who were using marijuana, PCP, and inhalants tended to evaluate themselves negatively in relation to their peers. "These findings would suggest that, at least with respect to marijuana, inhalants, and PCP, the extent to which the person positively evaluated him- or herself with respect to peers is significantly related to drug use" (Perez et al. 1980, 634).

Interestingly, a relationship of self-concept and drug use did not predict alcohol use. Age, sex, and the number of peers using alcohol were more predictive than self-concept was. The researchers draw on de Rios and Feldman (1977), who indicate that alcohol is generally well accepted within Hispanic culture. There are many occasions where the consumption of alcohol is expected and normative; the culture provides guidelines for the time, place, and amount of use.

A doctoral dissertation by Alterman (1985) compared measures of self-concept and locus of control (whether one responds more to internal or to external cues for behavior) of 148 Hispanic and Anglo children in the third and fourth grades. The effects of a substance abuse prevention program were evaluated, using the Coopersmith Self-Esteem Inventory and the Nowicki-Strickland Locus of Control Scale. Mean scores increased for all children, and there was a move toward more emphasis on internal control. Members of the experimental group (who used the prevention curriculum) improved their perceptions of how well they were liked by their classmates.

Native Americans

There are about 1.5 million persons of American Indian ancestry in the United States. They belong to hundreds of tribes representing distinct histories and cultural traditions that date back long before the European invasion of the continent. Roughly half of this group remain on reservations, located primarily in rural areas; the other half live in cities, primarily in the West and Midwest (Trimble, Padilla, and Bell 1987). The most extensive study of substance abuse among Native Americans was conducted by Oetting and Beauvais (1983) between 1975 and 1981. In their survey of Indian youth, they found that alcohol was the most popular drug, followed by marijuana, cigarettes, inhalants, stimulants, and cocaine. There were no significant findings concerning self-esteem in this research.

Mohatt (1972) provides a perspective on the use of alcohol in Native

American communities. In earlier days, an Indian warrior gained self-respect and an identity through accomplishments for the tribe. Brave deeds, hunting, and fighting were more than personal accomplishments; they contributed to the life and vitality of the Indian nation. But as the white culture moved in, a process of deculturation prevented the young warrior from acting in a way that gave him a sense of being effective for his community. Alcohol, introduced by whites, became a quasi-solution.

> He could drink until he was able to act in ways that proved to him and to others that he was indeed brave and to be respected; he could again feel the flow of strength in his veins. In this way tribal concerns were gradually overshadowed by the individual's desire for prestige and power. Such power was often not achieved by tribal mores and action, but through drinking large amounts of liquor. (1972, 271)

But the feelings of euphoria were only temporary. Although liquor may have induced feelings of power reminiscent of the successful hunt or battle, in the long run it has led to the disintegration of social controls and the demoralization of communities where heavy drinking is widespread.

A doctoral dissertation by Williams (1976) compares the self-concepts of alcoholic and nonalcoholic males of Indian and non-Indian ancestry, using scores on the Tennessee Self-Concept Scale. The subjects were divided into four groups of twenty-five persons each. There were two groups of alcoholic subjects, one Indian and one non-Indian; two groups of nonalcoholics were also differentiated by ancestry. The general finding was that the self-concept of alcoholics differed significantly from that of nonalcoholics. The factor of ancestry contributed far less to measured differences than the factor of alcoholism did. The self-concepts of the alcoholics emphasized negative attributes that led to a lack of self-acceptance, inadequate decision-making ability, and a weak sense of personal and family worth. Alcoholics also had psychologically deviant tendencies.

Graves (1973) studied the relationships between psychosocial variables, the rate of return to reservations, and drinking behavior among Navajo migrants to Denver. The study consistently found that when migrants were doing fairly well in Denver, earning wages above the group average, psychological variables were relatively unimportant in drinking behavior, and arrest rates were moderately low. But when migrants were doing poorly in terms of employment, the psychological variables became crucial. If they perceived the future as hopeless and felt powerless to bring about change, then they were likely to drink heavily and be picked up by the police. The description seems relevant to the concept of low and high self-esteem.

Several other studies have looked further at the relationship between economic strains and the coping functions of alcohol or drugs, although these studies do not focus specifically on Native Americans. Pearlin and Radabaugh (1976), for example, interviewed 2,300 people, a representative sample of the census area of Chicago. Level of self-esteem had a close relationship to level of income. Level of self-esteem was also closely related to educational attainment and to a sense of mastery. The group most lacking in economic resources and the opportunities for achievement associated with such resources also lacked the personal characteristics that are important in providing coping options. "The very people most entrapped by the process leading to the use of alcohol to control distress are also least in possession of a personality attribute that could aid their discovery of alternative ways of dealing with distress" (1976, 661). The authors conclude that an interlocking set of economic, social, and psychological conditions contributes to arousing anxiety and channeling behavior toward drinking as a means of coping.

Asian Pacific Americans

Asian Pacific Americans represent a wide number of different groups with different experiences, histories, and cultures. In fact, the differences among the thirty-two or more Asian Pacific groups are so complex that generalizations are usually oversimplifications. The current term *model minority* masks myriad problems, ranging from heavy drinking by certain groups, especially Japanese, Filipino, and Korean American males (Kitano et al. 1988) to the serious problems of drug abuse that have been described among youthful Asian Americans in Seattle–King County. Trimble, Padilla, and Bell (1987) quote from a report prepared by the Washington State Commission on Asian American Affairs:

> As the economy worsens and more Asians become unemployed, stresses mount which create emotional, familial, and social problems in our community. These problems have manifested themselves in a number of ways, ranging from an increase in family conflicts, child abuse, and alcoholism to more serious areas of emotional dysfunction such as suicide, depression, and psy-

chosis. . . . One of the most seriously affected populations is the Indochinese refugees. . . . The stress placed on this group is enormous. Faced with cutbacks . . . many of these refugees see no hope for the future. . . . Other Asian Pacific groups are facing similar difficulties. (Washington State Commission on Asian American Affairs, 1983, 115)

In traditional Asian cultures, individual efforts are submerged in group and family concerns, making the problem of assessing self-esteem among individuals very difficult. The concept of self-esteem might have a different meaning for those who identify with Asian cultures in which family and group esteem are more important than individual self-esteem. An old Japanese saying claims that "the nail that sticks out is the one most likely to be hammered" (a very loose translation). The individual with high self-confidence who speaks out and stands out risks incurring negative comments from the community ("Who does he think he is, a haole [white]?").

We could find no studies focusing specifically on Asian Americans, self-esteem, and the use of alcohol and drugs. An interview with a Japanese American ex-alcoholic may provide some insight into the relationship between alcohol and self-esteem, however. John, a nisei (second generation) and a member of Alcoholics Anonymous, felt that his past drinking had been related to peer group acceptance. He had found it difficult to be with other nisei; they were too "uptight" and would not loosen up. Instead, his favorite style was to go to a big-name Hollywood bar and order drinks for everybody. He got to know the waitresses and became a regular. Once he got the drinks down, he was able to talk to people and be friendly. This situation was especially gratifying to his feeling of confidence, to his sense of being an equal, and to his self-esteem (Kitano et al. 1985).

Differences Between the Sexes

Although this section has focused on studies of substance abuse among ethnic minorities, it is useful to briefly examine some research that deals with gender-based differences in patterns of drug and alcohol use.

Wilsnack and Beckman (1984), in discussing the use of alcohol and drugs among women who had been victims of sexual abuse, indicate that drugs may be used in an attempt to reduce feelings of guilt, shame, anger, and loss of self-esteem. Younger victims may express their inner turmoil through antisocial behavior, including both alcohol and drug use and indiscriminate sexual behavior. The pain and low self-esteem resulting from sexual abuse may drive some women into overtly self-destructive use of alcohol or drugs.

Gustafson (1988) analyzed thirty male-female couples, focusing on the relationship of alcohol consumption and power. Following the McClelland et al. (1972) model of power, this study hypothesized that persons characterized by high power needs and low activity inhibition would drink more heavily to achieve the expected increases in power. Results indicated that the subjects drank not to attain power, however, but because of strong dependency needs. By drinking excessively, a person can gratify dependency cravings without taking responsibility. In situations where the male lost some of his abilities because of intoxication, there was an expected change of dominance from the male to the female. There were no shifts in power when sober men interacted with intoxicated women.

Konovsky and Wilsnack (1982) studied the relationship between self-esteem and alcohol consumption among ninety-two married men and women between the ages of nineteen and fifty-two. Couples attended "wet" parties, where alcoholic beverages were served, and "dry" parties, where only soft drinks were available. The Tennessee Self-Concept Scale was used to measure self-esteem. The most striking finding was the different effects that drinking had on the self-esteem scores of women and men drinkers. Drinking did not have a clear-cut effect on men's self-esteem scores, but it significantly reduced feelings of self-esteem and self-satisfaction among women drinkers.

Several explanations were offered. One interpretation argued that because women reach higher blood alcohol levels than men do when drinking comparable amounts of alcohol, the women in the study may have experienced a greater physiological depressant effect from alcohol. A correlational analysis did not support this conclusion, however.

Another explanation was that drinking is more consistent with male roles, whereas it is viewed as deviant for females. Therefore, men at the party were behaving in ways congruent with masculine roles, whereas women perceived drinking as incongruent with their expected female roles. As a consequence, they may have experienced feelings of ambivalence and discomfort, which in turn were reflected in feelings of decreased self-esteem.

A final explanation, not necessarily in contradiction with the others, was that certain cocktail party behaviors, such as unwelcome or overly aggressive sexual advances by male drinking companions, may have increased feelings of tension and discomfort among the women drinkers.

Unwelcome sexual advances and increased male dominance may have reinforced women's sense of a lower status (lack of power), creating feelings of discomfort, distress, and lower self-esteem.

Self-Esteem

From our review, it is apparent that self-esteem is viewed in a number of different ways. From a sociocultural perspective, it is a dependent variable, that is, self-esteem is the result of a person's ethnic, social class, or gender group. Presumably, the reputation and status of one's primary reference group—be it an ethnic minority, a social class, a family, or even an athletic team—will result in high or low levels of self-esteem. Identifying with a baseball team that has just won a World Series makes us feel good, even if only temporarily.

We would label this feeling *general self-esteem*, which is the result of the past experiences and history of the individual, including attributes such as race and sex. Hoelter (1983) reports that in one comparison males scored higher on measures of self-esteem than females did, but that blacks scored higher than whites. It may be that a change in overall perception, such as moving from the devaluing experience of racism to the view that "black is beautiful," can affect one's level of general self-esteem. Brockner (1988) writes that the performance of individuals with low levels of general self-esteem is more easily influenced by external forces—that is, the locus of control is from the outside. Such people often lack self-confidence and have a high need for approval. Not liking themselves, they are especially dependent on the positive evaluation of others.

Another aspect of self-esteem is self-esteem that is in progress or in process. Individuals are perceived and judge themselves in relation to yet-to-be-fulfilled goals and activities, for example, going to college or working on an election. An actor's self-esteem may be "on hold" until the critical reviews are in. Negative reviews may not have much effect on an actor with a high level of general self-esteem, but they may be devastating to someone whose general self-esteem was already low.

Self-esteem is also used as an independent variable—that is, as the "cause" of behavior. An individual is said to behave in a particular manner because of a high or low level of self-esteem. Through knowledge of the variable, then, we can try to predict and understand behavior.

Some argue that the maintenance of one's self-esteem is a basic need, neither an independent nor a dependent variable. The need to "look good," both privately and publicly, is so pervasive that individuals will behave in a manner that maintains their self-esteem (Brockner 1988).

In our view, all these aspects of self-esteem are interrelated. General self-esteem affects goals and activities that are in process, and it also helps to determine everyday behavior. But there is no simple, linear relationship between the variables; being a member of a disadvantaged minority does not automatically lead to low self-esteem, nor is low self-esteem readily related to drug and alcohol use. Linear models interpreted in a mechanistic fashion tend to oversimplify the complexity of the problem.

In addition, the study of self-esteem in the current literature is plagued with serious problems. The concept of self-esteem is identified and defined in numerous ways. Techniques of measurement are far from standardized, and their level of comparability is uncertain. Problems of methodology and sampling undercut the usefulness of many studies. And a lack of conceptual and theoretical clarity is another obstacle yet to be overcome.

Self-Esteem, Drugs, and Alcohol

The most comprehensive view concerning the relationship between self-esteem and drug and alcohol use is put forward by Steffenhagen and Burns (1987), who contend that low levels of self-esteem are the cause, not the result, of deviant behavior. In other words, alcoholics or drug addicts behave as they do because of low self-esteem, rather than developing low self-esteem as the result of deviant behavior. This theory synthesizes and extends psychological and sociological perspectives into a single underlying factor, self-esteem, to explain drug and alcohol use. It postulates that an individual's reactions to his or her social environment are mediated by a sense of self-esteem.

> This theory, developed within a framework provided by Alfred Adler's individual psychology, places self-esteem at the apex of personality and assumes that individuals of any personality type may vary in self-esteem and that self-esteem itself, as well as distinctive styles of coping with the need for or lack of it, develops out of the social context in which given individuals are embedded. A lack of self-esteem is, thus, seen as the most important psychological variable in the etiology of deviance and/or personality maladjustment; the nurturance and development of an individual's self-esteem are the key factors in the rehabilitative process. (Steffenhagen and Burns 1987, 56)

Low levels of self-esteem are developed during socialization, through overpampering or its opposite, neglect. Self-esteem is viewed as sociodynamic: psychological correlates include high or low levels of self-esteem, goal orientation (socially useful or useless), and personality traits (normal or neurotic); sociological correlates include lifestyle (self-centered or contributive), peer group (supportive or nonsupportive), and social milieu (friendly or hostile).

Steffenhagen and Burns present a case to illustrate the theory. A young male drug abuser had come from a middle-class family, with a neurotic mother who overpampered him as a child. Although he always had a major difficulty with setting unrealistic goals, he excelled in school and was accepted by several graduate schools of dentistry. He dropped out of dentistry but did receive a master's degree in education. He was frustrated in many ways; his personality profile indicated a mildly neurotic individual. His major support system was his neurotic mother. He had already been exposed to drugs, because his father used medically prescribed drugs. Eventually, the young man's drug habit became so severe that he was beginning to lose friends. With a pampered lifestyle and goal aspirations that were unachievable, this individual had been placed in a position where his self-esteem had never developed adequately. A low level of self-esteem led to drug use (1987, 65).

Summary

There is little question that problems associated with drug and alcohol use have almost reached a "crisis stage" in the United States. The economic and social costs are enormous and affect every segment of society. Yet there is a paucity of good research, especially studies that could link the abuse of alcohol and drugs with self-esteem. What evidence there is remains inconsistent, and the following summary generalizations should be interpreted with caution.

• Empirical studies concerning the relationship between alcohol and drug abuse and self-esteem show mixed results. The tie appears stronger in some studies and in some theoretical models than in others. For example, Steffenhagen and Burns (1987) see low self-esteem as the single common denominator in the use of alcohol and drugs.

• Sociocultural models involve such variables as group reputation, identity, cohesion, power, dominated status, and morale. Models linking ethnic group, culture, and both group and individual self-esteem to the use of drugs and alcohol have yet to be systematically developed, and there is a consequent lack of empirical research.

The relationship between group reputation and individual self-esteem is difficult to trace; as Covington indicates, it is difficult to know whether group differences in self-esteem are a result of "intergroup differences in social or subcultural integration characteristics or whether variations stem from differences in the rates at which specific groups are able to translate these characteristics into heightened self-esteem" (1986, 123).

Most cross-cultural studies make little or no mention of self-esteem.

• There is a tie between the family and level of self-esteem. Descriptions of families that foster low self-esteem show that, on the one hand, children are ignored, unloved, and denigrated; on the other, they are indulged and overprotected so that their self-worth and self-esteem are affected. Studies of the children of alcoholics demonstrate the negative effects of inconsistent parenting on self-esteem.

• Individuals with low levels of self-esteem may be more prone to external influences, that is, to have an external locus of control. Brockner (1988) mentions plasticity and dependence on others for cues to behavior. Positive role models may be influential in shaping more desirable behaviors.

In general, we must conclude that alcohol and drug abuse stems from multiple sources and that there is no single "cause" of substance abuse. But self-esteem, although not directly linked to substance abuse in most research to date, may come close to providing a critical variable for further research, programs, policy, and treatment.

Bibliography

Albee, G. W. 1984. "Prologue: A Model for Classifying Prevention Programs." In *Readings in Primary Prevention of Psychopathology*, edited by J. M. Joffe, G. W. Albee, and L. D. Kelly, ix–xvii. Hanover, N.H.: University Press of New England.

Alcohol, Drug Abuse, and Mental Health Administration (ADAMHA). 1987. "ADAMHA Update." Fall. Washington, D.C.: ADAMHA.

Alcoholics Anonymous World Services. 1953. *Twelve Steps and Twelve Traditions.* New York: Alcoholics Anonymous World Services.

Alterman, T. 1985. "Self-Concept and Locus of Control in Hispanic and Anglo Third and Fourth Graders." *Dissertation Abstracts International* 46–B(4): 1353.

Babor, T. F., and J. H. Mendelson. 1986. "Ethnic/Religious Differences in the Manifestation and Treatment of Alcoholism." In *Alcohol and Culture: Comparative Perspectives from Europe and America*, edited by T. F. Babor, 46–59. New York: New York Academy of Sciences.

Bacon, M. K., H. Barry, and I. L. Child. 1965. "A Cross-Cultural Study of Drinking: II. Relation to Other Features of Culture." *Quarterly Journal of Studies on Alcohol*, Supplement no. 3 : 29–48.

Bales, R. F. 1946. "Cultural Differences in Rates of Alcoholism." *Quarterly Journal of Studies on Alcohol* 6 : 480–499.

Bandura, A. 1969. *Principles of Behavior Modification.* New York: Holt, Rinehart & Winston.

———. 1977. *Social Learning Theory.* Englewood Cliffs, N.J.: Prentice-Hall.

Baraga, D. 1978. "Self-Concept in Children of Alcoholics." *Dissertation Abstracts International* 39–B(1): 368.

Blauner, R. 1972. *Racial Oppression in America.* New York: Harper & Row.

Brockner, J. 1988. *Self-Esteem at Work.* Lexington, Mass.: D. C. Heath.

Cahalan, D. 1970. *Problem Drinkers: A National Survey.* San Francisco: Jossey-Bass.

———. 1982. "Epidemiology: Alcohol Use in American Society." In *Alcohol, Science, and Society Revisited*, edited by E. L. Gomberg, H. R. White, and J. A. Carpenter, 96–118. Ann Arbor: University of Michigan Press.

Cahalan, D., I. H. Cisin, and H. M. Crossley. 1969. *American Drinking Practices.* New Brunswick, N.J.: Rutgers Center of Alcohol Studies.

Cahalan, D., and R. Room. 1974. *Problem Drinking Among American Men.* Monograph no. 7. New Brunswick, N.J.: Rutgers Center of Alcohol Studies.

Child, I. L., M. K. Bacon, and H. Barry. 1965. "A Cross-Cultural Study of Drinking: I. Descriptive Measurements of Drinking Customs." *Quarterly Journal of Studies on Alcohol*, Supplement no. 3 : 1–28.

Clark, W., and L. Midanik. 1982. "Alcohol Use and Alcohol Problems Among U.S. Adults: Results of the 1979 National Survey." In *Alcohol Consumption and Related Problems*, 3–52. Alcohol and Health Monograph no. 1. DHHS Publication no. ADM 82–1190. Washington, D.C.: Government Printing Office.

Cohen, S. 1983. *The Alcoholism Problem: Selected Issues.* New York: Haworth Press.

Collins, L., G. A. Parks, and G. A. Marlatt. 1985. "Social Determinants of Alcohol Consumption: The Effects of Social Interaction and Model Status on the Self-Administration of Alcohol." *Journal of Consulting and Clinical Psychology* 53(2): 189–200.

Coopersmith, S. 1967. *The Antecedents of Self-Esteem.* San Francisco: Freeman.

Covington, J. 1986. "Self-Esteem and Deviance: The Effects of Race and Gender." *Criminology* 24(1): 105–138.

Davis, R. B. 1983. "Adolescents from Alcoholic Families: An Investigation in Self-Esteem, Locus of Control, and Knowledge and Attitudes Toward Alcohol." *Dissertation Abstracts International* 43–B(10): 3346.

de Rios, M. D., and D. F. Feldman. 1977. "Southern California Mexican American Drinking Patterns: Some Preliminary Observations." *Journal of Psychedelic Drugs* 9 : 151–158.

Epstein, E. J. 1977. *Agency of Fear: Opiates and Political Power in America.* New York: Putnam.

Gomberg, E. L. 1982a. "Alcoholism: Psychological and Psychosocial Aspects." In *Alcohol, Science, and Society Revisited,* edited by E. L. Gomberg, H. R. White, and J. A. Carpenter. Ann Arbor: University of Michigan Press.

———. 1982b. "Special Populations." In *Alcohol, Science, and Society Revisited,* edited by E. L. Gomberg, H. R. White, and J. A. Carpenter. Ann Arbor: University of Michigan Press.

Graves, T. D. 1973. "The Navajo Urban Migrant and His Psychological Situation." *Ethos* 1(3): 321–342.

Guglielmo, R., R. Polak, and A. P. Sullivan. 1985. "Development of Self-Esteem as a Function of Familial Reception." *Journal of Drug Education* 15(3): 277–283.

Gustafson, R. 1988. "Effects of Alcohol on Power in Social Interaction Between Man and Woman." *Journal of Studies on Alcohol* 49(1): 78–84.

Harper, F. 1976. *Alcohol Abuse and Black America.* Alexandria, Va.: Douglas.

Heath, D. B. 1982. "In Other Cultures, They Also Drink." In *Alcohol, Science, and Society Revisited,* edited by E. L. Gomberg, H. R. White, and J. A. Carpenter, 63–79. Ann Arbor: University of Michigan Press.

———. 1986. "Concluding Remarks." In *Alcohol and Culture: Comparative Perspectives from Europe and America,* edited by T. F. Babor, 234–238. New York: New York Academy of Sciences.

Hill, S. Y., S. R. Steinhauer, and J. Zubin. 1986. "Biological Markers for Alcoholism: A Vulnerability Model Conceptualization." In *Nebraska Symposium on Motivation: Alcohol and Addictive Behavior,* edited by P. C. Rivers. Lincoln: University of Nebraska Press.

Hoelter, J. W. 1983. "Factorial Invariance and Self-Esteem: Reassessing Race and Sex Differences." *Social Forces* 61(3): 834–846.

Horton, D. 1943. "The Functions of Alcohol in Primitive Societies: A Cross-Cultural Study." *Quarterly Journal of Studies on Alcohol* 4 : 199–220.

Jellinek, E. M. 1962. "Cultural Differences in the Meaning of Alcoholism." In *Society, Culture, and Drinking Patterns,* edited by D. J. Pittman and C. R. Snyder, 382–394. Carbondale: Southern Illinois University Press.

Kitano, H. 1985. *Race Relations.* Englewood Cliffs, N.J.: Prentice-Hall.

Kitano, H., I. Chi, C. K. Law, J. Lubben, and S. Rhee. 1988. "Alcohol Consumption by Japanese in Japan, Hawaii, and California." In *Cultural Influences and Drinking Patterns: A Focus on Hispanic and Japanese Populations,* edited by L. Towle and T. Harford, 99–133. Research Monograph no. 19. Rockville, Md.: U.S. Department of Health and Human Services.

Kitano, H., H. Hatanaka, W. Yeung, and S. Sue. 1985. "Japanese-American Drinking Patterns." In *The American Experience with Alcohol,* edited by L. A. Bennett and G. M. Ames, 335–357. New York: Plenum.

Konovsky, M., and S. C. Wilsnack. 1982. "Social Drinking and Self-Esteem in Married Couples." *Journal of Studies on Alcohol* 43(3): 319–333.

Lewis, M. W. 1985. "An Analysis of the Self-Concept Scores of Low-Income Black Alcoholics in Dissonant and Consonant Treatment Settings." *Dissertation Abstracts International* 46–B(4): 1324.

Lex, B. W. 1987. "Review of Alcohol Problems in Ethnic Minority Groups." *Journal of Consulting and Clinical Psychology* 55(3): 293–300.

Linsky, A. S., M. A. Straus, and J. P. Colby, Jr. 1985. "Stressful Events, Stressful Conditions, and Alcohol Problems in the United States: A Partial Test of Bales' Theory." *Journal of Studies on Alcohol* 46(1): 72–80.

McClelland, D. C., W. N. Davis, R. Kalin, and E. Wanner, eds. 1972. *The Drinking Man.* New York: Free Press.

McCord, W., and J. McCord. 1960. *Origins of Alcoholism.* Stanford, Calif.: Stanford University Press.

Marlatt, G. A., and J. R. Gordon. 1980. "Determinants of Relapse: Implications for the Maintenance of Behavior Change." In *Behavioral Medicine: Changing Health Lifestyles,* edited by P. O. Davidson and S. M. Davidson, 410–452. New York: Brunner/Mazel.

Martin, C. H. 1984. "The Relationship Between Level of Self-Concept and Drinking Patterns of Black Youths." *Dissertation Abstracts International* 46–A(2): 521.

Merton, R. K. 1957. *Social Theory and Social Structure.* New York: Free Press.

Miller, W. R. 1986. "Haunted by the *Zeitgeist:* Reflections on Contrasting Treatment Goals and Concepts of Alcoholism in Europe and the United States." In *Alcohol and Culture: Comparative Perspectives from Europe and America,* edited by T. F. Babor, 110–129. New York: New York Academy of Sciences.

Mohatt, G. 1972. "The Sacred Water: The Quest for Personal Power Through Drinking Among the Teton Sioux." In *The Drinking Man,* edited by D. C. McClelland, W. N. Davis, R. Kalin, and E. Wanner, 261–275. New York: Free Press.

National Institute on Alcohol Abuse and Alcoholism. 1979. *Alcohol and Health: Third Special Report to the U.S. Congress from the Secretary of Health, Education, and Welfare, June 1978.* Edited by E. P. Noble. DHEW Publication no. ADM 79–832. Washington, D.C.: Government Printing Office.

Oetting, E. R., and F. Beauvais. 1983. "Drug Use Among Native American Youth: A Summary of Findings (1975–1981)." Western Behavioral Studies, Colorado State University, Fort Collins.

O'Gorman, P. 1976. "Self-Concept, Locus of Control, and Perception of Father in Adolescent Homes With and Without Severe Drinking Problems." *Dissertation Abstracts International* 36–A(8): 5156.

Pearlin, L. J., and C. W. Radabaugh. 1976. "Economic Strains and the Coping Functions of Alcohol." *American Journal of Sociology* 82(3): 652–663.

Peele, S. 1985. *The Meaning of Addiction: Compulsive Experience and Its Interpretation.* Lexington, Mass.: Lexington Books.

Perez, R., A. Ramirez, R. Ramirez, and M. Rodriguez. 1980. "Correlates and Changes over Time in Drug and Alcohol Use Within a Barrio Population." *American Journal of Community Psychology* 8(6): 621–636.

Rees, C. D., and B. L. Wilborn. 1983. "Correlates of Drug Abuse in Adolescents: A Comparison of Families of Drug Abusers with the Families of Nondrug Abusers." *Journal of Youth and Adolescence* 12(1): 55–63.

Rosenberg, M. 1985. "Summary." In *Beginnings: The Social and Affective Development of Black Children,* edited by M. B. Spencer, G. K. Brookins, and W. R. Allen, 231–234. Hillsdale, N.J.: Erlbaum.

Segal, B. M. 1986. "The Soviet Heavy-Drinking Culture and the American Heavy-Drinking Subculture." In *Alcohol and Culture: Comparative Perspectives from Europe and America,* edited by T. F. Babor, 149–160. New York: New York Academy of Sciences.

Snyder, C. R. 1955. "Culture and Sobriety." *Quarterly Journal of Studies on Alcohol* 16: 701–742.

Steffenhagen, R. A. 1977. "Toward a Self-Esteem Theory of Drug Dependence: A Position Paper." *Journal of Alcohol and Drug Education* 22(2): 1–3.

Steffenhagen, R. A., and J. D. Burns. 1987. *The Social Dynamics of Self-Esteem.* New York: Praeger.

Steinglass, P. 1980. "A Life History Model of the Alcoholic Family." *Family Process* 19: 211–226.

———. 1982. "Alcoholism and the Family." In *Alcohol, Science, and Society Revisited,* edited by E. L. Gomberg, H. R. White, and J. A. Carpenter, 306–321. Ann Arbor: University of Michigan Press.

Stephens, R. C. 1985. "The Sociocultural View of Heroin Use: Toward a Role-Theoretic Model." *Journal of Drug Issues* 15(4): 433–446.

Straus, R. 1982. "The Social Costs of Alcohol in the Perspective of Change, 1945–1980." In *Alcohol, Science, and Society Revisited,* edited by E. L. Gomberg, H. R. White, and J. A. Carpenter, 134–148. Ann Arbor: University of Michigan Press.

Trimble, J. E., A. M. Padilla, and C. S. Bell. 1987. *Drug Abuse Among Ethnic Minorities.* DHHS Publication no. ADM 87–1474. Washington, D.C.: Department of Health and Human Services.

Vander Zanden, J. W. 1985. *Human Development.* New York: Knopf.

Washington State Commission on Asian American Affairs. 1983. "Report to the Governor." Olympia, Washington.

White, H. R. 1982. "Sociological Theories of the Etiology of Alcoholism." In *Alcohol, Science, and Society Revisited,* edited by E. L. Gomberg, H. R. White, and J. A. Carpenter, 205–232. Ann Arbor: University of Michigan Press.

Williams, J. R. 1976. "A Comparison of the Self-Concepts of Alcoholic and

Non-Alcoholic Males of Indian and Non-Indian Ancestry in Terms of Scores on the Tennessee Self-Concept Scale." *Dissertation Abstracts International* 36–A(9): 5844–5845.

Wilsnack, S. C., and L. J. Beckman. 1984. *Alcohol Problems in Women: Antecedents, Consequences, and Intervention.* New York: Guilford.

Woititz, J. G. 1977. "A Study of Self-Esteem in Children of Alcoholics." *Dissertation Abstracts International* 37–A(12): 7554.

———. 1978. "Alcoholism and the Family: A Survey of the Literature." *Journal of Alcohol and Drug Education* 23(2): 18–23.

Notes on Contributors

Bonnie Bhatti is a doctoral candidate at the School of Social Welfare, University of California, Berkeley, and a clinical social worker at the Palo Alto Medical Clinic in Fremont, California. She has several years of experience in both practice and research in the fields of child abuse and child welfare, and she has been a child abuse consultant in Canada and the United States.

Martin V. Covington is professor of psychology at the University of California, Berkeley, and research psychologist at the Institute of Personality Assessment and Research. He is senior author of the *Productive Thinking Program,* a course in learning to think developed for elementary school students. He is a recipient of the Berkeley Distinguished Teaching Award and is past president of the International Society for Test Anxiety Research.

Susan B. Crockenberg is professor of human development at the University of California, Davis. Her research has focused on development during infancy, both within the family and beyond, emphasizing how child and parent influence each other and how both are affected by various aspects of their social environment. The adaptation of teenagers to the role of mothers is an area of particular interest.

David Derezotes is a doctoral candidate at the School of Social Welfare, University of California, Berkeley, and project director of the High School CAPTA Evaluation Project at the Family Welfare Research Group, a research organization affiliated with the School of Social Welfare. He holds a Ph.D. in clinical psychology and has fifteen years of practice experience with children, youth, and families.

Walter M. Furman is director for administration of the Center for Child and Family Policy Studies at the School of Social Welfare, University of California, Los Angeles. He was formerly director of program evaluation for New York State's Office of Mental Health. He has been involved in applied research projects in education, aging, and, most recently, the social welfare areas of income maintenance and child protective services.

Elizabeth Kerst is a doctoral candidate in counseling psychology at the University of California, Los Angeles. Her primary research interest is in the field of substance abuse. She has worked in a therapeutic community for adolescent drug addicts and is interested in processes associated with recovery from addiction. She is an affiliate member of the American Psychological Association and a member of the American Association for Counseling and Development.

Seung-Ock Kim received a master's degree in sociology from Yonsei University in Korea and an MSW degree from the University of California, Berkeley. She is currently a doctoral candidate at the School of Social Welfare in Berkeley. She has studied the roles of personality and cultural influences in various social problems. Her current research interest focuses on drinking problems among Asian Americans.

Harry H. L. Kitano is professor of social welfare and sociology at the University of California, Los Angeles, and acting director of the Asian American Study Center at UCLA. He has held visiting professorships at the University of Bristol, the International Christian University in Japan, and the University of Hawaii, and he has been director of the University of California Tokyo Study Center in Tokyo.

Andrew M. Mecca is executive director of the California Health Research Foundation. He was appointed by Governor George Deukmejian to chair the California Task Force to Promote Self-Esteem and Personal and Social Responsibility. Author of nine books and numerous professional articles, Dr. Mecca has been a consultant to drug treatment and prevention programs in Australia, Thailand, India, the Pacific Rim, Europe, and the United States. He was chief of Alcohol and Drug Services in Marin County, California, for twelve years.

Suzanne M. Retzinger is a research sociologist at the University of California, Santa Barbara. She is the author of articles on conflict, emotions, and mental illness, and she has investigated communication processes that lead to the escalation of conflict and violence. She is currently involved in studying the peaceful resolution of disputes, mediation, and mediator training.

Michael T. Ryan brings a background in psychotherapy to his research and writing. He has worked on social service program evaluation for the National Institute of Justice, joining a concern for public policy with an interest in the social psychology of conflict. His current research focuses on the role of expressed emotion in the family interaction patterns of schizophrenic patients and on the role of neighborhood mediation programs in reducing community violence.

Thomas J. Scheff is professor of sociology at the University of California, Santa Barbara. He is the author of *Being Mentally Ill; Catharsis in Healing, Ritual, and Drama;* and the forthcoming *Microsociology: Discourse and Social Structure.* He is an associate of the state of California's Task Force on the Seriously Mentally Ill and is chair-elect of the section on the Sociology of Emotions, American Sociological Association.

Leonard Schneiderman is dean and professor at the School of Social Welfare, University of California, Los Angeles. He carried out a 1986 study of the Los Angeles County AFDC caseload—40 percent of the state's caseload—in preparation for the implementation of welfare reform (GAIN). He serves as a member of the Joint Select Task Force on the Changing Family, giving particular attention to families in economic peril. He has written extensively in the area of poverty and welfare reform.

Rodney Skager is professor of educational psychology at the Graduate School of Education, University of California, Los Angeles. His research focuses on the reasons people use alcohol and other drugs, on factors that account for "controlled" versus "abusive" use of such substances, and on the process of recovery for people who have become substance abusers. He is active professionally in drug and alcohol prevention programs and in intervention and recovery work.

Neil J. Smelser is University Professor of sociology at the University of California, Berkeley. He has conducted a wide range of research studies in various areas of social psychology and has supplemented his career in sociology by receiving training as a psychoanalyst at the San Francisco Psychoanalytic Institute. His publications include *Theories of Collective*

Behavior and *Personality and Social Systems* (edited with William T. Smelser).

Barbara A. Soby works with child victims as the coordinator of the Yolo County Victim/Witness Assistance Center, located in the district attorney's office in Woodland, California. She received her master's degree in child development in 1988 from the University of California, Davis, where she studied ethnic differences in support for pregnant teenagers.

Harry Specht is dean and professor at the School of Social Welfare, University of California, Berkeley. He has written extensively on the subjects of social policy and community organization. Most recently, he has studied social work practice, which is the subject of his latest book, *New Directions for Social Work Practice.*

John Vasconcellos is a twelve-term member of the California legislature and the author of the 1986 legislation creating the California Task Force to Promote Self-Esteem and Personal and Social Responsibility. He has been the chair of the Assembly Ways and Means Committee for ten years. He is the author of *A Liberating Vision: Politics for Growing Humans* and "A New Human Agenda: Toward Individual Self-Sufficiency."

Joseph Weber is a programmer analyst at MPR Associates, Inc., a San Francisco–based think tank specializing in public-sector educational research. He holds a master's degree in political-social psychology from the University of California, Los Angeles, and he was a staff analyst at the Center for Child and Family Policy Studies at UCLA for two years.

Index

Abbott, D., 279

Ability, perception of, 84–87, 95–97, 107; and academic performance, 84–87, 92, 93, 95–97, 98, 104; and competition, 98, 99, 104; equated with human value, 88; and failure, 89–91, 94, 98; as fixed (entity view of), 85, 99; as incremental, 97, 101, 107; and self-esteem, 75, 86–87, 88–91, 100; as source of status, 87, 89, 109. *See also* Competence, sense of

Abortion, and teenage pregnancy, 126, 131, 134, 135, 155

Academic performance, viii, xviii–xix, 5; and anxiety, 76, 93, 94; and autonomy, 105; behavioral model of, 81–82, 96–97; and causal attributions of success and failure, 76, 83, 84–88, 89–91, 92, 94, 96, 99, 100, 101, 105–106, 107; and competition, 22, 88, 94, 98–100, 101, 104, 110; effort exerted in, as threat to self-esteem, 89–91, 92, 96; emphasis on effort needed in, 101; and equity systems, 22, 101, 102–105; and expectations, 87, 91–92; and failure-accepting students, 93, 94, 95; failure avoidance in, 83, 84, 88–91, 92, 94, 99, 100, 110; and failure-avoiding students, 93, 94, 100; feedback concerning, 82; grades as motivation for, 81–82, 99; interactive model of, 81, 82–83, 84–86, 91–92, 93, 94; perception of ability and, 84–87, 92, 93,

95–97, 98, 104; perception of effort and, 84–85, 87–88, 92, 96–97, 101, 104; and procrastination, 89, 92; protection of self-worth as motivation for, 88–91, 93, 94, 98; redefining success in, 101; and self-esteem, 15, 22, 37, 73, 74–76, 78–80, 82–84, 86–87, 88–91, 94, 96–97, 106–107, 109, 153–154; and strategic thinking (skill training), 105–108; student-centered model of, 80, 83; and success-oriented students, 93–94; and teenage pregnancy, 131, 132, 133, 153–154; and teenage sexual behavior, 155; and test-taking, 91–92, 93, 94. *See also* Dropping out of school; Overstrivers; Social reform: and educational policy; Teachers; Underachievers

Adler, Alfred, 183, 319

Adler, L. O., 260, 279

Adolescents: alcohol use among, 58, 298, 299; drug use among, 58, 299, 300, 306; self-esteem of, 45, 133, 176, 258, 306; self-esteem of, and subsequent alcoholism, 261, 264; self-esteem and deviance among, 170–175, 268–270; suicide among, 58. *See also* Teenage parents; Teenage pregnancy

Ager, J. W., 140 (table), 141–142

Aggression: and alcohol and drug use, 272, 274, 277; and child abuse, 169; and frustration-aggression hypothesis,

Compositor: G & S Typesetters, Inc.
Text: 10/13 Sabon
Display: Sabon
Printer: Edwards Brothers, Inc.
Binder: Edwards Brothers, Inc.